Design for Dementia

Design for Dementia is written by an interdisciplinary team of professionals and academics whose aim is to present lessons learnt from the Dementia Demonstration House at the Building Research Establishment's Innovation Park. Known as Chris and Sally's House, the project represents a unique opportunity to show in practice what can be done to assist people living with dementia to continue to live at home and as part of the community with as much independence as possible. This book presents evidence based practical design guidance backed up by over 15 combined years of research by experienced professional designers.

Beginning with an introduction which provides the background to the global dementia epidemic to allow readers to gain a better understanding of the issues they must consider, the book then discusses how good design principles, planning and construction standards can be used to effectively respond to the dementia crisis. The detailed findings from research using Chris and Sally's House are presented and discussed, along with practical examples and success stories ranging from simple design features to the more complex use of sensors and automated ventilation.

The hope is that readers can apply the lessons learnt from Chris and Sally's House to successfully integrate solutions into the design of new or refurbished housing for the elderly and also that the tools and insights shared will inform the wider context of good housing design, as well as the spectrum of constraints and design standards which often apply. This book is important reading for architects, designers, engineers and project managers, but also anyone with an interest in learning about practical solutions to aid those with dementia to live well at home.

Bill Halsall is an architect and landscape architect, as well as the co-founder of Halsall Lloyd Partnership. He is also Honorary Visiting Industrial Fellow at Liverpool John Moores University, UK.

Mike Riley is Professor of Building Surveying and Director of the School of the Built Environment at Liverpool John Moores University, UK.

Eef Hogervorst is Professor of Biological Psychology and Director of Dementia Research at Loughborough University, UK. Previously she worked as a dementia researcher at Oxford and Cambridge University, having done her PhD at Maastricht University. She has published over 200 peer-reviewed papers, edited several dementia-related books and obtained over £10M funding for her research with collaborators. Eef is often invited for keynotes and public lectures to discuss her work.

Design for Dementia

Living Well at Home

Edited by Bill Halsall, Mike Riley and Eef Hogervorst

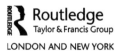

Routledge
Taylor & Francis Group

LONDON AND NEW YORK

Designed cover image: © Halsall Lloyd Partnership

First published 2024
by Routledge
4 Park Square, Milton Park, Abingdon, Oxon OX14 4RN

and by Routledge
605 Third Avenue, New York, NY 10158

Routledge is an imprint of the Taylor & Francis Group, an informa business

British Library Cataloguing-in-Publication Data
A catalogue record for this book is available from the British Library

Library of Congress Cataloging-in-Publication Data
Names: Halsall, Bill, editor. | Hogervorst, Eef, editor. | Riley, Mike, 1964– editor.
Title: Design for dementia : living well at home / edited by Bill Halsall, Eef Hogervost, and Mike Riley.
Description: Abingdon, Oxon ; New York, NY : Routledge, 2024. | Misspelled editor's name on CIP galley: should read Eef Hogervorst. | Includes bibliographical references and index.
Identifiers: LCCN 2023033862 (print) | LCCN 2023033863 (ebook) | ISBN 9781032306490 (hbk) | ISBN 9781032306483 (pbk) | ISBN 9781003306054 (ebk)
Subjects: LCSH: Dementia—Patients—Care—Case studies. | Dementia—Patients—Dwellings—Design and construction. | Health facilities—Design and construction. | Medical instruments and apparatus—Design and construction. | Health planning.
Classification: LCC RC521 .D48 2024 (print) | LCC RC521 (ebook) | DDC 616.8/31—dc23/eng/20231005
LC record available at https://lccn.loc.gov/2023033862
LC ebook record available at https://lccn.loc.gov/2023033863

ISBN: 978-1-032-30649-0 (hbk)
ISBN: 978-1-032-30648-3 (pbk)
ISBN: 978-1-003-30605-4 (ebk)

DOI: 10.1201/9781003306054

Typeset in Times New Roman
by Apex CoVantage, LLC

Contents

Foreword

Dementia is now a global epidemic, approaching 50 million people living with dementia, projected to rise to 75 million by 2050. Although we have become very aware of the issue in developed countries in recent years, not least because of its association with rapidly ageing populations, a majority of people living with dementia are to be found in the more populous low- and middle-income countries where access to social protection, support and care is very limited.

The emergent crisis in developed countries has been brought into sharp focus by the prevailing dominance of a model of medical and social care which is overdependent on hospitals and institutions at the expense of strengthening and reorienting domiciliary and community care, which is largely provided by families and friends. It has become clear that the current model is unsustainable in the medium term and that an urgent reappraisal is necessary in which there is a much better functional match between population health need and the buildings people call home, whether in private dwellings or long-stay social provision.

In tackling the challenge that faces us it is necessary to address the inherent fatalism which often surrounds discussion of the dementia group of conditions and extends from failure to appreciate that for a proportion of people living with dementia primary prevention is possible through policies that alleviate underlying social and economic conditions and behaviours to a lack of imagination when it comes to the design of appropriate living and neighbourhood environments. The prize to be achieved is significant increases in the length of time that people living with dementia may be able to live autonomously in familiar environments, together with improvements in the quality of life and wellbeing at each stage of illness and accompanying care pathways.

This latest offering by an extensive multi-disciplinary partnership with long experience of community architecture based on full community engagement joins up all the dots from academia and practice, with solid bridges into the worlds of medical and social care. It demystifies dementia in a jargon-free way, managing to be both comprehensive and detailed whilst also being accessible to the informed lay person and practitioner alike. It deserves to be widely read by all those involved in creating built environments fit for the future and has wider application, including to our approach to providing for other groups with neuro-diverse needs. Whilst this publication has come about largely from real life, bottom-up creative efforts in the United Kingdom, the messages it carries have important lessons globally in the current era of rapid urbanisation and the ongoing demographic transition in which ageing populations are becoming the norm.

Prof John R Ashton CBE
Former president of the UK Faculty of Public Health

Acknowledgements

The authors would like to gratefully acknowledge the support, assistance and contribution of the following people in the creation of this book:

A special thank-you to Prof John R Ashton CBE, former president of the UK Faculty of Public Health, not only for his contribution of the foreword but for his long-standing encouragement and support for this project.

Dr Robert G MacDonald for his contribution to Chapter 5 and for his original thinking, ideas and partnership working over many years.

Janice Macdonald, Interior Designer, HLP for her contribution to the quality graphic illustrations as well as her championing of Design for Dementia.

All the partners and staff of the Halsall Lloyd Partnership who have made their contributions and supported the Design for Dementia research project.

The staff at the Building Research Establishment, particularly David Kelly, Chris Hall and John O'Brien, who had the vision to invite the Halsall Lloyd Partnership and Loughborough University to put forward proposals for the Dementia Demonstration Project at their Innovation Park at Watford and who supported and contributed to the Chris and Sally's House project.

A special thank-you to all the members of the Dementia Action Alliance (DAA) and the Service Users Reference Forum (SURF) for all the help and enthusiasm which provided the initial inspiration for some of the research projects which form an important background to this book. They engaged and participated freely to share their experience so that the obstacles they face in their daily lives could be better understood by professionals and decision makers in the hope that the living environment for people with dementia can be more responsively designed now and in the future.

Rob Hughes for proofing the early drafts of the manuscript.

We are very grateful to Manisha Jain for her input to all the chapters on dementia she wrote during her PhD, as well as to Ahmad Aladawi, who provided input to these chapters too and his own on dementia and the indoor environment for his PhD, supported by Professor Malcolm Cook and Dr Ben M. Roberts. They worked so hard to get the final edits to us, just days before the submission. Manisha, Ahmad and Barbara Balocating Dunn are all supported by the Dunhill Medical Trust (DMT) to further develop their PhDs at Chris and Sally's House. We are indebted to the DMT for their generous support. Professor Sue Hignett was so helpful in providing her chapter within a few days of asking despite her incredibly busy schedule. Thank you.

Dom, thank you for cooking your amazing dinners, your support and input from the builder's perspective and your in-depth knowledge of part M. Sue, for your patience, generosity and support. Jules for continuous support, encouragement and good humour.

This work that forms the basis of Chapter 6 was supported by the Design Star Centre for Doctoral Training, Arts & Humanities Council (AHRC), www.designstar.org.uk/; Martin Habell, Adonika Brown, Rushcliffe Care Group, Halsall Lloyd Partnership, Building Research Establishment. Graphic design by Charlotte Jais and Zuli Galindo Estupiñan.

Author Profiles

Bill Halsall, *BA (Hons) B.Arch (Hons) L'pool, Architect, Dip LA (Dist) B'ham, CMLI*
Bill is a practicing architect, landscape architect and senior partner at the Halsall Lloyd Partnership.

His work is based on an inclusive philosophy, generating good design through participation and involvement of clients, communities and user groups. Tackling urban issues through promoting shared vision and consensus building between stakeholders, he has produced sustainable designs and masterplans with a high degree of ownership, commitment and deliverability.

Although a practitioner, there is a strong research element to his work. His approach is collaborative and participatory, working directly with the dementia community. He has participated in many seminars and conferences nationally and internationally and presented at over 20 events over the past few years on the subject of design for dementia. He brings practical expertise and experience to research initiatives and is Honorary Visiting Industrial Fellow at Liverpool John Moores University

During the past 10 years, together with Dr Robert G MacDonald of LJMU, he has co-authored three publications based on research into the design and adaptation of housing to accommodate the needs of people living with dementia: *Design for Dementia – A Guide*, *Design for Dementia – Research Projects* and *Design for Dementia – The International Dimension*. He is the architect for Chris and Sally's House – a demonstration project at the BRE's Innovation Park, Watford, based on this research.

Bill's involvement in inclusive and environmentally sustainable design continues to find expression through the creation of distinctive, innovative and evidence-based projects.

Eef Hogervorst

Eef Hogervorst holds a chair in Biological Psychology at Loughborough University, a Top 10 University in the UK. She also has visiting posts in Leicester and Nottingham, as well as at several Indonesian universities. Prior to this Eef worked as researcher at Oxford and Cambridge University. She is Director for Dementia Research at Loughborough. Eef has published over 200 peer-reviewed international publications and edited and contributed to several books related to dementia research. She is frequently invited to give keynotes at international conferences and regularly provides public lectures on dementia diagnoses, lifestyle change to prevent dementia and dementia-inclusive design. Eef is currently heading the INTERDEM task force in dementia-inclusive design of the lived environment which will result in an edited book by the same publisher with all renowned experts in this field (e.g. Bob Woods, Mary Marshall, Kevin Charras, Richard Fleming, etc.). With collaborators, she obtained over £10M funding for her research. Eef advises on several grant committees in the United Kingdom and United States and for the EU and is associate editor for several journals. She was part of the Loughborough group to be tendered for the refurbishment of Chris and Sally's House on the BRE site in Watford. Other experts from Loughborough contributing to this dementia-inclusive design were Prof Malcolm Cook (Civil and Building Engineering) and Prof Sue Hignett (Design School) from Loughborough University.

Mike Riley

Mike Riley is the Head of the School of Civil Engineering and Built Environment and Professor of Building Surveying at Liverpool John Moores University. He is also Visiting Professor in Building Surveying at University of Malaya and Amity University in Delhi. Mike has more than 30 years' experience in building surveying practice and construction and property education. He is a consultant to several national organisations in the United Kingdom and internationally, including Malaysia and Ghana.

Mike is the joint author of numerous textbooks in the field of construction technology and sustainability, and he has published many academic papers in the areas of building pathology, property management and building performance appraisal. In addition, he has presented papers and keynote addresses to prestigious international conferences and is a regular reviewer for several internationally renowned academic journals and conferences.

Mike obtained his first degree from Salford University (building surveying), followed by a master of science from Heriot-Watt University (building services engineering) and PhD from Liverpool John Moores University (building performance). He is a fellow of the Royal Institution of Chartered Surveyors, fellow of the Royal Institution of Surveyors Malaysia and senior fellow of the Higher Education Academy and is a chartered environmentalist.

Additional Contributors

Ahmad Aladawi

Ahmad is a highly accomplished PhD student at Loughborough University, passionate about creating innovative technologies for people with mental/physical disabilities. He holds a Master's degree with distinction in the Internet of Things (IoT) from Bournemouth University and a first-class honours degree in Computer Sciences. Ahmad has won many first-place prizes in competitions for his exceptional skills and talent in this field.

John Ashton, CBE

As a physician, psychiatrist and family doctor working in public health, John Ashton has spent almost 50 years working to heal the schism between science and the humanities. His work has included embracing collaboration with poetry, the arts and not least with the craft of architecture. This has included working with architects and communities on neighbourhood regeneration, the design for primary care premises, training the next generation of architects and designing housing and other buildings to optimise life with dementia. He contends that the crisis in medical care with an ageing population lies in large part in the failure to co-design living, supportive neighbourhoods. This requires a focus on the functioning of buildings that transcends the imperative of volume bricks and mortar that dominates current thinking. He sees architects and town planners as the conjoined twins of public health.

Malcolm Cook

Professor Malcolm Cook is Dean of the School of Architecture, Building and Civil Engineering. He is Professor of Building Performance Analysis and a member of the Building Energy Research Group. His research expertise lies in low-energy building design and the application of computational fluid dynamics (CFD) to natural ventilation. For over 25 years he worked with multi-disciplinary teams on the design and performance monitoring of some of the world's most innovative low-energy buildings. Over his research career, he led a combined research and enterprise portfolio totalling over £10m. Projects have included low-energy cooling and ventilation in India, the development of simulation models for thermal comfort and thermophysiological modelling, control systems for natural and hybrid ventilation and CFD modelling of natural ventilation. Recent work has involved assessing the effect of ventilation design and operation on the transmission risk of SARS-CoV-2 (Covid) and advising the government on the safe reopening of sports, arts and entertainment venues. He has speaking engagements at the CEPT University in India, Hong Kong University, Oklahoma State University and Lawrence Berkeley National Laboratory. He also serves on international advisory boards which have included the University of Antwerp, University of Applied Sciences Stuttgart, Karlsruhe University and Hong Kong University.

Sue Hignett

Professor Sue Hignett is Professor of Healthcare Ergonomics & Patient Safety at Loughborough University and a fellow of the Chartered Institute of Ergonomics and Human Factors (FCIEHF). Her academic interests focus on optimising human well-being and overall system performance with research on hospital and ambulance design, emergency response, staff wellbeing and patient safety (e.g., dementia, mobility and falls).

Manisha Jain

Manisha Jain has a background in psychology and obtained her BSc (Hons) and MSc from the University of Nottingham. She is currently undertaking her PhD at Loughborough University, where she is exploring exercise and technology in older adults and its applications for dementia.

Robert G MacDonald

Robert G MacDonald is an architect and public advisor, ARC NWC. He is President Emeritus of the Liverpool Architectural Society. Rob has researched and published about mental health, design for dementia and medical architecture. He leads an Art for Well Being course at the MerseyCare NHS Foundation Trust Life Rooms. In 2019 he was presented by Dr Phillip Hammond (BBC TV) with the DIMHN Recognition Award, and in 2014 he was recognised and honoured with the Roscoe Citizenship Award, which was presented by Lord David Alton.

Ben M. Roberts

Dr Ben M. Roberts researches thermal comfort, ventilation and overheating in temperate and tropical climates. Ben runs experiments in test houses, is involved in large international field trials and manages dynamic thermal model validation exercises. Ben recently completed the first evaluation of SMETER technologies and is now working in the United Kingdom and Ghana on a range of projects.

1 Introduction

The UK and Global Picture

Bill Halsall, Eef Hogervorst and Mike Riley

Introduction

The purpose of this book is to explore and review the role that design can play in assisting people living with dementia and their carers to live as well as possible, at home or in the right supportive environment, retaining their capacity for longer and maintaining as much autonomy and independence as possible.

There is clearly a role for design, and this field has been explored over many years by the University of Sterling and others, but dementia is a complex condition, and there are many different types and manifestations.

None of us can really imagine what the experience of dementia is. How can we really understand what the needs and aspirations of people living with dementia really are? How can we experience their world through their eyes, ears and other senses? There are simulators, and the experience is horrific, but we can't really know. We do know that people living with dementia are part of our society. It is estimated that in the UK between 70% and 80% of people living with dementia live at home, within our communities and using the same local facilities, neighbourhoods and town centres as everybody else.

Their experience is affected by the design of their homes and their environment. The way in which homes, facilities such as shops, parks and the built environment as a whole are designed affects the living experience of people with dementia as much as people with other physical and cognitive impairments which may be better recognised, such as sight- or hearing-impaired or physically disabled people in the community.

Because of the research that has been carried out over the past few decades, much is already known about design features which can help but also design features which can potentially create difficulty or even accidents causing injury and hospitalisation. However, apart from specialised projects, such as extra care schemes and specialist dementia facilities, there is not much evidence to suggest that this knowledge is permeating through to architects, planners or other designers.

Part of the aspiration of the authors is to disseminate knowledge and experience to professionals, students and others and to put forward ways in which consideration of dementia can be integrated into best practice and into the planning, design and construction process. Architects and designers have many other constraints and rules to negotiate and regulations to satisfy, and if there is to be significant progress towards creating a dementia-inclusive environment for all, then design for dementia best practice must be integrated into the design, development and construction process.

Dementia is a growing problem worldwide. It is characterised by a significant decline in brain function impacting the ability to live independently. People living with dementia require a high degree of care, especially as the disease advances. This level of care is costly, with the majority of these costs draining financial resources from the informal sector, as this is mainly carried by people with dementia and their families. Worldwide these costs exceeded USD 1.3 trillion in 2019 according to the World Health Organisation. In the UK institutionalised dementia care

DOI: 10.1201/9781003306054-1

cost is currently estimated at £1500–2000/week. Given a lack of trained personnel and high staff turnover, there would be advantages if people could stay in their own homes for as long as possible. As there is no effective long-term treatment yet available, supportive environments to allow people to maintain independence and dignity are crucially important. This philosophy of ageing in place is supported by most agencies working in the field of elderly care and was given new relevance in the recent COVID-19 crisis as a complementary resource to more institutional care models, potentially reducing care costs to the NHS and relieving the stress of carers and relatives.

Background

While there is a large amount of research into dementia, this tends to be based in specific research disciplines and may be inaccessible or unusable to those requiring practical assistance in coping with the experience of dementia – those living with dementia and their carers and families. The response to the dementia epidemic requires a broader response from a wider perspective and experience as well as an evidence-based approach. A multi-disciplinary team is required to deliver the joined-up approach needed. The results of research carried out by such teams should be disseminated to a wider audience, including local authorities, housing associations and other housing providers as well as communities and families.

In 2015, Bill Halsall of the Halsall Lloyd Partnership and Dr Robert G MacDonald of Liverpool John Moores University published *Design for Dementia – A Guide* and its companion, *Design for Dementia – Research Projects*. These publications were the result of a long research partnership between HLP and LJMU. Subsequently a third volume was published, *Design for Dementia – The International Dimension*.

This research was based on participatory work carried out in conjunction with Merseycare and the Dementia Action Alliance as well as other specialist academic staff at LJMU. As a result of this work, Bill Halsall and Robert G MacDonald became involved with the Building Research Establishment and the University of Loughborough in the collaborative research, design and construction of a Dementia Demonstration Project at the BRE's Innovation Park in Watford. Loughborough University, led by Prof Jacqui Glass from Civil and Building Engineering, tendered for the BRE call to develop a dementia-friendly home, and with an Enterprise grant from Loughborough University, a team was put together. This consisted of Prof Sue Hignett (a health care ergonomist) and Prof Hogervorst, a dementia specialist, with their PhD students Charlotte Jais and Jordan Elliott King to develop dementia personas to inform the design and to help develop home-based activity equipment, as well as to obtain patient and public involvement and engagement, and Prof Malcolm Cook with his PhD to investigate thermal modelling and automated assessment and regulation of the indoor environment of Chris and Sally's House. Later, Dunhill Medical Trust further funded the team with PhDs Barbara Balocating Dunn, an architect to help develop inclusive standards; Manisha Jain, a psychologist; and Ahmad Aladawi, a computer and indoor environment specialist to study the Chris and Sally's House further, aided by Ahmet Begde, a PhD and physiotherapist, who was funded by the Turkish government. Bill and Robert supported the PhDs throughout their journey with their input. Their contributions can be found throughout the book

The role of the University of Loughborough team has been to provide a rigorous evidence base for both the design of the demonstration project and this publication itself. This creative dynamic between academic rigour and practical professional expertise underpins the design of the dementia demonstration project and the conclusions of this publication.

Chris and Sally's House

A case study of this demonstration project is included in this publication. Chapters 6 and 7 and the lessons learnt from the project are incorporated into the design guidance of Chapter 10. The demonstration project became known as the Chris and Sally's House.

The Chris and Sally's House demonstration project at the Building Research Establishment, Watford, is an example of multi-disciplinary joined-up research and represents a unique opportunity to show in practice what can be done to assist people living with dementia, to sustain their capacity for longer and to continue to live as part of the community with as much independence as possible. The design implications outside of the house and the response required in public realm design and the planning of neighbourhoods will also be vital in ensuring that people living with dementia can participate fully in the life of the community. Most people living with dementia continue to live in their own homes and use the same facilities as everyone else.

Chris and Sally's House represents years of research into the potential of design to assist people living with dementia to sustain their capacity and live independently in their own homes for longer. Since its completion, Chris and Sally's House has received an estimated 25,000 visitors annually and caught the imagination of many concerned people and groups, nationally and internationally.

Usefulness of Design for Dementia – Living Well at Home

At the heart of this publication is a detailed source explaining the experience of the team and the evidence base as well as design guidance which may assist individual families or groups wishing to carry out the design of new dwellings or refurbishment projects on a small or large scale.

To be successfully integrated into the design of new or refurbished housing, the research base, as well as the lessons learnt and design guidance, should be accommodated into the wider context of housing design, as well as the spectrum of constraints and design standards which apply in the UK. To be of practical use, the design guidance is based in the experience of professional designers in the housing and health sectors.

Creating a record of Chris and Sally's House gives a lasting legacy for the demonstration project. It allows dissemination of the lessons learned to the wider dementia community. It provides design advice to individuals and groups and demonstrates the evidence base and project evolution. The book also records specialist elements of the research base, such as the use of sensors and automatically activated ventilation, the 'acti chair' and so on. It evaluates feedback from visitors and live research projects. As such, this manuscript can act as a textbook for future dementia-inclusive designers and architects and become a standard text on the subject of dementia-supportive design. The book can also act as resource for the many who will not be able to physically visit Chris and Sally's House in Watford. The book is for the lay public, local authorities, housing associations, families and carers dealing with the issues presented by living with dementia. Most of all, it is written in participation with people living with dementia and reflects their aspirations as well as the needs of their families and carers.

An Evidence-Based Approach

To fully get to grips with the design approach, we need to fully understand the context of dementia in the UK and globally and provide an evidence base for design decisions and methodologies.

Chapter 2 explores the impact of dementia within ageing societies, socially and in its cost to economies. It explains its effect on the human brain and on the lives of people living with it and their families and carers. The risk factors are described in detail, including genetic, environmental and lifestyle risks to individuals, as well as the context of the dementia epidemic.

Chapter 3 outlines the medical background, explaining the various causes of dementia and their effect. The behavioural and psychological symptoms are described in detail along with prevention strategies, exploring the use of new technologies. Ageing in place is a key concept, and the benefits of this strategy are summarised.

Chapter 4 develops these themes focusing on personal experience and health and wellbeing of people living with dementia. It describes the traditional medical model; the clustering of symptoms; and the interaction between an individual's biology, past experiences, and current environment. The person-centred care model is explained, including the value of reminiscence, individual activities and therapies such as massage and touch. Care provision in the UK is discussed, including the relative benefits of institutional care compared to care in the home.

Chapter 5 covers the role of engagement with the dementia community in generating better understanding of their requirements and aspirations in terms of design. Methodologies for design participation with people living with dementia are discussed, and outcomes from this type of action research are explained.

Chapter 6 introduces the personas, another approach to inclusive design, and details the evidence base for the design process used to develop the design options for Chris and Sally's House.

Chapter 7 is a detailed case study for the dementia demonstration project – Chris and Sally's House. It describes the interdisciplinary design process and the adaptive design scenarios which were developed. Through the appraisal of these adaptive design scenarios, a preferred solution evolved and was adopted for the physical conversion of the existing property into the demonstration project. It includes a design appraisal based on feedback from visitors and professional assessments.

Chapter 8 is a technical study which assesses the indoor environmental quality required by people living with dementia. This research identifies optimal indoor environmental parameters for people living with dementia and their carers. This research underpinned the environmental services design of Chris and Sally's House, with particular emphasis on achieving adequate ventilation in the context of dementia.

Chapter 9 demonstrates the role of post-occupation evaluation in delivering successful building performance. It covers the use of living labs to enhance the participatory element of evaluation, focusing on user-led co-creation as well as the applicability of other post-occupancy evaluation models.

Chapter 10 brings together all the lessons learnt in the form of design guidance, which explains design principles for dementia and illustrates them through practical examples within a spectrum of care scenarios. The design guide covers the public realm, including private gardens; built forms, including contextual siting and design of buildings for people living with dementia; and the private domain, developing themes of homeliness through interior design and explaining issues of perception and demonstrating how these can be addressed. Chapter 10 also sets the scene in terms of other UK-based design standards which may have to be negotiated to create fully integrated design solutions.

Chapter 11 discusses the way forward, including the concept of designing for dementia compatibility to create future flexibility and 'long life loose fit' solutions, as well as more specialist dementia-inclusive approaches. The use of new technology is explored both as an aid for communication and engagement and through the use of artificial intelligence and sensor technology. The implications of dementia-inclusive design for the industry and the supply chain are discussed, along with the implications for the NHS and the social care system. The idea of a regulatory framework to drive the adoption of dementia-inclusive design through planning frameworks is put forward. Chapter 11 also advocates the need for an aesthetic approach to design, with the aspiration to stimulate 'delight' as well as responding to the more practical aspects of design for dementia.

References

WHO, 2019. www.who.int/news-room/fact-sheets/detail/dementia [Accessed 06 Jan 2023].

2 The Impact of the Dementia Epidemic

Manisha Jain and Eef Hogervorst

Introduction

Dementia is a global phenomenon that is thought to affect millions of individuals worldwide. With the expected growth in patient numbers, dementia will have a ripple effect, impacting financial resources with high economic and human costs due to numerous aspects of dementia care. This chapter will discuss dementia the related costs in both low-middle income countries (LMICs) and high-income countries (HICs). The growth in dementia case numbers is expected to be highest in LMICs which are ill prepared, with few resources to combat this onslaught. We will briefly discuss the dementia journey and how it impacts the individual. The associated risk factors that can increase the likelihood of developing dementia are also reviewed. Further information regarding the medical background of dementia, including prevention of dementia, with its different symptoms and effects on cognition, activities of daily life, mood and behaviour can be found in Chapter 3.

Dementia Prevalence and Population Ageing

The proportion of older adults in the global population is increasing. By 2050, the number of adults aged 60 years and over is predicted to reach 2.1 billion worldwide (World Health Organisation 2022). Given the projected trends of population ageing and improved healthcare, it is expected that the rates of dementia will also increase, as age is considered the greatest known risk factor for dementia. Alzheimer's Disease International (ADI) and the World Health Organisation (WHO) have estimated that over 55 million individuals are currently living with dementia, with numbers almost doubling every 20 years, reaching 82 million in 2030 and 152 million in 2050 (Guerchet et al. 2020; World Health Organisation 2020; Alzheimer's Disease International 2023). In the United Kingdom (UK), it is estimated that 944,000 individuals are living with dementia, a figure that is predicted to exceed 1 million by 2025 (Luengo-Fernandez and Landeiro in prep, Wittenberg et al. 2019). UK costs are estimated at £25–35 billion per year, of which the majority is carried by family and people with dementia themselves (Wittenberg et al. 2019).

In recent decades, we have seen a significant increase in life expectancy, as a result of the decline in mortality rates associated with older age and better healthcare. With increased life expectancy comes an increased risk of medical illnesses that are linked with older age. As previously mentioned, dementia rates were predicted to increase worldwide (World Health Organisation 2020). However, the National Health Service (NHS) has indicated that recorded dementia diagnosis rates, including in those aged 65 years and over, decreased as of 31 December 2021 (NHS Digital 2022). These results should be considered with caution, as they were impacted by the COVID-19 pandemic, which would have likely affected the ability of those with dementia to obtain a diagnosis. While population ageing can be attributed to access to better healthcare, due to the effects of the COVID-19 pandemic, adults aged 50 years and over experienced greater barriers to health care access, such as postponing planned care or forgoing care for fear of infection

DOI: 10.1201/9781003306054-2

(Arnault et al. 2021). This was highlighted as the greatest for those who had the highest needs, who used healthcare services before the pandemic and especially the oldest individuals. Later data from the Office for National Statistics (ONS) stated that the leading cause of death in October 2022 was still dementia and Alzheimer's disease (AD), accounting for 11.6% of all deaths in England and 10.9% in Wales (Office for National Statistics 2022).

Despite this, the UK and other countries (e.g. the Netherlands, Scandinavia, USA) have shown a decrease in predicted numbers of dementia, and this may be due to better population health, including implementation of lifestyle changes related to dementia risk (cessation of smoking, exercising, better diets and monitoring cardiovascular health). This suggests that the implementation of protective factors, such as optimal environments that promote safe and healthy lifestyles, may reduce progression to high care needs, such as those associated with dementia. These protective factors are discussed in Chapter 3 in more detail.

It is expected that LMICs will suffer the brunt of population growth, as currently 60% of all individuals with dementia worldwide are thought to live in such countries (Alzheimer's Disease International and McGill University 2021). In these countries, there is a reduced capacity to deal with population growth, a lack of dementia awareness, reduced access to affordable healthcare services, underdeveloped dementia specialist services and a lack of culturally appropriate cognitive tests and other measurement tools (Comas-Herrera et al. 2016). It has been suggested that the number of individuals with dementia in LMICs is rising faster than in HICs, such as the UK, due to longer life expectancies and greater risk factor burden (Livingston et al. 2020). Such risk factors for dementia include lower educational attainment, midlife obesity, high blood pressure, diabetes, smoking, alcohol use and low physical activity but also the burden of communicable diseases such as HIV and other infectious diseases which can affect cognitive decline and dementia risk.

As LMICs also have limited resources, there is less access to education and specialist healthcare, higher levels of smoking and alcohol use and overall reduced awareness of public health (Mutumba and Schulenberg 2019; Walls et al. 2020). Consequently, this – in addition to population growth and ageing – may contribute to increased dementia risk in LMICs, with few resources to diagnose and manage symptoms. As such, dementia rates and risk may also be affected by cultural views that debate whether dementia is seen as a medical illness, a natural part of ageing, spirituality or religion (Owokuhaisa et al. 2020). Low-cost home environments could be particularly important for LMICs, and examples of such adaptations have been implemented in India (Nightingale care home in Bangalore) and Indonesia (Lawang care home) two decades ago. These countries had low-cost care provision, due to younger populations with lower pay for care, as compared to HICs where staff shortage is a significant issue in the provision of formal care. Low-cost technology is sought to offset this in HICs but requires more research in user acceptability and effectiveness. Japan and Singapore, with older populations, have done much work towards this type of care. However, more research needs to be done into individuals' home-based technology-supported care. This is discussed in more detail in the following paragraphs.

Cost of Dementia

Dementia poses a great burden on health and social care systems worldwide. As dementia rates, risk and population growth increases, so too does the economic and financial impact. Such costs consist of healthcare, which include medication, appointments, medical scans and screening. However, in the UK this is funded via direct taxation, and this may not be the case for other countries, where medical insurance may be required. Additionally, there are social care costs which cover home and residential care and informal unpaid care that is often provided by family and friends. This raises concern about the affordability, sustainability and adequacy of long-term dementia care, particularly as the cost of dementia increases with progressive dementia severity (Jönsson 2022). However, this becomes more critical as those with increased risk for more severe dementia and higher levels of care needs are associated with lower economic status (Hu et al. 2022).

The overall annual cost of dementia in England in 2019, using 2015 prices, was estimated to be £34.7 billion and projected to increase to £94.1 billion by 2040 (Wittenberg et al. 2019). Of this cost, healthcare accounts for 14%, which equates to £4.9 billion. In comparison, social (publicly and privately funded) and unpaid care accounts for 45% and 40%, equating to £15.7 billion and £13.9 billion, respectively. These percentages are approximately similar to what is seen when the cost is broken down for England, Scotland and Wales. The authors also highlight that these figures are projected to triple by 2040. Further research has specified the annual costs of dementia per person according to dementia severity. Average costs have been indicated as £24,400 for mild, £27,450 for moderate and £46,050 for severe dementia (Wittenberg, Knapp et al. 2019).

Additionally, recent estimates have been calculated for the cost of dementia in Europe. Using population representative data from the Survey of Health, Ageing, and Retirement in Europe from 2004–2017, supplemented with relevant information on caregiver wages and dementia prevalence, costs were calculated for 11 different countries (Meijer et al. 2022). The authors found that the mean annual direct out-of-pocket cost per person was the lowest in in the Czech Republic (€705), followed by Denmark and Sweden (€941 and €949, respectively). However, costs were highest in Austria, Belgium and Germany, amounting to over €1500. Overall, in all European countries within the analysis, the largest proportion of costs was accounted for by informal care.

On a global scale the WHO, in its Global Status on the Public Health Response to Dementia, estimated that the global cost associated with dementia care was $1.3 trillion in 2019 and was estimated to increase to $1.7 trillion by 2040 (The Lancet Public Health 2021). However, more recent findings have modelled projections and estimated the direct global spending that was attributable to dementia was $275 billion in 2019 (Velandia et al. 2022). The authors further estimated that this figure will reach $1.6 trillion by 2050 but could reach as high as $2.4 trillion.

Compared to HICs, studies on dementia costs in LMICs are fewer in number. The World Alzheimer Report 2015 indicated that while prevalence is higher in LMICs, costs are higher in HICs (Prince et al. 2015). It was suggested that this was due to lower wages and an increased proportion of unpaid informal care in LMICs. A recent study has been able to estimate the cost of dementia in LMIC, which also included lower-middle–income countries and upper-middle–income countries (Mattap et al. 2022). The findings estimated that the total national cost of dementia in 2017 was $148.2 billion, with the highest costs coming from upper-middle–income countries. More specifically, data from Peru indicated that frontotemporal dementia (FTD) had the highest costs compared to Alzheimer's disease and vascular dementia (VaD), whereas in Argentina, VaD had the highest costs compared to AD and FTD. Compared to HICs, LMIC costs are lower than what is seen in HICs. It can be understood that this is because of increased pressure and lack of capacity to deal with population growth and a lack of resources to deal with dementia diagnoses, treatment and management.

Overall, the results reported for HICs and LMICs indicate that dementia is indeed costly. However, on account of population ageing, these costs shall keep increasing, also in LMICs. It is anticipated that by 2050, the financial burden on healthcare systems in LMICs will be substantial, particularly in countries where dementia prevalence is highest and likely to continue rising (Velandia et al. 2022). Worldwide, it is evident that most dementia costs are incurred from informal care and indirect costs from unpaid care. It is becoming increasingly necessary to develop and implement cost-effective strategies to help manage dementia.

One such cost-effective solution is known as ageing in place or ageing in the home. This refers to older adults ageing in their own familiar environment, one in which they maintain their independence and sense of self (Pani-Harreman et al. 2021). It can be argued that ageing in place or in the home may be more cost effective because it does not incur the costs that formal nursing or residential care would (Horner and Boldy 2008; Pani-Harreman et al. 2021). It was estimated that 85% of older people prefer to stay at home. However, due to the additional needs of dementia,

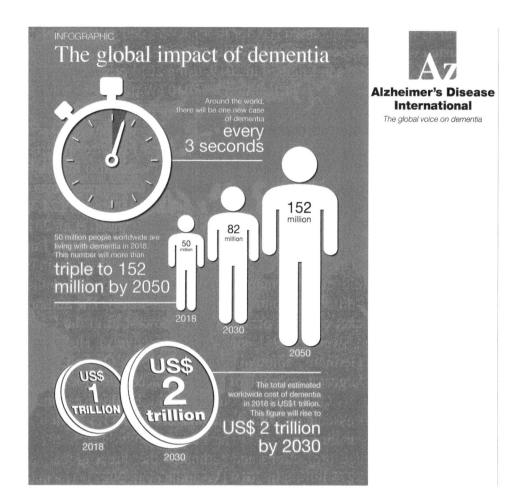

Figure 2.1 Global impact of dementia

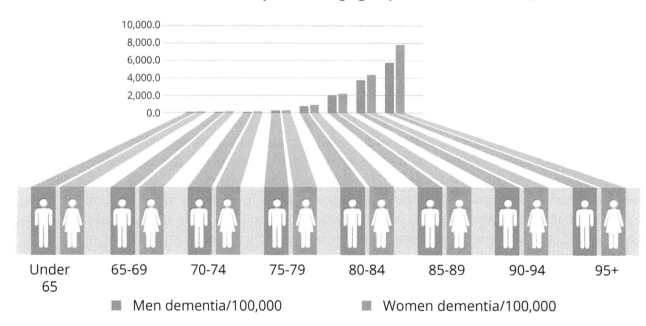

Figure 2.2 Deaths registered in 2019 in England and Wales due to dementia and Alzheimer's disease, by sex and age group/100,000 (ONS 2020)

particularly with activities of daily living (ADL), ageing in place and maintaining independence may not always be possible.

The economic and financial impact of dementia thus poses significant challenges for society, weighing heavily on the social and informal care sectors affecting both public and private budgets (Prince et al. 2014; Wittenberg, Knapp et al. 2019). Having recently entered the United Nations (UN) 'Decade of Healthy Ageing' (2021–2030), it is important to examine and develop research to help older adults age safely, comfortably and healthily. With the majority of older people choosing to stay at home, such research should look to determine cost-effective solutions for ageing in place facilitated by age and dementia friendly housing.

What Is Dementia and What Functions Does It Affect?

There is much overlap in cognitive decline between ageing and dementia. For instance, older people often have lower scores on free memory recall (e.g. of shopping list items), reduced speed of information processing and difficulty in working memory tasks with an additional load, such as dual tasking (Salthouse 1996; Hogervorst 1998; Silva-Fernandes et al. 2022). However, dementia is a pathological syndrome that is characterised by progressive cognitive decline, such as significant impairment of recent and remote memory, behaviour, thinking and planning, which affect the ability to perform activities of daily life. This causes high care costs. Dementia is not considered a normal part of ageing and is different from typical age-related decline. However, the presentation of symptoms is nuanced and can differ depending on the underlying cause. This will be discussed in Chapter 3. Cognitive decline can present as memory loss, language and communication impairments, attention and executive function (e.g. problem-solving and planning) dysfunction and visuospatial deficits. As a consequence, dementia impacts an individual's ability to engage with both basic and instrumental ADL, as well as social interactions.

Basic ADL (bADL) includes the fundamental skills that are required to maintain physical needs, such as personal hygiene, dressing, toileting, eating and transferring (Mlinac and Feng 2016). In comparison, instrumental ADL (iADL) are considered complex activities that are important for maintaining independence, such as cooking, managing finances and medication and grocery shopping (Mlinac and Feng 2016; Feger et al. 2020). iADL thus requires more cognitive input and will usually become apparent earlier in the disease, which can already be apparent in very mild dementia (Clinical Dementia Rating (CDR) 0.5), whereas bADL is usually affected in the moderate to severe stages of the morbidity (CDR stages 1–2) (Berg 1988; Maeshima et al. 2021).

The Diagnostic and Statistical Manual of Mental Disorders 5th Edition (DSM-5) refers to dementia as a major neurocognitive disorder (MNCD) as an update from its previous edition (American Psychiatric Association 2013). The DSM-5 highlights a set of diagnostic criteria that determine the presence of dementia or Major NCD symptoms and further criteria for the cause. For a diagnosis of dementia, the criteria indicate that an individual must have evidence of significant cognitive decline in one or more cognitive domains (complex attention, executive function, learning and memory, language, perceptual-motor or social cognition) determined by individual, informant, clinician and neuropsychological tests; have impairments in ADL; have impairments that do not exclusively occur in delirium (except for Lewy body dementia); and have impairments that are not better explained by another mental or physical disorder (such as depression or thyroid disorders, both common in older people). There is currently no effective long-term treatment for dementia. Recent medical developments still carry many side effects, are very costly and only have very small overall clinical effects.

As discussed, mild severity of symptoms denotes difficulties with iADL, whereas moderate dementia severity denotes difficulties with bADL and severe dementia highlights that the individual is fully dependent. This progression in support needed with everyday care and planning needs

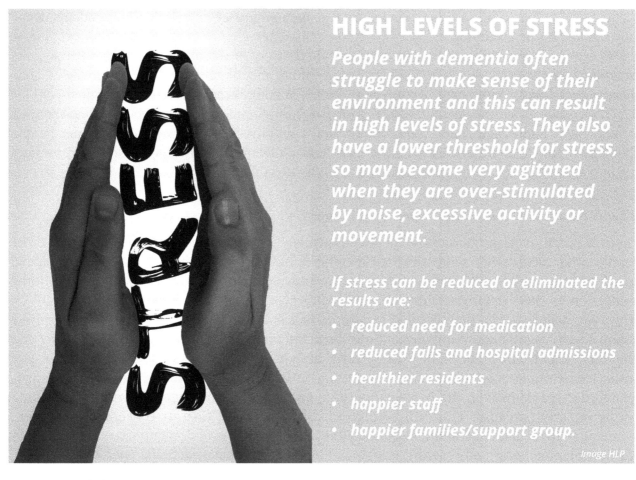

HIGH LEVELS OF STRESS

People with dementia often struggle to make sense of their environment and this can result in high levels of stress. They also have a lower threshold for stress, so may become very agitated when they are over-stimulated by noise, excessive activity or movement.

If stress can be reduced or eliminated the results are:

* *reduced need for medication*
* *reduced falls and hospital admissions*
* *healthier residents*
* *happier staff*
* *happier families/support group.*

Image HLP

Figure 2.3 High levels of stress

to be incorporated in age- and dementia-friendly design of environments. These environmental adaptations could significantly reduce dementia costs related to care. If these adaptations take into account the reduction of risk factors for dementia, costs could be further reduced.

Risk Factors for Dementia

Prevention of dementia is currently the only feasible approach to reduce growth in numbers of cases. This can be primary (over the lifespan); secondary (to prevent progression from mild cognitive impairment (MCI) to AD) and tertiary (to prevent progression from mild to moderate and severe dementia). There are numerous risk factors that contribute to the likelihood of developing dementia (Irving et al. 2020). Such factors can be genetic, environmental and lifestyle, all of which affect dementia risk, which will be discussed later in this chapter. Additionally, these risk factors can contribute to the development of different aetiologies of dementia, such as AD or VaD. Genetic factors are predisposed in an individual's genetics and can often result from genetic mutations. Environmental risk factors refer to the exposure to certain aspects or substances in one's environment that could potentially increase the risk for dementia. Last, lifestyle risk factors are often factors that can be modified through lifestyle choices. However, some of these factors can be governed by socioeconomic status, whereby an individual may not have the choice or the ability to alter their lifestyle decisions. Other demographic factors also cannot be (easily) altered. Age is universally considered the greatest risk factor for dementia, whereby after the age of 65 years, the risk of dementia increases (McCullagh et al. 2001). Low education is a major risk factor for dementia with an earlier onset. There is also a sex difference in dementia risk, as women are more likely to develop AD, whereas men are more likely to develop VaD (McCullagh et al. 2001; Podcasy and Epperson 2022).

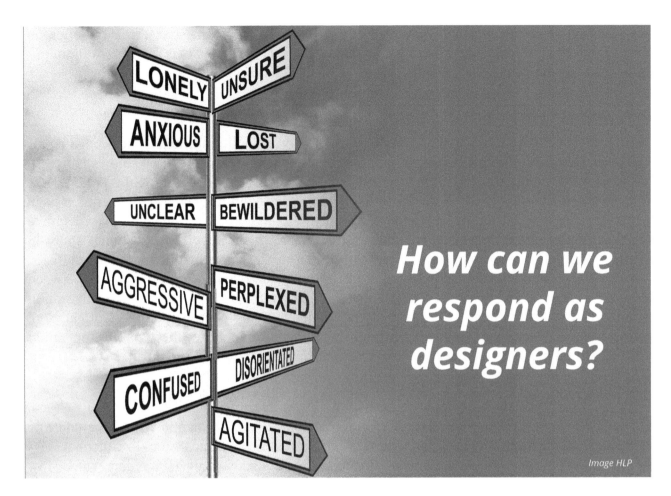

Figure 2.4 Experience of dementia

Genetic Risk Factors

The most well-established genetic risk factor is the gene for apolipoprotein E (APOE) and its variants (Mecocci and Boccardi 2021). This has been known as the Alzheimer's risk gene, which has differential effects on dementia risk, related to amyloid plaque build-up, which is toxic and a hallmark feature in Alzheimer's disease (Verghese et al. 2011). However, this gene can have variations in its DNA sequence at a specific location, and this can affect what the gene does. These variations also come in pairs, and whether the singular variations in the pair are the same or different can also affect what the gene does. In regard to AD, the APOE gene has a variation (known as ε4) that has been associated with increased dementia risk, while another variation (known as ε2) has been considered a protective factor, as dementia risk is decreased in these carriers (Verghese et al. 2011; Lourida et al. 2019).

Overall, the APOE gene is most associated with AD because it affects how the disease is started. However, there are other genetics that are associated with other types of dementia as well. For example, the heritability of FTD is accounted for by genes called progranulin (GRN), microtubule-associated protein tau (MAPT) and chromosome 9 open reading frame 72 (c9orf72).

It is likely that genetic risk factors interact with environmental and lifestyle factors, creating a vulnerability for disease. However, screening for genetic risk is not advised unless early onset AD is suspected with first-degree relatives with dementia onset before the age of 65. Early onset AD has a very high risk transfer in families. For the late-onset type, having both ε4 variations (a matching pair), which is considered rare, increases dementia risk by 9–15-fold (Yamazaki et al. 2019). Approximately 25% of people have one variation of the ε4 allele (not a matching pair, so coupled with ε3, for instance) and, dependent on ethnicity, will not necessarily develop AD in their lifetime. These variants increase dementia risk by 3–4-fold (Verghese et al. 2011; Heffernan et al. 2016; Gharbi-Meliani et al. 2021). Comparatively, it is estimated that 25–35% of individuals with AD do not carry the ε4 variation at all (Crean et al. 2011).

Environmental Risk Factors

The risk factors in one's environment can refer to air quality and pollution, metals and occupational-related exposures (Killin et al. 2016). Findings from a systematic review of 60 studies indicated that various environmental risk factors have been associated with dementia (Killin et al. 2016). High levels of nitrogen oxide were found to be associated with an increased dementia risk in two prospective cohort studies. The authors also highlighted that environmental tobacco smoke was associated with an increased risk of severe dementia in a large cross-sectional study in China. Aluminium was the most studied metal, with 16 studies investigating its negative effects. Larger, high-quality studies included in a systematic review found a positive association between aluminium presence and dementia risk. Temperature, in particular hypothermia and dehydration in hot and dry environments, can also worsen dementia symptoms, including disorientation, memory, visual function and planning. Monitoring the environment for these risk factors could be an important preventative intervention. Chapter 8 describes this in more detail.

Lifestyle Risk Factors

Numerous lifestyle and physical risk factors are associated with dementia. These include low educational attainment, hearing loss, hypertension, depression, diabetes, smoking, alcohol misuse, low or no physical activity, traumatic brain injury and social isolation (Baumgart et al. 2015). The 2020 Lancet Commission report categorised these risk factors according to the life stage in which they increase the risk of dementia (Livingston et al. 2020), and this was as follows: early life (education to promote cognitive reserve), midlife (hearing loss, hypertension, obesity, alcohol misuse and traumatic brain injury) and late life (physical inactivity, depression, smoking, social isolation, diabetes and air pollution). These modifiable factors taken together could prevent 40% of all dementia cases, which would reduce costs significantly (Livingston et al. 2020).

Previous research indicated that head trauma was not a risk factor for AD (Launer et al. 1999), but later research suggests that even mild head trauma can worsen dementia risk. Those with dementia are also at an increased fall risk (Meuleners et al. 2016). Without the reflex to buffer the effects of falls, head injury is often the result, leading to a worsening of symptoms. Environments should reduce fall risks with non-slip floors (particularly in wet rooms and around the bed), safe stairs with safety railing throughout and level flooring.

A large proportion of the risk factors stated previously are also implicated in cardiovascular health, and such factors can particularly lead to an increased risk of VaD. For example, midlife hypertension and obesity have been associated with an increased VaD but also AD risk (Fitzpatrick et al. 2009; Sharp et al. 2011). Engagement in physical activity has been shown to reduce the risk of VaD (Aarsland et al. 2010) and AD by acting on cardiovascular risk factors (e.g. reducing midlife hypertension and obesity). However, this can also occur through the stimulation of brain-derived nerve growth factor (BDNF, a molecule related to memory) to offset the loss of neuronal connectivity and through the promotion of muscle strength, flexibility and balance to reduce risk of falls reducing head injury (Hogervorst et al. 2012).

Most of these modifiable risk factors can be incorporated in aspects of the design of the environment to reduce dementia symptom onset and worsening at all stages of the prevention route (e.g. primary, secondary and tertiary prevention; see Chapter 3).

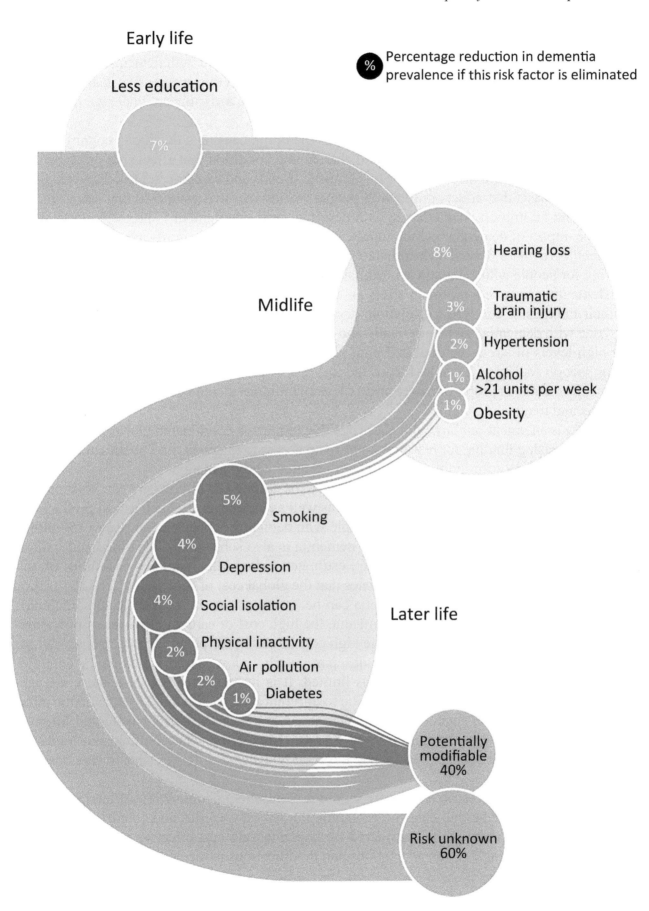

Figure 2.5 Risk factor infographic from Livingston et al. (2020)

Summary

This chapter provided an overview of the financial issues associated with dementia care. We also discussed the dementia journey and risk factors associated with this progressive change in function and dependency. The care of people with dementia poses a significant challenge for society and requires a multidisciplinary approach.

Dementia is a progressive condition that affects the brain, causing a decline in cognitive abilities, including memory. It is a complex and challenging condition that affects not only the individual with dementia but also their family members, friends and caregivers. Dementia is a global public health crisis that affects millions of people worldwide. It is estimated that there are currently around 50 million people living with dementia, and this number is projected to triple by 2050. The impact of dementia on individuals, families and society is significant and far reaching.

Dementia is a major burden on healthcare systems and economies. The direct and indirect costs of caring for people with dementia are estimated to be in the hundreds of billions of dollars globally. Dementia can have a profound effect on the social and emotional well-being of individuals and their families. It can lead to isolation, depression and a loss of independence. Caring for a loved one with dementia can be physically and emotionally demanding. Caregivers often experience high levels of stress, burnout and poor physical health. Dementia can also have a significant impact on society as a whole. It can lead to a loss of productivity and a strain on healthcare systems. Dementia disproportionately affects low and middle-income countries, where access to diagnosis and treatment is limited.

Dementia is an urgent public health challenge that requires a coordinated global response. This includes increasing funding for research, improving access to diagnosis and treatment and developing support services for individuals and families affected by dementia.

In the UK, the total cost of dementia is estimated to be around £26 billion per year. This includes direct costs, such as healthcare and social care, as well as indirect costs, such as lost productivity and informal care. The cost of caring for people with dementia is projected to rise to £50 billion by 2018. Globally, the economic impact of dementia is also substantial. The direct and indirect costs of caring for people with dementia are estimated to be in the hundreds of billions of dollars. The World Health Organisation estimates that the global cost of dementia reached $1 trillion by 2018. The economic impact of dementia can be attributed to a number of factors, including the increasing number of people with dementia, the high cost of care and the loss of productivity caused by the disease. Additionally, the high cost of caring for people with dementia can put a strain on healthcare systems and economies, particularly in low- and middle-income countries where access to diagnosis and treatment is limited. It is important to note that these are estimated costs, and the actual costs may vary due to different factors. Not only does dementia affect the expenditure of formal funding bodies, such as governments, but also private and informal care costs that are provided by families and friends. It is apparent that the financial impact of dementia is imbalanced between formal and informal budgets, as informal unpaid care costs are much higher.

Investing in dementia research and care would not only help people with dementia and their families but also could help to ease the economic burden on societies and countries. Offsetting dementia-related costs should be considered by implementing cost-effective solutions that can target risk factors through design adaptations and modifications in the environment.

References

Aarsland, D., Sardahaee, F.S., Anderssen, S., and Ballard, C., 2010. Is physical activity a potential preventive factor for vascular dementia? A systematic review, 14 (4), 386–395. https://doi.org/10.1080/13607860903586136.

Alzheimer's Disease International, 2023. Dementia statistics | Alzheimer's Disease International (ADI). www.alzint.org/about/dementia-facts-figures/dementia-statistics/ [Accessed 11 Jan 2023].

Alzheimer's Disease International and McGill University, 2021. World Alzheimer report 2021: Journey through the diagnosis of dementia. www.alzint.org/resource/world-alzheimer-report-2021/ [Accessed 11 Dec 2022].

American Psychiatric Association, DSM-5 Task Force, 2013. *Diagnostic and Statistical Manual of Mental Disorders*. 5th ed. American Psychiatric Publishing, Inc. https://doi.org/10.1176/appi. books.9780890425596.

Arnault, L., Jusot, F., and Renaud, T., 2021. Economic vulnerability and unmet healthcare needs among the population aged 50+ years during the COVID-19 pandemic in Europe. *European Journal of Ageing*, 19 (4), 811–825.

Baumgart, M., Snyder, H.M., Carrillo, M.C., Fazio, S., Kim, H., and Johns, H., 2015. Summary of the evidence on modifiable risk factors for cognitive decline and dementia: A population-based perspective. *Alzheimer's & Dementia*, 11 (6), 718–726.

Berg, L., 1988. Clinical dementia rating (CDR). *Psychopharmacology Bulletin*, 24 (4), 637–639.

Comas-Herrera, A., Guerchet, M., Karagiannidou, M., Knapp, M., and Prince, M., 2016. World Alzheimer report 2016: Improving healthcare for people living with dementia: Coverage, quality and costs now and in the future. www.alzint.org/resource/world-alzheimer-report-2016/ [Accessed 12 Dec 2022].

Crean, S., Ward, A., Mercaldi, C.J., Collins, J.M., Cook, M.N., Baker, N.L., and Arrighi, H.M., 2011. Apolipoprotein E ε4 prevalence in Alzheimer's disease patients varies across global populations: A systematic literature review and meta-analysis. *Dementia and Geriatric Cognitive Disorders*, 31 (1), 20–30.

Feger, D.M., Willis, S.L., Thomas, K.R., Marsiske, M., Rebok, G.W., Felix, C., and Gross, A.L., 2020. Incident instrumental activities of daily living difficulty in older adults: Which comes first? Findings from the advanced cognitive training for independent and vital elderly study. *Frontiers in Neurology*, 11, 1234.

Fitzpatrick, A.L., Kuller, L.H., Lopez, O.L., Diehr, P., O'Meara, E.S., Longstreth, W.T., and Luchsinger, J.A., 2009. Midlife and late-life obesity and the risk of dementia: Cardiovascular health study. *Archives of Neurology*, 66 (3), 336–342.

Gharbi-Meliani, A., Dugravot, A., Sabia, S., Regy, M., Fayosse, A., Schnitzler, A., Kivimäki, M., Singh-Manoux, A., and Dumurgier, J., 2021. The association of APOE ε4 with cognitive function over the adult life course and incidence of dementia: 20 years follow-up of the Whitehall II study. *Alzheimer's Research and Therapy*, 13 (1), 1–11.

Guerchet, M., Prince, M., and Prina, M., 2020. Numbers of people with dementia worldwide: An update to the estimates in the World Alzheimer Report 2015. www.alzint.org/resource/numbers-of-people-with-dementia-worldwide/ [Accessed 12 Dec 2022].

Heffernan, A.L., Chidgey, C., Peng, P., Masters, C.L., and Roberts, B.R., 2016. The neurobiology and age-related prevalence of the ε4 allele of apolipoprotein E in Alzheimer's disease cohorts. *Journal of Molecular Neuroscience*, 60 (3), 316–324.

Hogervorst, E., 1998. *Age-Related Cognitive Decline and Cognition Enhancers*. NeuroPsych Publishers: Maastricht.

Hogervorst, E., Clifford, A., Stock, J., Xin, X., and Stephan, B., 2012. Exercise to prevent cognitive decline and Alzheimer's disease: For whom, when, what, and (most importantly) how much? *Journal of Alzheimers Disease & Parkinsonism*, 2 (3), 1–3.

Horner, B., and Boldy, D.P., 2008. The benefit and burden of 'ageing-in-place' in an aged care community. *Australian Health Review*, 32 (2), 356–365.

Hu, B., Read, S., Wittenberg, R., Brimblecombe, N., Rodrigues, R., Banerjee, S., Dixon, J., Robinson, L., Rehill, A., and Fernandez, J.-L., 2022. Socioeconomic inequality of long-term care for older people with and without dementia in England. *Ageing & Society*, 1–21.

Irving, K., Hogervorst, E., Oliveira, D., and Kivipelto, M., 2020. *New Developments in Dementia Prevention Research State of the Art and Future Possibilities*. 1st ed. Routledge: London.

Jönsson, L., 2022. The personal economic burden of dementia in Europe. *The Lancet Regional Health – Europe*, 20, 100472.

Killin, L.O.J., Starr, J.M., Shiue, I.J., and Russ, T.C., 2016. Environmental risk factors for dementia: A systematic review. *BMC Geriatrics*, 16 (1), 1–28.

The Lancet Public Health, 2021. Reinvigorating the public health response to dementia. *The Lancet Public Health*, 6 (10), e696.

Launer, L.J., Andersen, K., Dewey, M.E., Letenneur, L., Ott, A., Amaducci, L.A., Brayne, C., Copeland, J.R.M., Dartigues, J.F., Kragh-Sorensen, P., Lobo, A., Martinez-Lage, J.M., Stijnen, T., and Hofman, A., 1999. Rates and risk factors for dementia and Alzheimer's disease. *Neurology*, 52 (1), 78–78.

Livingston, G., Huntley, J., Sommerlad, A., Ames, D., Ballard, C., Banerjee, S., Brayne, C., Burns, A., Cohen-Mansfield, J., Cooper, C., Costafreda, S.G., Dias, A., Fox, N., Gitlin, L.N., Howard, R., Kales, H.C., Kivimäki, M., Larson, E.B., Ogunniyi, A., Orgeta, V., Ritchie, K., Rockwood, K., Sampson, E.L., Samus, Q., Schneider, L.S., Selbæk, G., Teri, L., and Mukadam, N., 2020. Dementia prevention, intervention, and care: 2020 report of the lancet commission. *The Lancet*, 396 (10248), 413–446.

Lourida, I., Hannon, E., Littlejohns, T.J., Langa, K.M., Hyppönen, E., Kuźma, E., and Llewellyn, D.J., 2019. Association of lifestyle and genetic risk with incidence of dementia. *JAMA*, 322 (5), 430–437.

Luengo-Fernandez, R., and Landeiro, F., In preparation. The economic burden of dementia in the UK. https://dementiastatistics.org/statistics/numbers-of-people-in-the-uk-2/ [Accessed 22 Nov 2022].

Maeshima, S., Osawa, A., Kondo, I., Kamiya, M., Ueda, I., Sakurai, T., and Arai, H., 2021. Differences in instrumental activities of daily living between mild cognitive impairment and Alzheimer's disease: A study using a detailed executive function assessment. *Geriatrics & Gerontology International*, 21 (12), 1111–1117.

Mattap, S.M., Mohan, D., McGrattan, A.M., Allotey, P., Stephan, B.C.M., Reidpath, D.D., Siervo, M., Robinson, L., and Chaiyakunapruk, N., 2022. The economic burden of dementia in low- and middle-income countries (LMICs): A systematic review. *BMJ Global Health*, 7 (4), e007409. www.ncbi.nlm.nih.gov/pmc/articles/PMC8981345/ [Accessed 14 Dec 2022].

McCullagh, C.D., Craig, D., McIlroy, S.P., and Passmore, A.P., 2001. Risk factors for dementia. *Advances in Psychiatric Treatment*, 7 (1), 24–31.

Mecocci, P., and Boccardi, V., 2021. The impact of aging in dementia: It is time to refocus attention on the main risk factor of dementia. *Ageing Research Reviews*, 65, 101210. www.sciencedirect.com/science/article/pii/S1568163720303457?via%3Dihub [Accessed 16 Dec 2022].

Meijer, E., Casanova, M., Kim, H., Llena-Nozal, A., and Lee, J., 2022. Economic costs of dementia in 11 countries in Europe: Estimates from nationally representative cohorts of a panel study. *The Lancet Regional Health – Europe*, 20, 100445.

Meuleners, L.B., Fraser, M.L., Bulsara, M.K., Chow, K., and Ng, J.Q., 2016. Risk factors for recurrent injurious falls that require hospitalization for older adults with dementia: A population based study. *BMC Neurology*, 16 (1), 1–8.

Mlinac, M.E., and Feng, M.C., 2016. Assessment of activities of daily living, self-care, and independence. *Archives of Clinical Neuropsychology*, 31 (6), 506–516.

Mutumba, M., and Schulenberg, J.E., 2019. Tobacco and alcohol use among youth in low and middle income countries: A multi-country analysis on the influence of structural and micro-level factors. *Substance Use & Misuse*, 54 (3), 396.

NHS Digital, 2022. Recorded dementia diagnoses, January 2022 – GOV.UK. www.gov.uk/government/statistics/recorded-dementia-diagnoses-january-2022 [Accessed 11 Dec 2022].

Office for National Statistics, 2020. Statistical bulletin. Deaths registered in 2019 in England and Wales due to dementia and Alzheimer's disease, by sex, and age group/100,000. www.ons.gov.uk/peoplepopulationandcommunity/birthsdeathsandmarriages/deaths/bulletins/dementiaandalzheimersdiseasedeathsincludingcomorbiditiesenglandandwales/2019registrations#related-links [Accessed 11 Dec 2022].

Office for National Statistics, 2022. Monthly mortality analysis, England and Wales. www.ons.gov.uk/peoplepopulationandcommunity/birthsdeathsandmarriages/deaths/bulletins/monthlymortalityanalysisenglandandwales/latest [Accessed 11 Dec 2022].

Owokuhaisa, J., Rukundo, G.Z., Wakida, E., Obua, C., and Buss, S.S., 2020. Community perceptions about dementia in southwestern Uganda. *BMC Geriatrics*, 20 (1).

Pani-Harreman, K.E., Bours, G.J.J.W., Zander, I., Kempen, G.I.J.M., and van Duren, J.M.A., 2021. Definitions, key themes and aspects of 'ageing in place': A scoping review. *Ageing & Society*, 41 (9), 2026–2059.

Podcasy, J.L., and Epperson, C.N., 2022. Considering sex and gender in Alzheimer disease and other dementias. *Dialogues in Clinical Neuroscience*, 18 (4), 437–446.

Prince, M.A., Knapp, M., Guerchet, M., McCrone, P., Prina, M., Comas-Herrera, A., Wittenberg, R., Adelaja, B., Hu, B., King, D., Rehill, A., and Salimkumar, D., 2014. Dementia UK: Second edition – overview. Report.

Prince, M.A., Wimo, A., Guerchet, M., Gemma-Claire Ali, M., Wu, Y.-T., Prina, M., Yee Chan, K., and Xia, Z., 2015. World Alzheimer Report 2015: The global impact of dementia: An analysis of prevalence, incidence, cost and trends. www.alzint.org/u/WorldAlzheimerReport2015.pdf [Accessed 14 Dec 2022].

Salthouse, T.A., 1996. The processing-speed theory of adult age differences in cognition. *Psychological Review*, 103 (3), 403–428.

Sharp, S.I., Aarsland, D., Day, S., Sønnesyn, H., and Ballard, C., 2011. Hypertension is a potential risk factor for vascular dementia: Systematic review. *International Journal of Geriatric Psychiatry*, 26 (7), 661–669.

Silva-Fernandes, A., Cruz, S., Moreira, C.S., Pereira, D.R., Sousa, S.S., Sampaio, A., and Carvalho, J., 2022. Processing speed mediates the association between physical activity and executive functioning in elderly adults. *Frontiers in Psychology*, 13, 5242.

Velandia, P.P., Miller-Petrie, M.K., Chen, C., Chakrabarti, S., Chapin, A., Hay, S., Tsakalos, G., Wimo, A., and Dieleman, J.L., 2022. Global and regional spending on dementia care from 2000–2019 and expected future health spending scenarios from 2020–2050: An economic modelling exercise. *eClinicalMedicine*, 45.

Verghese, P.B., Castellano, J.M., and Holtzman, D.M., 2011. Apolipoprotein E in Alzheimer's disease and other neurological disorders. *The Lancet Neurology*, 10 (3), 241–252.

Walls, H., Cook, S., Matzopoulos, R., and London, L., 2020. Advancing alcohol research in low-income and middle-income countries: A global alcohol environment framework. *BMJ Global Health*, 5 (4), e001958.

Wittenberg, R., Hu, B., Barraza-Araiza, L.F., and Funder, A.R., 2019. CPEC Working Paper 5 The projections were produced using an updated version of a model developed by CPEC at LSE for the Modelling Outcome and Cost Impacts of Interventions for Dementia (MODEM) study. www.modem-dementia.org.uk [Accessed 11 Dec 2022].

Wittenberg, R., Hu, B., Barraza-Araiza, L.F., and Rehill, A., 2019. Projections of older people with dementia and costs of dementia care in the United Kingdom, 2019–2040. *CPEC Working Paper*, 5 (Nov), 1–79.

Wittenberg, R., Knapp, M., Hu, B., Comas-Herrera, A., King, D., Rehill, A., Shi, C., Banerjee, S., Patel, A., Jagger, C., and Kingston, A., 2019. The costs of dementia in England. *International Journal of Geriatric Psychiatry*, 34 (7), 1095–1103.

World Health Organisation, 2020. Dementia. www.who.int/news-room/fact-sheets/detail/dementia [Accessed 15 Nov 2022].

World Health Organisation, 2022. Ageing and health. www.who.int/news-room/fact-sheets/detail/ageing-and-health [Accessed 15 Nov 2022].

Yamazaki, Y., Zhao, N., Caulfield, T.R., Liu, C.C., and Bu, G., 2019. Apolipoprotein E and Alzheimer disease: Pathobiology and targeting strategies. *Nature Reviews Neurology*, 15 (9), 501.

3 The Medical Background of Dementia

Manisha Jain, Ahmad Aladawi and Eef Hogervorst

Introduction

Dementia is a pathology in the brain that causes deterioration in memory function, behaviour, thinking and the ability to perform daily tasks, which results in increased dependency on others (WHO 2022). This is different from normal ageing, which varies from successful ageing to the manifestation of issues with memory and the slowing down of performance on complex tasks (Hogervorst 1998).

As outlined in the previous chapter, there are nearly 50 million people with dementia globally, and this number will increase by 10 million each year. In the UK, there are 850,000 people living with dementia, and 80% live in their own homes. This number is expected to exceed 1 million by 2025 (Wittenberg et al. 2019). The total National Health Service cost of dementia in the UK is £36.7 billion, and since the number of those with dementia will increase, the cost is expected to reach £59.2 billion by 2030 (Wittenberg et al. 2019).

Most of this cost is carried by those with dementia and their carers themselves and is related to the movement into more formal care, such as nursing homes. A carer is a family member, friend or anyone who looks after the patient and helps them with their daily needs, supports them and improves their health and well-being. A carer can be an older person who does not have dementia, as at Chris and Sally's House (Jais et al. 2019) or family members, a friend, a neighbour or a formally paid carer.

With more younger people also moving away from home in LMICs, there are fewer carers, and the need for dementia-friendly housing and guidelines for its optimal design is growing. By achieving this optimal design, not only will the cost be reduced, but it will also widen the horizon to include people with dementia in society and make them independent, healthy and more comfortable. How much care and the type of care people need is affected by the type of dementia and where someone is in their dementia journey

The Dementia Journey: Causes of Dementia

Dementia has many types which, in the early stages, differentially affect cognitive ability of the patient and impact individuals' ability to perform activities of daily living, in particular instrumental activities of daily living such as cooking, dressing, shopping and banking differently (Cloutier et al. 2021). In later stages, these differences in functional ability become smaller and most individuals with dementia in the moderate-severe stages will have multiple cognitive impairments impacting their ability to live independently and thus the design of their homes. As dementia progresses and symptoms worsen in later stages, individuals may experience difficulty with basic ADL such as continence and eating.

Dementia has different clinical manifestations as a result of its underlying causes, and its onset can be gradual and progressive or sudden. However, at all stages, there is a need for adaptive

DOI: 10.1201/9781003306054-3

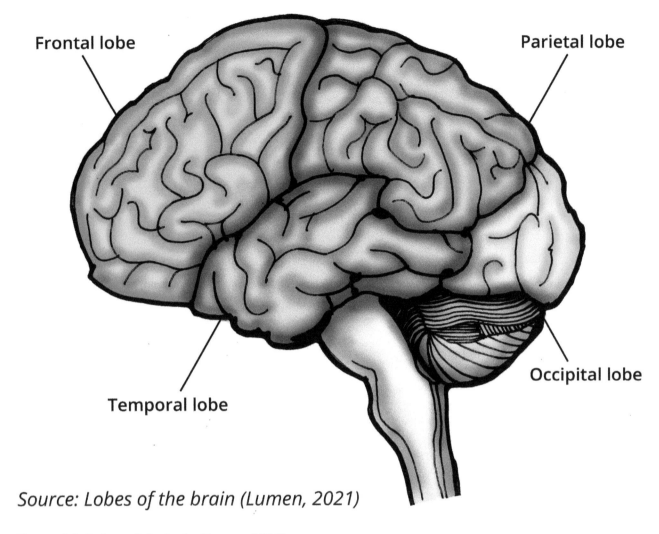

Frontal lobe

Parietal lobe

Occipital lobe

Temporal lobe

Source: Lobes of the brain (Lumen, 2021)

Figure 3.1 Lobes of the brain (Lumen 2021)

design and environments. In addition, in this chapter, we will discuss preventative strategies for different manifestations and stages of dementia and how design can support these endeavours.

Mild Cognitive Impairment

Before people reach the dementia stage, the prodromal stage (also known as a precursor stage) of mild neurocognitive disorder, with cognitive loss having little to no impact on ADL, was previously defined as mild cognitive impairment (MCI) (Petersen et al. 1999; Petersen 2000). Cognitive decline that is greater than what is typical of older age, such as performance on cognitive tests outside of 1.5 SD of the mean (Petersen et al. 2001; Petersen 2004; Portet et al. 2006), but does not affect ADL may be indicative of MCI. The prevalence of MCI has been estimated to range between <1% and 42% in the older adult population. However, this figure is dependent on the classification criteria used and setting (Petersen et al. 1999; Ward et al. 2012; Sachdev et al. 2015; Petersen 2016; Richardson et al. 2019).

The diagnostic criteria for MCI are similar to that of dementia; however, there is a more modest cognitive decline in one or more of the six cognitive domains. These domains are memory and learning, language, executive function, complex attention, social cognition and perceptual and motor function. Importantly, these cognitive deficits do not interfere with an individual's capacity for independence in ADL. For example, most iADL remain intact, but there may be a need for

The Alzheimer's Continuum

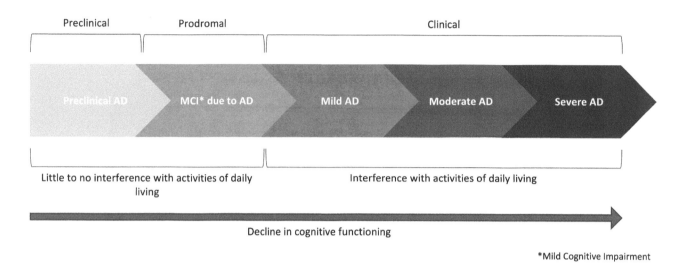

Figure 3.2 Infographic of MCI and AD

Source: Manisha Jain

extra accommodations for completing the more complex tasks. MCI can be further classified into two types, amnestic (aMCI) or non-amnestic (naMCI). In aMCI, memory impairments are often predominant and are frequently considered the precursor stage of Alzheimer's disease (Grundman et al. 2004; Csukly et al. 2016). In comparison, naMCI is characterised by impairment in cognitive domains other than memory (Csukly et al. 2016). However, the DSM-5 does not differentiate between amnestic and non-amnestic for an MCI diagnosis (Sachs-Ericsson and Blazer 2014), which is called a minor neurocognitive disorder.

Annual conversion rates indicate that 10–15% of MCI cases will convert to dementia, and more specifically to AD (Petersen et al. 1999; Chen et al. 2022). It is probable that aMCI cases are more likely to convert to AD with impairments in memory (Sachs-Ericsson and Blazer 2014). Comparatively, naMCI may be more likely to convert to dementia with Lewy body disease, a type of dementia that is discussed later in this chapter (Ferman et al. 2013). However, this does not mean that MCI cases will always convert to dementia, as some cases of MCI can revert to normal or near-normal cognitive functioning (Koepsell and Monsell 2012; Overton et al. 2019). In our study in Oxford, 25% of aMCI reverted back to normal cognitive functioning over a 2–3-year follow-up (Schrijnemaekers et al. 2007) As aMCI is more common than dementia in the over 65s, age-friendly design needs to incorporate the continuum of potential cognitive issues impacting independence, such as memory loss, but also perceptuomotor, planning, language and communication issues.

Alzheimer's Disease

Alzheimer's disease is the most common cause of dementia amongst the older adult population (Gaugler et al. 2016), accounting for 50–80% of all dementia cases (Hogervorst et al. 2003; Gaugler et al. 2016; Deb et al. 2017). AD is a progressive neurodegenerative disease that is largely characterised by progressive memory impairment, accompanied later by an overall decline in other areas of cognition (Deture and Dickson 2019). The hallmark pathology of

AD is attributed to amyloid plaques outside of cells and neurofibrillary tangles of tau proteins inside cells, causing a neuronal loss in function (Knowles et al. 1999; Deture and Dickson 2019; Tiwari et al. 2019). However, the build-up of plaques and tangles can also be observed in the ageing brain even without dementia (Sengoku 2020). AD is also associated with widespread cerebral atrophy, whereby the brain shrinks. This shrinkage has been shown to start within areas of the brain known as the medial temporal lobes and fusiform gyrus, and then eventually spreading to the posterior temporal lobes and parietal lobes before reaching the frontal lobes (Whitwell 2010). The shrinkage of certain areas in the brain that govern certain cognitive abilities means these end up deteriorating. For example, atrophy in the frontal lobes could cause a decline in executive function, which could cause issues with problem-solving, planning and self-monitoring of behaviour.

According to the DSM-5, diagnostic criteria for dementia caused by AD are outlined as:

- Insidious onset and gradual progression of impairment in one or more cognitive domains decline in memory and learning and decline in at least one other domain based on neuropsychological tests.
- Progressive decline without an extended plateau.
- No mixed aetiology and no other disorder or disease that can better explain the symptoms.

However, finding pure AD (without other pathology such as vascular lesions or Lewy bodies) is very rare at post-mortem (Hogervorst et al. 2003). The symptoms of AD can often present as memory loss, difficulty in planning, impairments in spatial awareness, language difficulty, confusion with time or place, misplacing items and mood or personality disturbances (Gaugler et al. 2016).

Additionally, in the earlier stages of the disease, individuals may experience difficulty with iADL. However, in more advanced stages, they may also need help with bADL. For example, an individual with prodromal AD (aMCI) or transitioned into AD may begin to experience a decline in their ability to manage their finances or do grocery shopping and prepare meals (iADL), whereas an individual with moderate or severe AD would require assistance with their fundamental basic needs (bADL) (Marshall et al. 2012). To further elaborate, due to the memory impairments that arise with AD, an individual may find difficulty in remembering the steps in the recipe to prepare a meal or may forget to turn the stove off, which could lead to dangerous and potentially life-threatening situations. This experience may differ compared to an individual who has a different cause of dementia, for example, frontotemporal dementia, whereby memory remains largely intact for a long period of time. The DSM-5 indicates that in AD, social cognition and procedural memory can remain relatively untouched for extended periods of time; however, degradation in these areas can affect iADL and social interactions, potentially leading to neglect, poor health and isolation.

Vascular Dementia

Vascular dementia (VaD) is considered the second most common cause of dementia, accounting for approximately 20% of cases (Wolters and Ikram 2019; Dumurgier and Sabia 2021). The cause of VaD is attributable to cerebrovascular pathologies, affecting cerebral vessels which can limit oxygen and nutrient supply to cells (Iadecola 2013). This can occur most commonly from significant cerebrovascular diseases, which can include strokes (multi- and singular infarcts) and microvascular disease, among others. There are also vascular risk factors which include cardiovascular disease, diabetes, hypertension and atrial fibrillation (Gannon et al. 2019; Papanastasiou et al. 2021). However, there is the possibility of the co-occurrence of AD and VaD, often referred to as mixed dementia, whereby both pathologies can coexist (Zekry et al. 2002).

The diagnostic criteria for VaD from the DSM-5 are highlighted as:

- Cognitive deficits temporarily related to one or more cerebrovascular events;
- Cognitive decline is prominent in complex attention and executive function;
- Presence of cerebrovascular disease from examination and neuroimaging;
- It is not better explained by another brain disease or systemic disorder.

VaD can often occur with a sudden onset, which may be temporarily linked to a cerebral or cardiovascular event. Cognitive symptoms can include memory and executive impairment, as well as language and communication deficits. In other instances, memory loss can occur suddenly or in a stepwise approach following a stroke or other cerebrovascular event. Further symptoms can include slurred speech, stroke-related impairments, incontinence, visual impairments and unsteady gait (Venkat et al. 2015).

Due to the causes of VaD various ADL may be greatly affected, especially due to post-stroke deficits and/or other underlying illnesses. Memory is often more preserved in VaD than in AD, with planning and executive functions including changed social behaviour being more affected (Hogervorst et al. 2003). However, there is limited research on the functional ability of those with VaD, and this may be due to clinical differences among patient subgroups (Boyle and Cahn-Weiner 2004; Cipriani et al. 2020). People with VaD may experience significant limitations in their bADL, even more so than those with AD, including bathing, dressing, eating and transferring. (Gure et al. 2010). However, this is often caused by the effects of vascular lesions on motor systems and not the actual dementia process.

Comparatively, iADL are most often affected in VaD because of executive function impairments, such as planning or problem-solving, and later memory impairments develop further reducing ability in iADL (Cipriani et al. 2020). This would affect their ability to do their own grocery shopping and manage medication, finances, travel and cooking. With limitations in both bADL and iADL, daily carer assistance may be required. While it has be posited that functional ability differs between VaD and AD, authors have claimed that while the nature of ADL deficits remain the same, it is the rate of progression that is different between these types of dementia (Boyle and Cahn-Weiner 2004). For example, it was indicated that ADL decline is slower amongst VaD than AD, with iADL deteriorating first before bADL.

Dementia With Lewy Bodies

Dementia with Lewy bodies (DLB) is considered the third most common cause of dementia and the second most common neurodegenerative disorder following AD, accounting for 10–20% of cases (Zaccai et al. 2005; Mueller et al. 2017). However, recent research quantified this type as only 4.2% of all dementia cases based on a clinical population of the National Health Service (NHS) secondary care services in the UK (Kane et al. 2018). DLB pathology is characterised by the accumulation of aggregated α-synuclein proteins, called Lewy bodies, located in the brain stem, neocortical areas and limbic system (McKeith 2002; Mueller et al. 2017; Rezaie et al. 1996). However, DLB is usually co-morbid with AD pathology (McKeith 2004; Outeiro et al. 2019) and rarely occurs by itself at post-mortem confirmation (Hogervorst et al. 2003).

The diagnostic criteria for DLB according to the DSM-5 are indicated as:

- Insidious onset and gradual progression which meets a combination of core and suggestive diagnostic features.

- The core features of DLB are as follows:

  - Fluctuating cognition with pronounced impairments in attention and alertness (which are very similar to signs of delirium; see previously).
  - Well-formed visual hallucinations.
  - Spontaneous features of parkinsonism, with onset after cognitive decline (otherwise this would be Parkinson's disease with dementia).
- The suggestive features of DLB are:

  - Meets the criteria for rapid eye movement sleep behaviour disorder and neuroleptic sensitivity.

For a probable diagnosis, there must be a presentation of two core features or one suggestive and one or more core features. For a possible diagnosis, this must be one core feature or one or more suggestive features.

Individuals with DLB present with various cognitive, neuropsychiatric and motor symptoms. As highlighted by the DSM-5 criteria, there can be spontaneous fluctuations in arousal and attention, with examples being daytime drowsiness, disengagement and blank stares (Chin et al. 2019). Those with DLB have also been shown to have visuospatial deficits measured by cognitive assessments, such as included in the Mini-Mental Status Examination (MMSE) (Folstein et al. 1975), whereby the pentagon-copying test in the MMSE is a valid predictive tool for DLB (Caffarra et al. 2013; Cagnin et al. 2015; Chin et al. 2019).

Visual hallucinations which are well formed and detailed are considered a hallmark characteristic of DLB, whereby up to 80% of individuals are affected (Taylor et al. 2011; Mehraram et al. 2022). While visual hallucinations are the most common, those with DLB may also experience auditory hallucinations, with prevalence rates ranging from 18–43% (Piggott et al. 2007; Suárez-González et al. 2014; Eversfield and Orton 2019). Such auditory hallucinations are either verbal or non-verbal and include human voices and animate and inanimate sounds (Eversfield and Orton 2019). However, when misdiagnosed as old-age psychiatric disorders, antipsychotic medication can worsen the prognosis. Individuals with DLB also experience motor symptoms such as spontaneous parkinsonian features such as rigidity, bradykinesia and tremors, but also gait instability and increased risk of falls (Jellinger and Korczyn 2018; Taylor et al. 2020).

Due to the nature of the symptoms experienced by those with DLB, it is expected that there is decreased functional ability affecting both bADL and iADL. As such, the combination of types of symptoms and limited functional ability can lead to a diminished quality of life (QoL). Results from the Lewy Body Dementia Association (LBDA) caregiver survey have indicated that more than 90% of those with DLB were unable to perform certain iADL, such as cooking and shopping, and more than 60% needed assistance with bADL (McKeith et al. 2005; Zweig and Galvin 2014). In addition, due to sensitivity to hallucinations, care must be given to the environment to reduce stimuli (e.g. patterned wallpaper or floors, noisy white goods) that can elicit these. The memory disorders usually develop at a later stage, while language (word finding) and executive dysfunction develop earlier than in AD.

Frontotemporal Dementia

Frontotemporal dementia is considered a rarer cause of dementia symptoms and is the second-leading cause early onset dementia following AD, most commonly affecting individuals aged 45–65 years (Ratnavalli et al. 2002; Snowden et al. 2002). FTD accounted for an average of 10.2% of dementia cases from prevalence studies in adults aged <65 years, in comparison to an average of 2.7% in adults aged >65 years (Hogan et al. 2016). Overall, it is characterised by behaviour, language and executive function deficits as a result of progressive degeneration, neuronal loss and the shrinkage of the frontal and temporal lobes (Warren et al. 2013; Bang et al. 2015). Such deficits form the basis of the types of FTD, namely the behaviour variant (bvFTD) and language variant, known as primary progressive aphasia (PPA). PPA is specified into three further variants, non-fluent, semantic and logopenic (Gorno-Tempini et al. 2011).

According to the DSM-5, the diagnostic criteria for FTD are indicated as:

- an insidious onset and gradual progression;
- relative sparing of learning and memory and perceptual motor function. However, it highlights different criteria for the variants of FTD.
- For bvFTD, the criteria suggest that there should be three or more of the following behavioural symptoms:

  - Disinhibition.
  - Apathy or inertia.
  - Loss of sympathy or empathy.
  - Perseverative, stereotyped, compulsive or ritualistic behaviours.
  - Hyperorality or dietary changes.
  - Pronounced decline in social cognition and/or executive function.

- Comparatively, for the language variant, there is:

  - Pronounced decline in language ability, such as speech production, word finding, object naming, grammar and word comprehension.

While there are separate criteria for the variants of FTD, the DSM-5 indicates that an individual may present with both.

The symptoms presented by an individual with bvFTD are often categorised in the behavioural domain; however, there are also deficits in executive function and personality changes. Apathy is considered a common symptom, presenting itself as a lack of motivation and interest, particularly in previous hobbies, self-care and personal responsibilities, all of which can lead into social isolation (Piguet et al. 2011). Additionally, disinhibition typically coexists with apathy that can cause socially inappropriate behaviour, sexual disinhibition and impulsivity. Such impulsivity can instigate risk-taking behaviours such as gambling, which has been linked with bvFTD (Manes et al. 2010).

In comparison, the language variant of FTD or PPA describe the gradual dissolution of language function (Mesulam 2001). Non-fluent PPA, which can often be combined with agrammatism, is characterised by slow non-fluent, effortful speech with lengthy pauses, utterances and inconsistent sound errors (Grossman 2012; Bang et al. 2015). Semantic PPA is characterised by difficulty in word-finding for people, places and objects (particularly for low-frequency words) and word comprehension (Laforce 2013; Bang et al. 2015). Logopenic PPA is characterised by speech fluency that is interrupted by long pauses for word finding and impaired repetition (Gorno-Tempini et al. 2011; Laforce 2013).

Those with FTD can experience limited functional ability in numerous ADL. However, the way in which such ADL are affected differ from what is seen with other types of dementia. The results of a longitudinal study demonstrated that apathy played a strong role in functional disability in both bvFTD and the semantic variant of PPA; however, apathy and stereotypical behaviours were associated with increased functional disability in those with bvFTD (O'Connor et al. 2016).

Additionally, recent findings have highlighted that those with bvFTD experienced mild impairment in bADL and moderate impairment in iADL (Musa Salech et al. 2022). The authors further indicated that apathy and disinhibition played a significant role in bADL function, whereas apathy, executive function, and emotion recognition contributed to iADL function. These results are further corroborated, whereby after controlling for age, gender, ethnicity, education, and symptom duration, those with bvFTD had greater deficits in iADL compared to the semantic and non-fluent variants of PPA (Moheb et al. 2017). Overall, research has suggested that those with bvFTD experience greater difficulty with ADL in comparison to those with the language variant or PPA. The latter would more affect social interactions but could include issues with, for instance, shopping.

Mixed Dementia

Experiencing more than one disease that affects the functionality of the patient's brain and cognitive ability is known as mixed dementia (MD) (Tayler et al. 2021). For instance, the patient might have symptoms from both Alzheimer's disease and VaD or Alzheimer's disease and Lewy body dementia. Sometimes the patient has symptoms from more than two types of dementia, such as having symptoms from Alzheimer's disease, VaD and Lewy body dementia combined (Tayler et al. 2021). The majority of dementias at pathological confirmation are mixed dementias (Hogervorst et al. 2003). Other types of dementia, such as HIV-associated dementia (HAND) and Korsakov dementia, are less common overall (APA 2013).

Ultimately, finding multiple pathologies (e.g., amyloid plaques and white matter disease or infarcts and Lewy bodies) is most common at death when the dementia diagnosis is confirmed (Hogervorst et al. 2003).

Behavioural and Psychological Symptoms of Dementia

People with dementia not only experience the symptoms highlighted previously but also behavioural and psychological symptoms, as already outlined in FTD.

Behavioural and psychological symptoms of dementia (BPSD) represent the heterogenous non-cognitive symptoms that are subjectively experienced by an individual with dementia (of any cause) that can affect mood, thought, perception, motor activity and personality (Cerejeira et al. 2012). This can present as aggression, anxiety, depression, delusions, hallucinations, wandering, apathy and sleep disturbances, among others (Cerejeira et al. 2012; Feast et al. 2016). The most frequent BPSD were irritability, apathy and agitation (Baharudin et al. 2019).

BPSD can be caused due to disturbances and discomfort in an individual's environment, within themselves (such as mood), pain, personal hygiene and care, medication, other medical illnesses, stress and sensory stimulation. BPSD manifestations can also be exacerbated in the late afternoon and evening, known as 'sundowning', a phenomenon that is well known among healthcare providers and often leads to carer burn-out (Canevelli et al. 2016). Light could potentially help these symptoms (Hanford and Figueiro 2013; Onega and Pierce 2020). Due to the chronic and progressive nature of dementia, it is expected that BPSD will get worse over time. As such, the worsening of BPSD can lead to institutionalisation (the movement into more formal care), as dependency levels and needs become too costly and complex to be dealt with in the home (Hancock et al. 2006; Orrell et al. 2007).

Results of a systematic review and meta-analysis highlighted that poorer cognitive function and BPSD were frequently associated with the increased risk of admission into a nursing home (Toot et al. 2017). However, as said, BPSD is also linked psychological distress in caregivers (Borsje et al. 2016). For example, it has been demonstrated that aggression, agitation and apathy were most distressing for caregivers (Feast et al. 2016). Nevertheless, recent research has questioned professional caregiver burnout, as no association between care home staff burnout level and staff turnover was established (Costello et al. 2020). The authors suggested that this should be further examined at an individual level and how this affects individuals' home care. It has been suggested that grief and resilience-focused interventions that specially target practical and emotional aspects should be implemented to ensure caregiver well-being (Gilsenan et al. 2022).

Such instances of BPSD can arise due to biological, psychological and environmental disturbances that can lead to unmet needs (Tible et al. 2017). An unmet need is described as a problem whereby an individual is not receiving the necessary solutions to meet the need. More specifically, the unmet needs model postulates that presentations of BPSD arise due to an individual's inability to meet their needs because of an increased difficulty in communicating and expressing these needs (Cohen-Mansfield and Werner 1995; Cohen-Mansfield et al. 2015). Consequently, the unmet needs of those with dementia, particularly in nursing homes, cause BPSD. Unmet needs have been associated with reduced quality of life, higher levels of depression and anxiety and increased behavioural problems (Slade et al. 2005; Hancock et al. 2006; Hoe et al. 2006). Research has also indicated that increased unmet needs were found in the absence of daytime activities, company and behaviour that contributed to BPSD (Ferreira et al. 2017). Environments should thus provide opportunities to engage in meaningful activities to offset these needs. However, more recent findings have shown that self-reported unmet needs from those with mild to moderate dementia did not always lead to need-related distress (Minyo and Judge 2022). Personalised approaches are important in assessing the needs and distress of both those with dementia and their carers (Cohen-Mansfield et al. 2015).

Prevention Strategies

With no cure for dementia, prevention strategies are key areas of focus to reduce the increase in numbers of people afflicted. As outlined, the prevention of dementia can be considered using three categorical prevention strategies: primary, secondary and tertiary (Irving et al. 2020; Lee et al. 2022; Maki 2021). Primary prevention aims to prevent a disease before it manifests. Secondary prevention aims to prevent further symptoms of the disease within the earliest stages, and tertiary prevention aims to delay the progression and improvement of symptoms post-diagnosis. According to these categories, dementia prevention can only occur during the primary and secondary stages; however, by the tertiary stage, it is important to focus on delaying further progression and maintaining cognition. Which preventative efforts should be done at which stage is discussed in more detail in the following sections.

Physical Activity

There is growing evidence that has suggested that modifying these risk factors and psychosocial interventions can reduce the risk of dementia and prevent or slow the progression of cognitive decline. One such example is physical exercise, whereby physical inactivity has been considered a late-life risk factor (Duan et al. 2018; McDermott et al. 2019; Livingston et al. 2020). Findings from Australia demonstrate that physical inactivity was related to the largest proportion of dementia cases, creating a compelling argument for investments in risk factor reduction programmes, particularly for physical exercise (Ashby-Mitchell et al. 2017). Optimistically, recent reviews have demonstrated that physical exercise interventions, such as aerobic and anaerobic exercise, can improve global cognitive functioning, as well as memory and executive functioning, in those with Alzheimer's disease and MCI (Guitar et al. 2018; Jia et al. 2019; Loprinzi et al. 2019; Biazus-Sehn et al. 2020). Additionally, physical activity was associated with a lower incidence of dementia, suggesting a protective role (Iso-Markku et al. 2022). Physical activity has also been associated with slowed cognitive decline across 6 years of participant engagement (Li et al. 2022). The engagement of physical activity at the primary and secondary prevention stages could prove beneficial in protecting cognition (see previous discussion on possible mechanisms).

However, not all research is consistent with these findings. Other reviews have indicated that the evidence is insufficient to conclude the efficacy of exercise on cognition (Brasure et al. 2018; Li et al. 2020). This has been suggested due to the large variance in exercise interventions, such as delivery methods, intensity, frequency and duration, as well as the lack of standardised measurement tools for cognitive domains (Cammisuli et al. 2018). With such differences between the interventions, direct comparisons to determine efficacy can be difficult to achieve with confidence. Furthermore, methodological variances, such as small sample sizes recruited for exercise interventions, can influence the statistical power of the findings and therefore affect the reliability of the results and hinder further interpretations.

Physical activity has also been shown to influence BPSD. Physical activity has been shown to be a beneficial non-pharmacological intervention to help manage BPSD in those with dementia (Kouloutbani et al. 2022). More specifically, it was highlighted that repetitive aerobic exercise three to five times a week was found to have a positive effect on BPSD.

As discussed earlier, functional ability declines with dementia, and this can cause limitations in both bADL and iADL. However, findings have indicated that physical activity can also have positive effects of ADL. Multicomponent physical activity interventions, which combined endurance, strength and balance, have been demonstrated to improve physical functioning and bADL compared to progressive resistance training (Blankevoort et al. 2010). Furthermore, a review conducted by members of our team also demonstrated that physical activity, and more specifically multicomponent exercise, had a reported improvement in ADL for those with dementia and MCI (Begde et al. 2021). This has been corroborated by another systematic review and meta-analysis whereby home-based physical activity had a medium to large effect size on ADL (de Almeida et al. 2020). Nevertheless, not all findings are supportive of this, as a recent review highlighted that aerobic and multicomponent training had no effect on ADL (Steichele et al. 2022). A common problem that is associated with physical activity research is the heterogeneity that is seen across studies. Therefore, results should be considered with this in mind.

Overall, physical activity has been demonstrated to improve global cognition, memory, executive functioning, BPSD and ADL. However, in the design and implementation stage of exercise interventions, there are numerous factors that should be considered, for example, dementia severity, as this will affect an individual's ability to engage in exercise due to decline in cognition and functional ability. Additionally, gait instability needs to be addressed and accounted for, as those with dementia are often at increased risk for falls, and this can also be exacerbated by issues with visual and perceptual functioning. Furthermore, older adults with dementia may also have other illnesses, such as cardiovascular illnesses and effects of stroke on motor ability, that may be even more prevalent in VaD. Such factors must be addressed to develop a safe training intervention that can help in numerous areas that are associated with dementia.

Technology Use

Modern technological advances have allowed for the development of various information and communication technologies (ICTs) that have multiple applications to dementia.

This can include monitoring, prompting, socialising, maintaining functionality, exercising and leisure. Technologies that can aid in such ways can help those with dementia to maintain their independence and perhaps support ageing in place.

Technologies that have been developed to support ageing in place are known as cognitive assistive technologies that can aid with ADL (Intille 2004; Mihailidis et al. 2008). An example of such technologies has been seen in Cognitive Orthosis for Assisting Activities at Home (COACH) (Mihailidis et al. 2008). This technology was developed to aid and prompt those with dementia to wash their hands and take them through the procedure using verbal and visual prompts (Astell et al. 2019). Other cognitive assistive technologies have been adapted into smart homes, and an example of this has been demonstrated in the Gloucester Smart Home (Orpwood et al. 2004). This was a prototype of a home designed for those with dementia that have been fitted with stove and bath monitors, item locators and a digital message board that can provide verbal and visual prompts for medication reminders. This type of technology can help those with dementia with their iADL, which may be more useful for someone with MCI or mild dementia. However, an individual with more severe dementia may require more assistance, as they may have limitations with bADL, and therefore this technology might not be entirely useful when dementia advances. This is because those who need help with bADL are considered more dependent, and this technology seemed to only address iADL support. Addressing the issues with bADL, an assistive technology has been developed, known as the development of a responsive emotive sensing system (DRESS) prototype, to help those with dementia with the bADL of dressing (Burleson et al. 2018). This prototype has been developed to detect various clothing items and aid in dressing, with the future developments of the prototype being planned to determine dressing progress and generate prompts. Nevertheless, DRESS is still currently in development before being implemented amongst a dementia population.

Technology has also been shown to help those with dementia to socialise and maintain relationships with family and friends. Devices such as tablets, smartphones, computers and laptops can provide a means for communication, as well as multitasking other activities such as browsing the internet, using social media and even banking. Previous research has highlighted that Skype communication was useful for those with dementia to talk with their nurse as well as their family, which was rated using a questionnaire by their caregivers (Hori et al. 2009). A more recent study examined Skype and landline telephone usage among those with dementia in nursing homes in Australia over 12 months (van der Ploeg et al. 2016). While the results were not significant, the authors found that Skype calls using a tablet lasted longer than telephone conversations and operationalised agitation behaviours reduced during Skype calls compared to telephone. These findings demonstrate that using technology to connect individuals with dementia to their family and friends has the potential to increase happiness and reduce BPSD, loneliness and social isolation (National Institute of Aging 2019).

The COVID-19 pandemic has undoubtedly brought on a new digital era, whereby people all over the world have been connecting and communicating using various technologies and the internet, particularly in times of lockdown. A recent qualitative analysis of the technology experiences of those with dementia during the pandemic have demonstrated positive perspectives (Talbot and Briggs 2022). The participants highlighted that technology had helped them in their everyday life, such as using Google maps on their smartphone during their walks and doing online shopping. Additionally, they found that using technology for social communication made it more accessible without the need for travel. It has also been highlighted that using technology has helped them learn new skills and engage in exercise. However, participants also stated that using technology can be cognitively demanding and tiring. This experience is one that is frequently noticed – and this may be because older adults have a lack of technology experience and knowledge as well as different attitudes towards technology, cognitive function and related demographic characteristics (Czaja et al. 2006). Despite this, there are potential positive uses of technology for older adults with dementia in more recent times, such as for prompting and social interaction. However, it also demonstrates areas which need addressing for making these technologies more suitable and accessible for older adults and those with dementia.

Technological devices, such as smartphones, tablets and laptops, have been increasingly used in physical activity training. However, such devices are not limited to this and can also include gaming consoles and virtual reality. While it has been largely established that physical activity could be effective for improving various symptoms associated with dementia, additive technologies to supplement such training may provide further stimulation and perhaps add a cognitive element to the exercise. Numerous technology-based or computerised physical activity interventions have demonstrated effective improvement global cognition, memory and executive function in those with dementia and MCI (Ge et al. 2018; Zhang et al. 2019; Wang et al. 2022). Furthermore, a recent 3-month home-based clinical trial examined the effects of a portable exergame, known as the interactive Physical and Cognitive Exercise System (iPACES), tested by individuals who had MCI (Anderson-Hanley et al. 2018). Participants engaged with an interactive screen which presented a virtual bike path and used an under-table elliptical pedaller. The results demonstrated an improvement in executive function and delayed verbal memory.

However, as discussed previously, technology usage among older adults can be difficult, even more so for those with dementia. Unfamiliarity can cause agitation and confusion, which could affect adherence. Additionally, cognitive impairments can impede their ability to learn new technologies and remember how to use them. Findings from a qualitative study examined barriers and facilitators to exercise training using motion-based technology from a gaming console (Ladekjær Larsen et al. 2022). The authors found that using a technological device for training was a source of both autonomy and conflict. It was also observed that there was a lack of social exposure, in comparison to training as a group in a centre, and participants' relatives indicated that this may not be suitable for someone with dementia, as they experience increased loneliness.

Overall, technologies can provide positive effects across a wide range of activities for those with dementia. However, they should be carefully designed for individuals with dementia, as they can also cause negative experiences. Therefore, different technological solutions should be targeted to different individuals depending on their wants and needs. This should be taken into account particularly when designing and adapting homes to be age and dementia friendly and integrating technology. Technology should be designed with those with dementia in mind, ensuring that usability is suitable for someone with reduced cognitive function, functional ability and other morbidities, as well as for different dementia severities. Technology use may be more suitable for individuals with MCI or mild dementia; however, those with more severe dementia may have trouble with technology engagement.

Ageing in Place

To encourage and support ageing in place for older adults, there are various factors that must be considered to ensure that a space is safe, engaging and effective at what it intends to do. As mentioned, ageing in place refers to ageing in one's familiar environment whereby independence and sense of self is maintained (Pani-Harreman et al. 2021). Ageing in a familiar environment can also help to maintain an individual's sense of autonomy, personhood and quality of life. Additionally, it can also be posited that as moving into different and new environments can often cause those with dementia to experience agitation, confusion and aggression, the maintenance of a stable and familiar environment may also help with BPSD. Nevertheless, functional ability and independence can be difficult to uphold as a result of limited ADL ability and cognitive decline. There should be consideration in how environments are designed and optimised to ensure that various needs are met.

The majority of houses today are not suitable to support ageing in place, as they may not have appropriate adaptations to support older adults living in their own environments. Housing may need to be updated and designed to be dementia friendly in ways that take into consideration the various symptoms and functional abilities of those with dementia. Such considerations that are translated into design could be spatial navigation, visual access, layout complexity, patterns and colours (Wiener and Pazzaglia 2021). For example, a good open layout can help with wayfinding and ensure visual access to key areas of the home such as the bathroom. Furthermore, changes to visual perception can alter how colours and pattern are perceived, whereby dark colours can appear to be holes and patterns may appear to be moving. However, the engagement of prevention strategies within a dementia-friendly environment, such as exercise and technology use, should also be considered for ageing in place. For example, technology could be integrated into home design to create an intuitive and easily accessible interface for older adults that could be optimised for ADL, such as prompting for medication or for water intake, as well as for engagement in exercise.

Nevertheless, due to the progressive nature of dementia and declines in cognition and ADL, formal care may be required, as the needs of an individual with severe dementia can become too great. However, the same principles as highlighted for ageing in place can also be adapted for use within formal care group settings.

Summary

Dementia is predicted to affect millions worldwide in both HICs and LMICs. Due to increasing global population growth and ageing, it is anticipated that there will be parallel rises in dementia rates and costs. Many initiatives have been established to address rising dementia rates using holistic approaches to manage various aspects of dementia, including stigma, care, risk factors, equality and treatment of symptom progression, among others. The UN's Decade of Healthy Ageing (2021–2030) demonstrates a global collaboration to establish and drive research for healthy ageing that can impact the lives of older adults with dementia and reduce risk through prevention at all levels. More importantly, the Decade of Healthy Ageing has highlighted that a key Decade Action Area is age-friendly environments. As there is no cure for dementia, prevention strategies may provide an effective way of managing dementia progression and symptoms. Such strategies can be established with physical exercise, technology use and supportive dementia-friendly environments that can support ageing in place.

References

American Psychiatric Association, 2013. Diagnostic and statistical manual of mental disorders. 5th ed. https://doi.org/10.1176/appi.books.9780890425596.

Anderson-Hanley, C., Stark, J., Wall, K.M., Vanbrakle, M., Michel, M., Maloney, M., Barcelos, N., Striegnitz, K., Cohen, B.D., and Kramer, A.F., 2018. The interactive physical and cognitive exercise system (iPACESxsTM): Effects of a 3-month in-home pilot clinical trial for mild cognitive impairment and caregivers. *Clinical Interventions in Aging*, 13, 1565–1577.

Ashby-Mitchell, K., Burns, R., Shaw, J., and Anstey, K.J., 2017. Proportion of dementia in Australia explained by common modifiable risk factors. *Alzheimer's Research and Therapy*, 9 (1), 1–8.

Astell, A.J., Bouranis, N., Hoey, J., Lindauer, A., Mihailidis, A., Nugent, C., and Robillard, J.M., 2019. Technology and dementia: The future is now. Dementia and geriatric cognitive disorders. www.karger.com/Article/FullText/497800 [Accessed 15 Dec 2022].

Baharudin, A.D., Din, N.C., Subramaniam, P., and Razali, R., 2019. The associations between behavioral-psychological symptoms of dementia (BPSD) and coping strategy, burden of care and personality style among low-income caregivers of patients with dementia. *BMC Public Health*, 19 (4), 1–12.

Bang, J., Spina, S., and Miller, B.L., 2015. Frontotemporal dementia. *The Lancet*, 386 (10004), 1672–1682.

Begde, A., Jain, M., Hogervorst, E., and Wilcockson, T., 2021. Does physical exercise improve the capacity for independent living in people with dementia or mild cognitive impairment: An overview of systematic reviews and meta-analyses. *Aging and Mental Health*, 2022 (12), 2317–2327.

Biazus-Sehn, L.F., Schuch, F.B., Firth, J., and Stigger, F. de S., 2020. Effects of physical exercise on cognitive function of older adults with mild cognitive impairment: A systematic review and meta-analysis. *Archives of Gerontology and Geriatrics*. https://pubmed.ncbi.nlm.nih.gov/32460123/ [Accessed 14 Dec 2022].

Blankevoort, C.G., van Heuvelen, M.J.G., Boersma, F., Luning, H., de Jong, J., and Scherder, E.J.A., 2010. Review of effects of physical activity on strength, balance, mobility and ADL performance in elderly subjects with dementia. *Dementia and Geriatric Cognitive Disorders*, 30 (5), 392–402.

Borsje, P., Hems, M.A.P., Lucassen, P.L.B.J., Bor, H., Koopmans, R.T.C.M., and Pot, A.M., 2016. Psychological distress in informal caregivers of patients with dementia in primary care: Course and determinants. *Family Practice*, 33 (4), 374–381.

Boyle, P.A., and Cahn-Weiner, D., 2004. Assessment and prediction of functional impairment in vascular dementia. *Expert Review of Neurotherapeutics*, 4 (1), 109–114.

Brasure, M., Desai, P., Davila, H., Nelson, V.A., Calvert, C., Jutkowitz, E., Butler, M., Fink, H.A., Ratner, E., Hemmy, L.S., McCarten, J.R., Barclay, T.R., and Kane, R.L., 2018. Physical activity interventions in preventing cognitive decline and Alzheimer-type dementia a systematic review. *Annals of Internal Medicine*. https://pubmed.ncbi.nlm.nih.gov/29255839/ [Accessed 14 Dec 2022].

Burleson, W., Lozano, C., Ravishankar, V., Lee, J., and Mahoney, D., 2018. An assistive technology system that provides personalized dressing support for people living with dementia: Capability study. *JMIR Medical Informatics*, 6 (2), e21. https://medinform.jmir.org/2018/2/e21, 6 (2), e5587 [Accessed 18 Dec 2022].

Caffarra, P., Gardini, S., Dieci, F., Copelli, S., Maset, L., Concari, L., Farina, E., and Grossi, E., 2013. The qualitative scoring MMSE pentagon test (QSPT): A new method for differentiating dementia with Lewy body from Alzheimer's disease. *Behavioural Neurology*, 27 (2), 213–220.

Cagnin, A., Bussè, C., Jelcic, N., Gnoato, F., Mitolo, M., and Caffarra, P., 2015. High specificity of MMSE pentagon scoring for diagnosis of prodromal dementia with Lewy bodies. *Parkinsonism & Related Disorders*, 21 (3), 303–305.

Cammisuli, D.M., Innocenti, A., Fusi, J., Franzoni, F., and Pruneti, C., 2018. Aerobic exercise effects upon cognition in Alzheimer's disease: A systematic review of randomized controlled trials. *Archives Italiennes de Biologie*, 156 (1–2), 54–63.

Canevelli, M., Valletta, M., Trebbastoni, A., Sarli, G., D'Antonio, F., Tariciotti, L., de Lena, C., and Bruno, G., 2016. Sundowning in dementia: Clinical relevance, pathophysiological determinants, and therapeutic approaches. *Frontiers in Medicine*, 3 (DEC), 73. www.ncbi.nlm.nih.gov/pmc/articles/PMC5187352/ [Accessed 20 Dec 2022].

Cerejeira, J., Lagarto, L., and Mukaetova-Ladinska, E.B., 2012. Behavioral and psychological symptoms of dementia. *Frontiers in Neurology*, 3. https://pubmed.ncbi.nlm.nih.gov/22586419/ [Accessed 20 Dec 2022].

Chen, Y., Qian, X., Zhang, Y., Su, W., Huang, Y., Wang, X., Chen, X., Zhao, E., Han, L., and Ma, Y., 2022. Prediction models for conversion from mild cognitive impairment to Alzheimer's disease: A systematic review and meta-analysis. *Frontiers in Aging Neuroscience*, 14, 137.

Chin, K.S., Teodorczuk, A., and Watson, R., 2019. Dementia with Lewy bodies: Challenges in the diagnosis and management. *Australian and New Zealand Journal of Psychiatry*, 53 (4), 291–303.

Cipriani, G., Danti, S., Picchi, L., Nuti, A., and di Fiorino, M., 2020. Daily functioning and dementia. *Dementia & Neuropsychologia*, 14 (2), 93.

Cloutier, S., Chertkow, H., Kergoat, M.J., Gélinas, I., Gauthier, S., and Belleville, S., 2021. Trajectories of decline on instrumental activities of daily living prior to dementia in persons with mild cognitive impairment. *International Journal of Geriatric Psychiatry*, 36 (2), 314–323.

Cohen-Mansfield, J., Dakheel-Ali, M., Marx, M.S., Thein, K., and Regier, N.G., 2015. Which unmet needs contribute to behavior problems in persons with advanced dementia? *Psychiatry Research*, 228 (1), 59.

Cohen-Mansfield, J., and Werner, P., 1995. Environmental influences on agitation: An integrative summary of an observational study. 10 (1), 32–39. http://dx.doi.org/10.1177/153331759501000108.

Costello, H., Cooper, C., Marston, L., and Livingston, G., 2020. Burnout in UK care home staff and its effect on staff turnover: MARQUE English national care home longitudinal survey. *Age and Ageing*, 49 (1), 74–81.

Csukly, G., Sirály, E., Fodor, Z., Horváth, A., Salacz, P., Hidasi, Z., Csibri, É., Rudas, G., and Szabó, Á., 2016. The differentiation of amnestic type MCI from the non-amnestic types by structural MRI. *Frontiers in Aging Neuroscience*, 8 (MAR), 52.

Czaja, S.J., Charness, N., Fisk, A.D., Hertzog, C., Nair, S.N., Rogers, W.A., and Sharit, J., 2006. Factors predicting the use of technology: Findings from the Center for Research and Education on Aging and Technology Enhancement (CREATE). *Psychology and Aging*, 21 (2), 333.

de Almeida, S.I.L., Gomes Da Silva, M., and Marques, A.S.P. de D., 2020. Home-based physical activity programs for people with dementia: Systematic review and meta-analysis. *Gerontologist*. https://academic.oup.com/gerontologist/article/60/8/e600/5681706 [Accessed 14 Dec 2022].

Deb, A., Thornton, J.D., Sambamoorthi, U., and Innes, K., 2017. Direct and indirect cost of managing Alzheimer's disease and related dementias in the United States. *Expert Review of Pharmacoeconomics & Outcomes Research*, 17 (2), 189.

Deture, M.A., and Dickson, D.W., 2019. The neuropathological diagnosis of Alzheimer's disease. *Molecular Neurodegeneration*, 14 (1), 1–18.

Duan, Y., Lu, L., Chen, J., Wu, C., Liang, J., Zheng, Y., Wu, J., Rong, P., and Tang, C., 2018. Psychosocial interventions for Alzheimer's disease cognitive symptoms: A Bayesian network meta-analysis. *BMC Geriatrics*, 18 (1).

Dumurgier, J., and Sabia, S., 2021. Life expectancy in dementia subtypes: Exploring a leading cause of mortality. *The Lancet Healthy Longevity*, 2 (8), e449–e450.

Eversfield, C.L., and Orton, L.D., 2019. Auditory and visual hallucination prevalence in Parkinson's disease and dementia with Lewy bodies: A systematic review and meta-analysis. *Psychological Medicine*, 49 (14), 2342–2353.

Feast, A., Moniz-Cook, E., Stoner, C., Charlesworth, G., and Orrell, M., 2016. A systematic review of the relationship between behavioral and psychological symptoms (BPSD) and caregiver well-being. *International Psychogeriatrics*, 28 (11), 1761–1774.

Ferman, T.J., Smith, G.E., Kantarci, K., Boeve, B.F., Pankratz, V.S., Dickson, D.W., Graff-Radford, N.R., Wszolek, Z., Gerpen, J. van, Uitti, R., Pedraza, O., Murray, M.E., Aakre, J., Parisi, J., Knopman, D.S., and Petersen, R.C., 2013. Nonamnestic mild cognitive impairment progresses to dementia with Lewy bodies. *Neurology*, 81 (23), 2032.

Ferreira, A.R., Martins, S., Dias, C., Simões, M.R., and Fernandes, L., 2017. Behavioral and psychological symptoms: A contribution for their understanding based on the unmet needs model. *European Psychiatry*, 41 (S1), S657–S657.

Folstein, M.F., Folstein, S.E., and McHugh, P.R., 1975. 'Mini-mental state'. A practical method for grading the cognitive state of patients for the clinician. *Journal of Psychiatric Research*, 12 (3), 189–198.

Gannon, O.J., Robison, L.S., Custozzo, A.J., and Zuloaga, K.L., 2019. Sex differences in risk factors for vascular contributions to cognitive impairment & dementia. *Neurochemistry International*, 127, 38–55.

Gaugler, J., James, B., Johnson, T., Scholz, K., and Weuve, J., 2016. Alzheimer's disease facts and figures. *Alzheimer's & Dementia*, 12 (4), 459–509.

Ge, S., Zhu, Z., Wu, B., and McConnell, E.S., 2018. Technology-based cognitive training and rehabilitation interventions for individuals with mild cognitive impairment: A systematic review. *BMC Geriatrics*, 18 (1), 1–19.

Gilsenan, J., Gorman, C., and Shevlin, M., 2022. Explaining caregiver burden in a large sample of UK dementia caregivers: The role of contextual factors, behavioural problems, psychological resilience, and anticipatory grief. www.tandfonline.com/doi/abs/10.1080/13607863.2022.2102138 [Accessed 11 Dec 2022].

Gorno-Tempini, M.L., Hillis, A.E., Weintraub, S., Kertesz, A., Mendez, M., Cappa, S.F., Ogar, J.M., Rohrer, J.D., Black, S., Boeve, B.F., Manes, F., Dronkers, N.F., Vandenberghe, R., Rascovsky, K., Patterson, K., Miller, B.L., Knopman, D.S., Hodges, J.R., Mesulam, M.M., and Grossman, M., 2011. Classification of primary progressive aphasia and its variants. *Neurology*, 76 (11), 1006–1014.

Grossman, M., 2012. The non-fluent/agrammatic variant of primary progressive aphasia. *The Lancet Neurology*, 11 (6), 545–555.

Grundman, M., Petersen, R.C., Ferris, S.H., Thomas, R.G., Aisen, P.S., Bennett, D.A., Foster, N.L., Jack, C.R., Galasko, D.R., Doody, R., Kaye, J., Sano, M., Mohs, R., Gauthier, S., Kim, H.T., Jin, S., Schultz, A.N., Schafer, K., Mulnard, R., van Dyck, C.H., Mintzer, J., Zamrini, E.Y., Cahn-Weiner, D., and Thal, L.J., 2004. Mild cognitive impairment can be distinguished from Alzheimer disease and normal aging for clinical trials. *Archives of Neurology*, 61 (1), 59–66.

Guitar, N.A., Connelly, D.M., Nagamatsu, L.S., Orange, J.B., and Muir-Hunter, S.W., 2018. The effects of physical exercise on executive function in community-dwelling older adults living with Alzheimer's-type dementia: A systematic review. *Ageing Research Reviews*. https://pubmed.ncbi.nlm.nih.gov/30102996/ [Accessed 20 Dec 2022].

Gure, T.R., Kabeto, M.U., Plassman, B.L., Piette, J.D., and Langa, K.M., 2010. Differences in functional impairment across subtypes of dementia. *The Journals of Gerontology Series A: Biological Sciences and Medical Sciences*, 65A (4), 434.

Hancock, G.A., Woods, B., Challis, D., and Orell, M., 2006. The needs of older people with dementia in residential care. *International Journal of Geriatric Psychiatry*, 21 (1), 43–49.

Hanford, N., and Figueiro, M., 2013. Light therapy and Alzheimer's disease and related dementia: Past, present, and future. *Journal of Alzheimer's Disease: JAD*, 33 (4), 913.

Hoe, J., Hancock, G., Livingston, G., and Orrell, M., 2006. Quality of life of people with dementia in residential care homes. *The British Journal of Psychiatry*, 188 (5), 460–464.

Hogan, D.B., Jetté, N., Fiest, K.M., Roberts, J.I., Pearson, D., Smith, E.E., Roach, P., Kirk, A., Pringsheim, T., and Maxwell, C.J., 2016. The prevalence and incidence of frontotemporal dementia: A systematic review. *Canadian Journal of Neurological Sciences*, 43 (S1), S96–S109.

Hogervorst, E., Bandelow, S., Combrinck, M., Irani, S., and Smith, A.D., 2003. The validity and reliability of 6 sets of clinical criteria to classify Alzheimer's disease and vascular dementia in cases confirmed post-mortem: Added value of a decision tree approach. *Dementia and Geriatric Cognitive Disorders*, 16 (3), 170–180.

Hori, M., Kubota, M., Ando, K., Kihara, T., Takahashi, R., and Kinoshita, A., 2009. [The effect of videophone communication (with Skype and webcam) for elderly patients with dementia and their caregivers]. Gan to Kagaku ryoho. *Cancer & Chemotherapy*, 36 Suppl 1, 36–38.

Iadecola, C., 2013. The pathobiology of vascular dementia. *Neuron*, 80 (4), 844–866.

Intille, S.S., 2004. A new research challenge: Persuasive technology to motivate healthy aging. *IEEE Transactions on Information Technology in Biomedicine*, 8 (3), 235–237.

Irving, K., Hogervorst, E., Oliveira, D., and Kivipelto, M., 2020. *New Developments in Dementia Prevention Research: State of the Art and Future Possibilities*. 1st ed. Routledge: London.

Iso-Markku, P., Kujala, U.M., Knittle, K., Polet, J., Vuoksimaa, E., and Waller, K., 2022. Physical activity as a protective factor for dementia and Alzheimer's disease: Systematic review, meta-analysis and quality assessment of cohort and case – control studies. *British Journal of Sports Medicine*, 56 (12), 701–709.

Jais, C., et al., 2019. Chris and Sally's House: Adapting a home for people living with dementia (innovative practice). *Dementia and Geriatric Cognitive Disorders*, 20 (2), 770–778. https://doi.org/10.1177/1471301219887040.

Jellinger, K.A., and Korczyn, A.D., 2018. Are dementia with Lewy bodies and Parkinson's disease dementia the same disease? *BMC Medicine*, 16 (1), 1–16.

Jia, R.X., Liang, J.H., Xu, Y., and Wang, Y.Q., 2019. Effects of physical activity and exercise on the cognitive function of patients with Alzheimer disease: A meta-analysis. *BMC Geriatrics*, 19 (1), 181.

Kane, J.P.M., Surendranathan, A., Bentley, A., Barker, S.A.H., Taylor, J.P., Thomas, A.J., Allan, L.M., McNally, R.J., James, P.W., McKeith, I.G., Burn, D.J., and O'Brien, J.T., 2018. Clinical prevalence of Lewy body dementia. *Alzheimer's Research and Therapy*, 10 (1), 1–8.

Knowles, R.B., Wyart, C., Buldyrev, S.V., Cruz, L., Urbanc, B., Hasselmo, M.E., Stanley, H.E., and Hyman, B.T., 1999. Plaque-induced neurite abnormalities: Implications for disruption of neural networks in Alzheimer's disease. *Proceedings of the National Academy of Sciences*, 96 (9), 5274–5279.

Koepsell, T.D., and Monsell, S.E., 2012. Reversion from mild cognitive impairment to normal or near-normal cognition: Risk factors and prognosis. *Neurology*, 79 (15), 1591–1598.

Kouloutbani, K., Venetsanou, F., Markati, A., Karteroliotis, K.E., and Politis, A., 2022. The effectiveness of physical exercise interventions in the management of neuropsychiatric symptoms in dementia patients: A systematic review. *International Psychogeriatrics*, 34 (2), 177–190.

Ladekjær Larsen, E., Waldorff, F.B., Hansen, H.P., and la Cour, K., 2022. Home-based training technology for persons with dementia: A qualitative study of barriers and facilitators for mobility-based training at home. *BMC Geriatrics*, 22 (1), 1–10.

Laforce, R., 2013. Behavioral and language variants of frontotemporal dementia: A review of key symptoms. *Clinical Neurology and Neurosurgery*, 115 (12), 2405–2410.

Lee, J., Howard, R.S., and Schneider, L.S., 2022. The current landscape of prevention trials in dementia. *Neurotherapeutics*, 19 (1), 228–247.

Li, B., Liu, C., Wan, Q., and Yu, F., 2020. An integrative review of exercise interventions among community-dwelling adults with Alzheimer's disease. *International Journal of Older People Nursing*, 15 (1), e12287.

Li, C., Ma, Y., Hua, R., Zheng, F., and Xie, W., 2022. Long-term physical activity participation trajectories were associated with subsequent cognitive decline, risk of dementia and all-cause mortality among adults aged ≥50 years: A population-based cohort study. *Age and Ageing*, 51 (3).

Livingston, G., Huntley, J., Sommerlad, A., Ames, D., Ballard, C., Banerjee, S., Brayne, C., Burns, A., Cohen-Mansfield, J., Cooper, C., Costafreda, S.G., Dias, A., Fox, N., Gitlin, L.N., Howard, R., Kales, H.C., Kivimäki, M., Larson, E.B., Ogunniyi, A., Orgeta, V., Ritchie, K., Rockwood, K., Sampson, E.L., Samus, Q., Schneider, L.S., Selbæk, G., Teri, L., and Mukadam, N., 2020. Dementia prevention, intervention, and care: 2020 report of the Lancet Commission. *The Lancet*, 396 (10248), 413–446.

Loprinzi, P.D., Blough, J., Ryu, S., and Kang, M., 2019. Experimental effects of exercise on memory function among mild cognitive impairment: Systematic review and meta-analysis. *Physician and Sports Medicine*. https://pubmed.ncbi.nlm.nih.gov/30246596 [Accessed 18 Dec 2022].

Lumen, 2021. Biology for majors. https://courses.lumenlearning.com/wm-biology2/chapter/brain/ [Accessed 11 Jan 2023].

Maki, Y., 2021. Ikigai interventions for primary, secondary, and tertiary prevention of dementia. *Aging and Health Research*, 1 (3), 100026. www.sciencedirect.com/science/article/pii/S266703212100024X [Accessed 20 Dec 2022].

Manes, F.F., Torralva, T., Roca, M., Gleichgerrcht, E., Bekinschtein, T.A., and Hodges, J.R., 2010. Frontotemporal dementia presenting as pathological gambling. *Nature Reviews Neurology*, 6 (6), 347–352.

Marshall, G.A., Amariglio, R.E., Sperling, R.A., and Rentz, D.M., 2012. Activities of daily living: Where do they fit in the diagnosis of Alzheimer's disease? *Neurodegenerative Disease Management*, 2 (5), 483.

McDermott, O., Charlesworth, G., Hogervorst, E., Stoner, C., Moniz-Cook, E., Spector, A., Csipke, E., and Orrell, M., 2019. Psychosocial interventions for people with dementia: A synthesis of systematic reviews. *Aging and Mental Health*. www.tandfonline.com/doi/full/10.1080/13607863.2017.1423031 [Accessed 12 Dec 2022].

McKeith, I.G., 2002. Dementia with Lewy bodies. *The British Journal of Psychiatry*, 180 (2), 144–147.

McKeith, I.G., 2004. Dementia with Lewy bodies. *Dialogues in Clinical Neuroscience*, 6 (3), 333–341.

McKeith, I.G., Dickson, D.W., Lowe, J., Emre, M., O'Brien, J.T., Feldman, H., Cummings, J., Duda, J.E., Lippa, C., Perry, E.K., Aarsland, D., Arai, H., Ballard, C.G., Boeve, B., Burn, D.J., Costa, D., del Ser, T., Dubois, B., Galasko, D., Gauthier, S., Goetz, C.G., Gomez-Tortosa, E., Halliday, G., Hansen, L.A., Hardy, J., Iwatsubo, T., Kalaria, R.N., Kaufer, D., Kenny, R.A., Korczyn, A., Kosaka, K., Lee, V.M.Y., Lees, A., Litvan, I., Londos, E., Lopez, O.L., Minoshima, S., Mizuno, Y., Molina, J.A., Mukaetova-Ladinska, E.B., Pasquier, F., Perry, R.H., Schulz, J.B., Trojanowski, J.Q., and Yamada, M., 2005. Diagnosis and management of dementia with Lewy bodies. *Neurology*, 65 (12), 1863–1872.

Mehraram, R., Peraza, L.R., Murphy, N.R.E., Cromarty, R.A., Graziadio, S., O'Brien, J.T., Killen, A., Colloby, S.J., Firbank, M., Su, L., Collerton, D., Taylor, J.P., and Kaiser, M., 2022. Functional and structural brain network correlates of visual hallucinations in Lewy body dementia. *Brain*, 145 (6), 2190–2205.

Mesulam, M.M., 2001. Primary progressive aphasia. *Annals of Neurology*, 49 (4), 425–432.

Mihailidis, A., Boger, J.N., Craig, T., and Hoey, J., 2008. The COACH prompting system to assist older adults with dementia through handwashing: An efficacy study. *BMC Geriatrics*, 8 (1), 1–18.

Minyo, M.J., and Judge, K.S., 2022. Perceived unmet need and need-related distress of people living with dementia. *Gerontology and Geriatric Medicine*, 8. www.ncbi.nlm.nih.gov/pmc/articles/PMC9149624/ [Accessed 20 Dec 2022].

Moheb, N., Mendez, M.F., Kremen, S.A., and Teng, E., 2017. Executive dysfunction and behavioral symptoms are associated with deficits in instrumental activities of daily living in frontotemporal dementia. *Dementia and Geriatric Cognitive Disorders*, 43 (1–2), 89–99.

Mueller, C., Ballard, C., Corbett, A., and Aarsland, D., 2017. The prognosis of dementia with Lewy bodies. *The Lancet Neurology*, 16 (5), 390–398.

Musa Salech, G., Lillo, P., van der Hiele, K., Méndez-Orellana, C., Ibáñez, A., and Slachevsky, A., 2022. Apathy, executive function, and emotion recognition are the main drivers of functional impairment in behavioral variant of frontotemporal dementia. *Frontiers in Neurology*, 12, 2384. https://pubmed.ncbi.nlm.nih.gov/35095710/ [Accessed 22 Dec 2022].

National Institute of Aging, 2019. Social isolation, loneliness in older people pose health risks. www.nia.nih.gov/news/social-isolation-loneliness-older-people-pose-health-risks [Accessed 31 May 2022].

O'Connor, C.M., Clemson, L., Hornberger, M., Leyton, C.E., Hodges, J.R., Piguet, O., and Mioshi, E., 2016. Longitudinal change in everyday function and behavioral symptoms in frontotemporal dementia. *Neurology Clinical Practice*, 6 (5), 419–428.

Onega, L.L., and Pierce, T.W., 2020. Use of bright light therapy for older adults with dementia. *BJPsych Advances*, 26 (4), 221–228.

Orpwood, R., Gibbs, C., Adlam, T., Faulkner, R., and Meegahawatte, D., 2004. The Gloucester smart house for people with dementia – user-interface aspects. *Designing a More Inclusive World*, 237–245.

Orrell, M., Hancock, G., Hoe, J., Woods, B., Livingston, G., and Challis, D., 2007. A cluster randomised controlled trial to reduce the unmet needs of people with dementia living in residential care. *International Journal of Geriatric Psychiatry*, 22 (11), 1127–1134.

Outeiro, T.F., Koss, D.J., Erskine, D., Walker, L., Kurzawa-Akanbi, M., Burn, D., Donaghy, P., Morris, C., Taylor, J.P., Thomas, A., Attems, J., and McKeith, I., 2019. Dementia with Lewy bodies: An update and outlook. *Molecular Neurodegeneration*, 14 (1).

Overton, M., Pihlsgård, M., and Elmståhl, S., 2019. Diagnostic stability of mild cognitive impairment, and predictors of reversion to normal cognitive functioning. *Dementia and Geriatric Cognitive Disorders*, 48 (5–6), 317–329.

Pani-Harreman, K.E., Bours, G.J.J.W., Zander, I., Kempen, G.I.J.M., and van Duren, J.M.A., 2021. Definitions, key themes and aspects of 'ageing in place': A scoping review. *Ageing & Society*, 41 (9), 2026–2059.

Papanastasiou, C.A., Theochari, C.A., Zareifopoulos, N., Arfaras-Melainis, A., Giannakoulas, G., Karamitsos, T.D., Palaiodimos, L., Ntaios, G., Avgerinos, K.I., Kapogiannis, D., and Kokkinidis, D.G., 2021. Atrial fibrillation is associated with cognitive impairment, all-cause dementia, vascular dementia, and Alzheimer's disease: A systematic review and meta-analysis. *Journal of General Internal Medicine*, 36 (10), 3122–3135.

Petersen, R.C., 2000. Mild cognitive impairment or questionable dementia? *Archives of Neurology*, 57 (5), 643–644.

Petersen, R.C., 2004. Mild cognitive impairment as a diagnostic entity. *Journal of Internal Medicine*, 256 (3), 183–194.

Petersen, R.C., 2016. Mild cognitive impairment. *Continuum* (Minneapolis, MN), 22 (2 Dementia), 404–418.

Petersen, R.C., Doody, R., Kurz, A., Mohs, R.C., Morris, J.C., Rabins, P.V., Ritchie, K., Rossor, M., Thal, L., and Winblad, B., 2001. Current concepts in mild cognitive impairment. *Archives of Neurology*, 58 (12), 1985–1992.

Petersen, R.C., Smith, G.E., Waring, S.C., Ivnik, R.J., Tangalos, E.G., and Kokmen, E., 1999. Mild cognitive impairment: Clinical characterization and outcome. *Archives of Neurology*, 56 (3), 303–308.

Piggott, M.A., Ballard, C.G., Rowan, E., Holmes, C., McKeith, I.G., Jaros, E., Perry, R.H., and Perry, E.K., 2007. Selective loss of dopamine D2 receptors in temporal cortex in dementia with Lewy bodies, association with cognitive decline. *Synapse* (New York, N.Y.), 61 (11), 903–911.

Piguet, O., Hornberger, M., Mioshi, E., and Hodges, J.R., 2011. Behavioural-variant frontotemporal dementia: Diagnosis, clinical staging, and management. *The Lancet Neurology*, 10 (2), 162–172.

Portet, F., Ousset, P.J., Visser, P.J., Frisoni, G.B., Nobili, F., Scheltens, P., Vellas, B., and Touchon, J., 2006. Mild cognitive impairment (MCI) in medical practice: A critical review of the concept and new diagnostic procedure. Report of the MCI working group of the European consortium on Alzheimer's disease. *Journal of Neurology, Neurosurgery, and Psychiatry*, 77 (6), 714.

Ratnavalli, E., Brayne, C., Dawson, K., and Hodges, J.R., 2002. The prevalence of frontotemporal dementia. *Neurology*, 58 (11), 1615–1621.

Rezaie, P., Cairns, N.J., Chadwick, A., and Lantos, P.L., 1996. Lewy bodies are located preferentially in limbic areas in diffuse Lewy body disease. *Neuroscience Letters*, 212 (2), 111–114.

Richardson, C., Stephan, B.C.M., Robinson, L., Brayne, C., and Matthews, F.E., 2019. Two-decade change in prevalence of cognitive impairment in the UK. *European Journal of Epidemiology*, 34 (11), 1085–1092.

Sachdev, P.S., Lipnicki, D.M., Kochan, N.A., Crawford, J.D., Thalamuthu, A., Andrews, G., Brayne, C., Matthews, F.E., Stephan, B.C.M., Lipton, R.B., Katz, M.J., Ritchie, K., Carrière, I., Ancelin, M.L., Lam, L.C.W., Wong, C.H.Y., Fung, A.W.T., Guaita, A., Vaccaro, R., Davin, A., Ganguli, M., Dodge, H., Hughes, T., Anstey, K.J., Cherbuin, N., Butterworth, P., Ng, T.P., Gao, Q., Reppermund, S., Brodaty, H., Schupf, N., Manly, J., Stern, Y., Lobo, A., Lopez-Anton, R., Santabárbara, J., Zimmerman, M., Derby, C., Leung, G.T.Y., Chan, W.C., Polito, L., Abbondanza, S., Valle, E., Colombo, M., Vitali, S.F., Fossi, S., Zaccaria, D., Forloni, G., Villani, S., Christensen, H., MacKinnon, A., Easteal, S., Jacomb, T., Maxwell, K., Bowman, A., Burns, K., Broe, A., Dekker, J., Dooley, L., de Permentier, M., Fairjones, S., Fletcher, J., French, T., Foster, C., Nugent-Cleary-Fox, E., Gooi, C., Harvey, E., Helyer, R., Hsieh, S., Hughes, L., Jacek, S., Johnston, M., McCade, D., Meeth, S., Milne, E., Moir, A., O'Grady, R., Pfaeffli, K., Pose, C., Reuser, L., Rose, A., Schofield, P., Shahnawaz, Z., Sharpley, A., Thompson, C., Queisser, W., Wong, S., Mayeux, R., Brickman, A., Luchsinger, J., Sanchez, D., Tang, M.X., Andrews, H., Marcos, G., De-La-Cámara, C., Saz, P., Ventura, T., Quintanilla, M.A., and Lobo, E., 2015. The prevalence of mild cognitive impairment in diverse geographical and ethnocultural regions: The COSMIC collaboration. *PLoS One*, 10 (11), e0142388.

Sachs-Ericsson, N., and Blazer, D.G., 2014. The new DSM-5 diagnosis of mild neurocognitive disorder and its relation to research in mild cognitive impairment. 19 (1), 2–12. https://doi.org/10.1080/136078 63.2014.920303.

Schrijnemaekers, A.M.C., de Jager, C.A., Hogervorst, E., and Budge, M.M., 2007. Cases with mild cognitive impairment and Alzheimer's disease fail to benefit from repeated exposure to episodic memory tests as compared with controls. 28 (3), 438–455. http://dx.doi.org/10.1080/13803390590935462.

Sengoku, R., 2020. Aging and Alzheimer's disease pathology. *Neuropathology*, 40 (1), 22–29.

Slade, M., Leese, M., Cahill, S., Thornicroft, G., and Kuipers, E., 2005. Patient-rated mental health needs and quality of life improvement. *The British Journal of Psychiatry*, 187 (3), 256–261.

Snowden, J.S., Neary, D., and Mann, D.M.A., 2002. Frontotemporal dementia. *The British Journal of Psychiatry*, 180 (2), 140–143.

Steichele, K., Keefer, A., Dietzel, N., Graessel, E., Prokosch, H.U., and Kolominsky-Rabas, P.L., 2022. The effects of exercise programs on cognition, activities of daily living, and neuropsychiatric symptoms in community-dwelling people with dementia – a systematic review. *Alzheimer's Research and Therapy*, 14 (1), 1–13.

Suárez-González, A., Serrano-Pozo, A., Arroyo-Anlló, E.M., Franco-Macías, E., Polo, J., García-Solís, D., and Gil-Néciga, E., 2014. Utility of neuropsychiatric tools in the differential diagnosis of dementia with Lewy bodies and Alzheimer's disease: Quantitative and qualitative findings. *International Psychogeriatrics*, 26 (3), 453–461.

Talbot, C.V., and Briggs, P., 2022. The use of digital technologies by people with mild-to-moderate dementia during the COVID-19 pandemic: A positive technology perspective. 21 (4), 1363–1380. https://doi.org/10.1177/14713012221079477.

Tayler, H., Miners, J.S., Güzel, Ö., MacLachlan, R., and Love, S., 2021. Mediators of cerebral hypoperfusion and blood-brain barrier leakiness in Alzheimer's disease, vascular dementia and mixed dementia. *Brain Pathology*, 31 (4), e12935.

Taylor, J.P., Firbank, M., Barnett, N., Pearce, S., Livingstone, A., Mosimann, U., Eyre, J., McKeith, I.G., and O'Brien, J.T., 2011. Visual hallucinations in dementia with Lewy bodies: Transcranial magnetic stimulation study. *The British Journal of Psychiatry*, 199 (6), 492.

Taylor, J.P., McKeith, I.G., Burn, D.J., Boeve, B.F., Weintraub, D., Bamford, C., Allan, L.M., Thomas, A.J., and O'Brien, J.T., 2020. New evidence on the management of Lewy body dementia. *The Lancet Neurology*, 19 (2), 157–169.

Tible, O.P., Riese, F., Savaskan, E., and von Gunten, A., 2017. Best practice in the management of behavioural and psychological symptoms of dementia. *Therapeutic Advances in Neurological Disorders*, 10 (8), 297.

Tiwari, S., Atluri, V., Kaushik, A., Yndart, A., and Nair, M., 2019. Alzheimer's disease: Pathogenesis, diagnostics, and therapeutics. *International Journal of Nanomedicine*, 14, 5541.

Toot, S., Swinson, T., Devine, M., Challis, D., and Orrell, M., 2017. Causes of nursing home placement for older people with dementia: A systematic review and meta-analysis. *International Psychogeriatrics*, 29 (2), 195–208.

van der Ploeg, E.S., Eppingstall, B., and O'Connor, D.W., 2016. Internet video chat (Skype) family conversations as a treatment of agitation in nursing home residents with dementia. *International Psychogeriatrics*, 28 (4), 697–698.

Venkat, P., Chopp, M., and Chen, J., 2015. Models and mechanisms of vascular dementia. *Experimental Neurology*, 272, 97.

Wang, Y.Y., Yang, L., Zhang, J., Zeng, X.T., Wang, Y., and Jin, Y.H., 2022. The effect of cognitive intervention on cognitive function in older adults with Alzheimer's disease: A systematic review and meta-analysis. *Neuropsychology Review*, 32 (2), 247–273.

Ward, A., Arrighi, H.M., Michels, S., and Cedarbaum, J.M., 2012. Mild cognitive impairment: Disparity of incidence and prevalence estimates. *Alzheimer's & Dementia*, 8 (1), 14–21.

Warren, J.D., Rohrer, J.D., and Rossor, M.N., 2013. Frontotemporal dementia. *BMJ*, 347 (7920). www.bmj.com/content/347/bmj.f4827 [Accessed 14 Dec 2022].

Whitwell, J.L., 2010. Progression of atrophy in Alzheimer's disease and related disorders. *Neurotoxicity Research*, 18 (3–4), 339–346.

Wiener, J.M., and Pazzaglia, F., 2021. Ageing- and dementia-friendly design: Theory and evidence from cognitive psychology, neuropsychology and environmental psychology can contribute to design guidelines that minimise spatial disorientation. *Cognitive Processing*, 22 (4), 715–730.

Wittenberg, E., et al., 2019. *Projections of Older People with Dementia and Costs of Dementia Care in the United Kingdom 2019–2040*. London School of Economics: London.

Wolters, F.J., and Arfan Ikram, M., 2019. Epidemiology of vascular dementia. *Arteriosclerosis, Thrombosis, and Vascular Biology*, 39 (8), 1542–1549.

World Health Organisation Factsheet on Dementia, 2022. www.who.int/news-room/fact-sheets/detail/dementia [Accessed 11 Jan 2023].

Zaccai, J., McCracken, C., and Brayne, C., 2005. A systematic review of prevalence and incidence studies of dementia with Lewy bodies. *Age and Ageing*, 34 (6), 561–566.

Zekry, D., Hauw, J.J., and Gold, G., 2002. Mixed dementia: Epidemiology, diagnosis, and treatment. *Journal of the American Geriatrics Society*, 50 (8), 1431–1438.

Zhang, H., Huntley, J., Bhome, R., Holmes, B., Cahill, J., Gould, R.L., Wang, H., Yu, X., and Howard, R., 2019. Effect of computerised cognitive training on cognitive outcomes in mild cognitive impairment: A systematic review and meta-analysis. *BMJ Open*, 9 (8), e027062.

Zweig, Y.R., and Galvin, J.E., 2014. Lewy body dementia: The impact on patients and caregivers. *Alzheimer's Research and Therapy*, 6 (2), 1–7.

4 Personal Experiences of Dementia

Eef Hogervorst and Manisha Jain

Introduction

In the previous chapter we described behavioural and psychological symptoms associated with dementia (BPSD), which particularly impact care needs and are thought to lead to carer burnout, requiring institutionalisation of people with dementia. Ideally institutionalisation needs to be avoided, as many people rapidly deteriorate once they leave their familiar surroundings to be moved to traditional care homes. In addition, in Europe, a lack of professional nursing and care staff has led to recruitment difficulties in hospitals and care homes. New models of how we regard and address these behaviours and psychological symptoms in dementia need to be explored, and this may also improve staff retention and quality of life in those with dementia. In this chapter, we describe how person-centred approaches to BPSD are different from the medical model and the implications this has for age- and dementia-friendly design.

With regard to physical health, while cardiovascular disease risk factors play an important role in midlife, such as abdominal obesity, high blood pressure and high cholesterol, these were all found to reverse 1–2 years before the onset of dementia (Hogervorst 2018). This reversal in physiological risk factors could be due to people living with dementia forgetting to eat, with resultant frailty or loss of body mass, which can impact risk of falls, as described in the previous chapter. In this chapter we focus on the personal experience of people with dementia and their mental health and well-being. This person-centred care model is in contrast to the traditional medical model, which is described in the following paragraph.

The Traditional Medical Model

The medical model uses a traditional directive and prescriptive approach with medical treatment approaches for BPSD. In this model (Cloak and Khalili 2022), BPSD are seen as emotional, perceptual and behavioural disturbances that are similar to those seen in psychiatric disorders and which assume groupings of symptoms.

Individual BPSD are thus often classified into five domains:

1. Cognitive/perceptual (delusions, hallucinations).
2. Motor (e.g., pacing, wandering, repetitive movements, physical aggression).
3. Verbal (e.g., yelling, calling out, repetitive speech, verbal aggression).
4. Emotional (e.g., euphoria, depression, apathy, anxiety, irritability).
5. Vegetative (disturbances in sleep and appetite).

These symptoms can occur as a result of dementia pathology and can occur early in the dementia journey. Some symptoms are thought to cluster together resulting in typologies, but statistical support for these groupings is variable, and some studies find that symptoms

DOI: 10.1201/9781003306054-4

cluster together in different ways. For instance, in an EU multi-centre study, (Petrovic et al. 2007), 96% of people with dementia were found to have at least one BPSD symptom. Apathy and depression were found most frequently (60%) followed by irritability, anxiety and agitation (all around 41–45% of this sample). In this study, clustering of symptoms was seen as follows:

1. Psychosis (irritability, agitation, hallucinations and anxiety)
2. Mood lability (depression, disinhibition, but also elation)
3. Psychomotor behaviours (strange motor behaviour and delusions)
4. Instinctual behaviours (appetite disturbance, sleep disturbance and apathy).

These identified statistical clusters were substantially different from each another. However, while EU-wide, this was a cross-sectional, relatively small study from memory clinic practices, which may include people at different (earlier) stages of their dementia journey but still living in communities.

Another meta-analysis (van der Linde et al. 2014), including different dementia settings and people living with different dementia severities, investigated clustering of BPSD over 62 studies and found consistency in the following groupings:

1. *Hyperactivity*: irritability and aggression, sometimes also including aberrant motor behaviour, disinhibition, anxiety or euphoria.
2. *Affective symptoms*: dysphoria and anxiety, sometimes also including apathy, hallucinations or sleeping problems.
3. *Psychosis*: delusions and hallucinations, sometimes also including sleeping problems or aberrant motor behaviour.
4. Euphoria, sometimes also including *disinhibition*.
5. Symptoms that did not show consistent results in cluster analyses include apathy, eating disturbances, night-time behaviour disturbances, disinhibition and aberrant motor behaviour.

The differences that are seen in the clustering of BPSD may be because individual symptoms do not always occur together or even occur in the same timescale of a person's life. This variation may explain the differences in the clusters of BPSD within and between people with dementia.

Depression, for instance, while often found to be co-morbid with early cognitive decline and dementia, is also a significant risk factor for dementia, occurring years before dementia onset (Byers and Yaffe 2011; Cantón-Habas et al. 2020). Depression in the medical model is often treated with medication (e.g. SSRIs). Other psychotherapeutic approaches, such as cognitive behavioural therapy, are thought to be less effective once people develop dementia and have less cognitive ability to evaluate their emotions, thoughts and behaviours. However, findings from a recent systematic review (Watt et al. 2021) demonstrated that non-pharmacological interventions, such as cognitive stimulation combined with exercise and social interaction, were more efficacious at reducing symptoms of depression among those with dementia than using antidepressant medication.

The medical model is biopsychosocial and suggests that the symptoms are the result of the interactions between an individual's biology, prior experiences and current environment. As outlined, BPSD are usually medically treated with pharmaceuticals within this model. However, it is also recognised within this medical model that personality (neuroticism), previous trauma, communication issues and environmental factors (e.g., environmental indoor temperature or other sensory over-or under-stimulation) can also all affect BPSD.

Environmental contributions to BPSD recognised in the medical model can be:

1. Unmet needs (e.g., for food, fluid, companionship).
2. Behavioural/learning (e.g., when unwanted behaviour is unwittingly reinforced, such as by only providing attention when a patient calls out).
3. Patient-environment mismatch (e.g., when a caregiver's expectations exceed a patient's capability).

As such, discomfort (pain, illness) and delirium are checked first, with a full medical review including brain scans for tumours and medication taken, to reduce symptoms associated with morbidity and toxicity (e.g. overuse of medication or medication interacting together to result in BPSD). Then, the risk to patients themselves and others is established to investigate care needs. A history and observation of BPSD need to be done by the hospital or care home staff (when, what, circumstances) and baselines of symptoms need to be established with questionnaires and other instruments (BEHAVE-AD, NPI, etc). In this model, the guidance is focused on a 'one size fits all' approach.

Cloak and Khalili (2022) also mentioned that in most medical guidelines, there is no inclusion of caregiver training with correct responses to discomfort (e.g. to check for constipation, pain, etc.):

> unmet needs, or attempts to communicate; of creating soothing environments with optimal levels of stimulation; and responding to patients in ways that de-escalate problematic behaviours (e.g., distraction, giving patients clear instructions and simple choices, not rewarding the behaviours)

This caregiver training is very much part of the person-centred approach (see the following).

This comment also highlights the tension in developing design, where home design must include opportunity for expression of personal needs and preferences, while home design guidelines for people with dementia need to sketch a 'one size fits all approach', that is, creating homes that benefit independent living for people with dementia and their carers.

Another review suggested that non-pharmaceutical therapies, including the aforementioned caregiver training, could reduce agitation and use of antipsychotic medication. This is important, as such medication can increase drowsiness and fall risk. For instance, aromatherapy, bright light therapy to reduce circadian disturbances, massage and multisensory stimulation and reminiscence therapy (in which patients are engaged in reviewing their past via conversation, journaling and photographs) can all help with BPSD (Ballard et al. 2020). Multi-sensory therapy can include exposure to pets, robotics or using other game-like approaches (Park et al. 2020; Petersen et al. 2017). These elements can be included in the 'one-size fits all approach' for design guidelines, as they benefit most people, for example, with dementia and those exhibiting neurodiversity.

There is only anecdotal evidence for the effectiveness for agitation, and it includes, for instance, giving patients simple tasks to perform, such as folding laundry or using busy quilts (lap quilts with attached interesting objects such as zippers, Velcro, beads, ties, etc.) and weighted blankets (similar to those used to calm children with pervasive developmental disorders). A clinical trial in Minnesota is currently underway to evaluate the latter (ClinicalTrials.gov ID NCT03643991).

Many of these non-pharmacological treatments are also part of the person-centred care approach, but, as stated, these often assume 'one size fits all' in the medical model.

The Person-Centred Care Model

Person-centred care (PCC) was developed by Professor Tom Kitwood at the University of Bradford in the late 1980s (Fazio et al. 2018). The model focuses on people's individual needs, independence, self-esteem and quality of life. The model embraces privacy, partnership, choice, dignity, respect and rights as its other core values. Universal needs are attachment, comfort, identity, inclusion, occupation and love, but individual needs require a multi-disciplinary approach which include support for participation in activities that can affect BPSD.

Activities That Impact Design and Benefit Individual Symptoms of BPSD

A recent review and meta-analyses of 30 studies (Lee et al. 2022). used personalised approaches (i.e., asking people what they would like to do, what they used to like to do and what they currently want to engage with as equal partners) which can impact design needs. In this review, reminiscence therapy showed a moderate effect size, while music therapy and multisensory stimulation had a small effect size on BPSD. In this review, reminiscence and music therapy were also found to alleviate depression. The authors wrote that perhaps 'music therapy distracts people from their unpleasant emotions . . . allows for the expression of people's current emotions' . . . (Chu et al. 2014), and that 'reminiscence therapy uses empathy and interactions with others through the re-experience of past memories to help people with their problems' (Hsieh et al. 2010; Aşiret and Kapucu 2016; Lopes et al. 2016; Scales et al. 2018), 'expressing one's thoughts or feelings through the remaining memory (i.e., reminiscence therapy) could be a meaningful activity to persons living with dementia; it might promote their self-understanding through communication with others and further improves ego-integrity by reconstructing their memories' (Lee et al. 2022).

Music therapy includes design needs, such as a soundproof music room and instruments (e.g. piano) or at least a good sound and audio system that can be used via Alexa or other easy-to-implement systems. Multi-sensory therapy could possibly include moveable soft furnishings, fixed furnishings with different textures or spaces for pets or robot pets to provide these stimuli without much need for additional space but with a need for safety and useability checks. For reminiscence therapy, props can be used as part of the décor, such as pictures and objects. Other reviews (Ballard et al. 2020) also investigated individual BPSD symptoms (i.e. behaviours and moods reflecting unmet needs as outcomes such as aggression, depression and agitation) to investigate whether particular activities (which may impact design needs) are actually beneficial in reducing these symptoms.

This review discussed benefits of person-centred physical and cognitive activities (especially walking, gardening and social interaction). Many studies have shown that being outdoors in nature exposed to green or blue spaces can improve mood, alertness and calm and have overall health benefits.

Reminiscence (using video, photos, life storytelling, using props with another person or by using pictures and photos as decorations in the home), in the aforementioned review (Ballard et al. 2020), helped reduce agitation and depression in six of the seven studies reviewed. Partners for these activities (if not present) could be accessed via online systems, which would require internet access and simple-to-use setups. These systems could also be useful for validation therapy. Validation therapy is based on acceptance of individual reality and the personal truth of another's experience and incorporates specific techniques (Neal and Barton Wright 2003). Validation therapy reduced agitation and apathy in two small trials, while music therapy reduced agitation and anxiety but not depression. Exercise also reduced BPSD but not depression. Our ACTI chair in the Chris and Sally home is an example of safe home-based exercise which could help promote well-being, independence and cognitive function such as memory (Hogervorst et al. 2012). We and others also previously found that loneliness played a huge part in increasing the risk of dementia (Rafnsson et al. 2020) and that quality interactions are very important to reduce the risk of severe cognitive decline. Doing activities with other people in groups (Hogervorst et al. 2012), possibly online with easy-to-use instructions, can help support older people living alone.

With regard to other individual activities and therapies, massage and touch were also shown in a meta-analyses of 11 studies of 526 people to reduce physical and verbally aggressive behaviour (but not mood, such as anxiety, sadness or anger). However, the overall quality of the small studies included in this analysis was low (Wu et al. 2017). Costs of spa salon and hairdresser visits or arranging home visits by massage therapists or hairdressers may be high, but a resulting reduction of aggressive behaviour can result in significant savings. This may be due to less need for formal medical visits to assess and prescribe sedative medication. Sedative medication can reduce quality of life and, as stated, increase the risk for falls and secondary morbidity that may require hospitalisation and reduce lifespan. Using massage and touch to reduce aggression would also decrease carer burn-out and institutionalisation and reduce the risk of aggressive or other types of assault on staff, furniture and residents and older people's abuse of those being cared for. However, to our knowledge, no such cost-benefit analyses have been performed.

In sum, music, reminiscence, multi-sensory activity, exercise and aromatherapy were possibly most useful for BPSD, and design to promote these activities should be implemented in homes. Homes should allow space for these activities and perhaps the inclusion of props in the design to facilitate these activities. This can also be implemented in group settings, such as care homes. However, design adaptations may need to be in place to accommodate various group sizes and relative needs.

Tools to Identify Individual Needs, Capabilities and Preferences for PCC

Our persona approach to guide design is discussed in more detail in Chapter 6. However, here we discuss tools to engage with people to identify their needs, capabilities and preferences. Briefly, the persona approach was developed to encompass a cluster of symptoms and experiences of dementia which can be used in the design process. This approach demonstrates the range of experiences, the good and bad days, and how this should be included in design.

The Applied Cognition, Technology and Interaction Group (ACTING) meeting was held on March 31, 2022, with various stakeholders and all members, including Professor Tom Dening (old age psychiatrist and BPSD expert), various other clinicians and care providers, academics, researchers and Mencap staff. Mencap is the UK charity for people with a learning disability. We discussed whether clusters of BPSD should be further developed into personas, distinct in symptomatology and corresponding to specific design and care needs. The focus group thought this could lead to further stigmatisation of people with dementia and may be the direct opposite approach from the person-centred model. This approach was rejected as not useful, despite there being some statistical evidence for BPSD persona grouping, as discussed previously.

The Loughborough Social Sciences team, in particular Dr Saul Albert and Professor Elizabeth Peel, use an applied research method called conversation analysis (Antaki 2011) which uses anonymised video and audio recording to study how people interact with each other and with design/technology. This approach could be used to qualitatively analyse how BPSD can be prevented by carers to improve quality of life and empower both carers and people with dementia in care and at home. This team also used a 'walking and talking' interview technique (Elliott-King 2020), which was employed to walk with people living with dementia, their carers and other stakeholders in and around the Chris and Sally house to obtain in-depth qualitative feedback about the design implementations.

Another person-based approach from Miami-based researchers is called the Preferences for Every Day Living Inventory (PELI), which helps rank what is important to people, with information on their background, personality, family, work and activities enjoyed. This can be put on a card and travel with the person's walker or wheelchair to quickly give personalised key information on needs (Scripps Gerontology Center 2019). A similar, but more advanced, free and

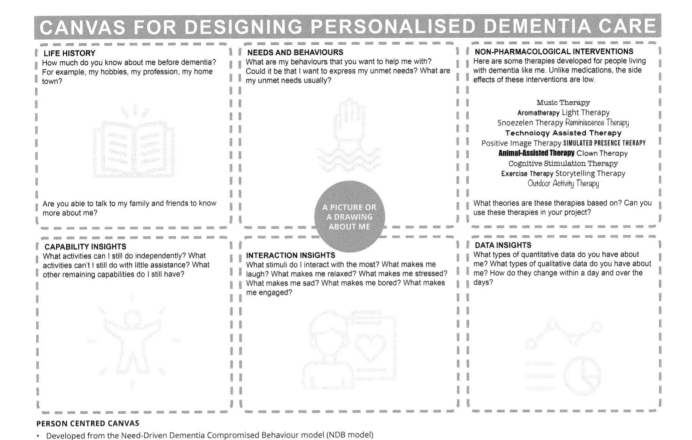

CANVAS FOR DESIGNING PERSONALISED DEMENTIA CARE

LIFE HISTORY
How much do you know about me before dementia? For example, my hobbies, my profession, my home town?

Are you able to talk to my family and friends to know more about me?

NEEDS AND BEHAVIOURS
What are my behaviours that you want to help me with? Could it be that I want to express my unmet needs? What are my unmet needs usually?

A PICTURE OR A DRAWING ABOUT ME

NON-PHARMACOLOGICAL INTERVENTIONS
Here are some therapies developed for people living with dementia like me. Unlike medications, the side effects of these interventions are low.

Music Therapy
Aromatherapy Light Therapy
Snoezelen Therapy Reminiscence Therapy
Technology Assisted Therapy
Positive Image Therapy SIMULATED PRESENCE THERAPY
Animal-Assisted Therapy Clown Therapy
Cognitive Stimulation Therapy
Exercise Therapy Storytelling Therapy
Outdoor Activity Therapy

What theories are these therapies based on? Can you use these therapies in your project?

CAPABILITY INSIGHTS
What activities can I still do independently? What activities can't I still do with little assistance? What other remaining capabilities do I still have?

INTERACTION INSIGHTS
What stimuli do I interact with the most? What makes me laugh? What makes me relaxed? What makes me stressed? What makes me sad? What makes me bored? What makes me engaged?

DATA INSIGHTS
What types of quantitative data do you have about me? What types of qualitative data do you have about me? How do they change within a day and over the days?

PERSON CENTRED CANVAS
- Developed from the Need-Driven Dementia Compromised Behaviour model (NDB model)
- Systematic review on non-pharmacological interventions for dementia care
- Established after investigation of the three design approaches *(i.e. Ergonomics in Aging, Co-design, and Data-enabled Design)*

g.wang-2@tudelft.nl

Figure 4.1 Person-centred canvas

available tool for co-design for people with dementia is Know Me, which was developed with the Technical University of Delft (TU) (Wang et al. 2021). The system includes capabilities, needs and preferences for activities and how this can be implemented in design. This system can be used online with resources available or by using hard copy cards (see subsequently). However, the tool was only tested in students without actual live exposure to those with dementia, so it still requires further assessment of its validity for a person-centred design approach.

Care Provision in the UK – Institutional Care Provision Versus Care in the Home

The majority of people living with dementia prefer to stay at home (Alzheimer's Society and YouGov 2014; Alzheimer's Society 2016). While many good initiatives have focused on improving the quality of care homes (Irving et al. 2020), currently governmental reductions in social and healthcare budgets resulting in significant staff shortages highlight the need for better personal home care. 'Better' is defined here through high quality of life, independence and safety for people living with dementia and a reduced carer burden, as well as a reduced load for primary formal care, such as GP and home visits by GP, health visitors and nursing staff. Taking into account the personalised needs of people living with dementia, our design should thus also include personalised preferences for activities in people's homes.

Summary

Activities that worked to reduce agitation and depression in people living with dementia included music, multisensory and reminiscence therapy. For aggressive and disinhibited behaviour, massage and touch therapy were shown to be beneficial, but this would require visits, potentially from third parties specialising in this, or carer training. To our knowledge, cost-benefit analyses have not been officially performed, but the benefits could be assessed via reduction of costs (medical visits, medication, damage to property, carer burn-out and institutionalisation) and improved quality of life for both people with dementia and their carers as assessed using quality of life (e.g. with the ED5Q or SF36) to calculate QALY, which is a traditionally used benefit measure in cost-benefit analyses.

For care homes that use the person-centred approach, a cost-benefit analysis has been done. For instance, in the WHELD study (Ballard et al. 2020), using the person-centred approach with optimal design in care homes to promote person-centred evidence-based activities was found to save up to £4740–£2000 per care home over a 9-month period due to a reduced need for medical/GP visits and improved quality of life of residents. It resulted in less agitation in particular and also promoted staff well-being, which would ultimately be likely to result in reduced staff turnover (Ballard et al. 2020). This study showed that using these person-centred approaches does not increase costs over benefits. Future work should provide such cost-benefit analyses for individual homes.

References

Alzheimer's Society, 2016. Fix dementia care hospitals. www.alzheimers.org.uk/sites/default/files/migrate/downloads/fix_dementia_care_-_hospitals.pdf [Accessed 20 Dec 2022].

Alzheimer's Society and YouGov, 2014. Dementia 2014: Opportunity for change. www.alzheimers.org.uk/sites/default/files/migrate/downloads/dementia_2014_opportunity_for_change.pdf [Accessed 20 Dec 2022].

Antaki, C., 2011. *Applied Conversation Analysis. Applied Conversation Analysis.* Palgrave Macmillan: London.

Aşiret, G.D., and Kapucu, S., 2016. The effect of reminiscence therapy on cognition, depression, and activities of daily living for patients with Alzheimer disease. *Journal of Geriatric Psychiatry and Neurology*, 29 (1), 31–37.

Ballard, C., Orrell, M., Moniz-Cook, E., Woods, R., Whitaker, R., Corbett, A., Aarsland, D., Murray, J., Lawrence, V., Testad, I., Knapp, M., Romeo, R., Zala, D., Stafford, J., Hoare, Z., Garrod, L., Sun, Y., McLaughlin, E., Woodward-Carlton, B., Williams, G., and Fossey, J., 2020. Improving mental health and reducing antipsychotic use in people with dementia in care homes: The WHELD research programme including two RCTs. *Programme Grants for Applied Research*, 8 (6), 1–98.

Byers, A.L., and Yaffe, K., 2011. Depression and risk of developing dementia. *Nature Reviews. Neurology*, 7 (6), 323.

Cantón-Habas, V., Rich-Ruiz, M., Romero-Saldaña, M., and Carrera-González, M.D.P., 2020. Depression as a risk factor for dementia and Alzheimer's disease. *Biomedicines*, 8 (11), 1–15.

Chu, H., Yang, C.Y., Lin, Y., Ou, K.L., Lee, T.Y., O'Brien, A.P., and Chou, K.R., 2014. The impact of group music therapy on depression and cognition in elderly persons with dementia: A randomized controlled study. *Biological Research for Nursing*, 16 (2), 209–217.

Cloak, N., and Khalili, Y., 2022. Behavioral and psychological symptoms in dementia. *StatPearls.* www.ncbi.nlm.nih.gov/books/NBK551552/ [Accessed 22 Dec 2022].

Elliott-King, J., 2020. Factors affecting assessment, uptake and adherence to physical activities in people with dementia: An inclusive approach. https://repository.lboro.ac.uk/articles/thesis/Factors_affecting_assessment_uptake_and_adherence_to_physical_activities_in_people_with_dementia_an_inclusive_approach/11993496 [Accessed 19 Dec 2022].

Fazio, S., Pace, D., Flinner, J., and Kallmyer, B., 2018. The fundamentals of person-centered care for individuals with dementia. *The Gerontologist*, 58 (suppl_1), S10–S19. https://doi.org/10.1093/GERONT/GNX122.

Hogervorst, E., Clifford, A., Stock, J., Xin, X., and Bandelow, S., 2012. Exercise to prevent cognitive decline and Alzheimer's disease: For whom, when, what, and (most importantly) how much? *Journal of Alzheimers Disease & Parkinsonism*, 2, e117. doi: 10.4172/2161-0460.1000e117 [Accessed 20 Dec 2022].

Hogervorst, E., Oliveira, D., and Brayne, C., 2018. Lifestyle factors and dementia: Smoking, exercise and diet. *New Developments in Dementia Prevention Research*. 1st ed. Routledge: London, 29–46.

Hsieh, C.J., Chang, C., Su, S.F., Hsiao, Y.L., Shih, Y.W., Han, W.H., and Lin, C.C., 2010. Reminiscence group therapy on depression and apathy in nursing home residents with mild-to-moderate dementia. *Journal of Experimental & Clinical Medicine*, 2 (2), 72–78.

Irving, K., Hogervorst, E., Oliveira, D., and Kivipelto, M., 2020. *New Developments in Dementia Prevention Research State of the Art and Future Possibilities*. 1st ed. Routledge: London.

Lee, K.H., Lee, J.Y., and Kim, B., 2022. Person-centered care in persons living with dementia: A systematic review and meta-analysis. *The Gerontologist*, 62 (4), e253–e264.

Lopes, T.S., Afonso, R.M.L.B.M., and Ribeiro, Ó.M., 2016. A quasi-experimental study of a reminiscence program focused on autobiographical memory in institutionalized older adults with cognitive impairment. *Archives of Gerontology and Geriatrics*, 66, 183–192.

Neal, M., and Barton Wright, P., 2003. Validation therapy for dementia. *Cochrane Database of Systematic Reviews*, 2010 (1). https://doi.org/10.1002/14651858.CD001394/MEDIA/CDSR/CD001394/IMAGE_N/NCD001394-CMP-003-02.PNG.

Park, S., Bak, A., Kim, S., Nam, Y., Kim, H.S., Yoo, D.H., and Moon, M., 2020. Animal-assisted and pet-robot interventions for ameliorating behavioral and psychological symptoms of dementia: A systematic review and meta-analysis. *Biomedicines*, 8 (6).

Petersen, S., Houston, S., Qin, H., Tague, C., and Studley, J., 2017. The utilization of robotic pets in dementia care. *Journal of Alzheimer's Disease*, 55 (2), 569.

Petrovic, M., Hurt, C., Collins, D., Burns, A., Camus, V., Liperoti, R., Marriott, A., Nobili, F., Robert, P., Tsolaki, M., Vellas, B., Verhey, F., and Byrne, E., 2007. Clustering of behavioural and psychological symptoms in dementia (BPSD): A European Alzheimer's Disease Consortium (EADC) study. *Acta Clinica Belgica*, 62, 426–432. https://doi.org/10.1179/acb.2007.062.

Rafnsson, S.B., Orrell, M., D'Orsi, E., Hogervorst, E., and Steptoe, A., 2020. Loneliness, social integration, and incident dementia over 6 years: Prospective findings from the English longitudinal study of ageing. *The Journals of Gerontology. Series B, Psychological Sciences and Social Sciences*, 75 (1), 114–124.

Scales, K., Zimmerman, S., and Miller, S.J., 2018. Evidence-based nonpharmacological practices to address behavioral and psychological symptoms of dementia. *The Gerontologist*, 58 (suppl_1), S88–S102.

Scripps Gerontology Center, 2019. Preferences for everyday living inventory (PELI) project partners with Ohio nursing homes to improve residents' quality of life – Miami University. www.miamioh.edu/cas/academics/centers/scripps/news-events/2019/02/peli-pal-2-2019.html [Accessed 26 Jan 2023].

van der Linde, R.M., Dening, T., Matthews, F.E., and Brayne, C., 2014. Grouping of behavioural and psychological symptoms of dementia. *International Journal of Geriatric Psychiatry*, 29 (6), 562–568. https://doi.org/10.1002/GPS.4037.

Wang, G., Albayrak, A., Hogervorst, E., and van der Cammen, T.J.M., 2021. Know-me: A toolkit for designing personalised dementia care. *International Journal of Environmental Research and Public Health 2021*, 18 (11), 5662.

Watt, J.A., Goodarzi, Z., Veroniki, A.A., Nincic, V., Khan, P.A., Ghassemi, M., Lai, Y., Treister, V., Thompson, Y., Schneider, R., Tricco, A.C., and Straus, S.E., 2021. Comparative efficacy of interventions for reducing symptoms of depression in people with dementia: Systematic review and network meta-analysis. *BMJ*, 372.

Wu, J., Wang, Y., and Wang, Z., 2017. The effectiveness of massage and touch on behavioural and psychological symptoms of dementia: A quantitative systematic review and meta-analysis. *Journal of Advanced Nursing*, 73 (10), 2283–2295.

5 Engagement and Participation in the Dementia Community

Bill Halsall and Robert G MacDonald

Introduction

The person-centred care model described in the last chapter focuses on individual needs and outlined some of the design factors involved. Bill Halsall and Dr Robert G MacDonald carried out direct design engagement with people living with dementia and their carers and health professionals to gain insight into the issues that they are confronted with in their living environment and to explore how designers can help to create more conducive internal and external environments which can assist people living with dementia to live well at home.

Design Engagement

Designing 'with' people living with dementia as well as 'for' them is a fundamental proposition of this book. People with dementia experience the world in a different way to other people. Their cognition is impaired. Design can help them to better navigate the exterior public realm and their interior domain. Getting design right for people living with dementia can assist in helping them to retain their capacity for longer and to live independently in their own homes and neighbourhoods.

Familiarity with surroundings is recognised as a key to reducing symptoms and loss of function associated with the condition of dementia. By implication, if people can remain in their own homes in their own neighbourhoods, then the disorientation, confusion and anxiety of a move to a new environment can be eliminated or at least postponed.

Through engagement and participation with people living with dementia and their carers and health professionals, we hope to understand their needs, requirements and aspirations more clearly and hopefully put this knowledge and understanding into the design and development of new care homes, extra care schemes and remodelling projects as well as interior adaptations. Externally the design of the built environment can also be modified to take account of the experience of people living with dementia as well as the needs of other users such as the blind and partially sighted and physically disabled people.

But how can we approach the objective of engaging and consulting with people living with dementia? Direct questions may get nowhere because being confronted with making decisions may be stressful and people with dementia may not be equipped to respond in the usual way. Exercises carried out by Dr Robert G MacDonald and Bill Halsall focused on techniques which engaged conversation, building trust and confidence through sharing experience and stimulating the senses with hands-on approaches, which invite reminiscence or stories (Halsall and MacDonald 2015).

We have tried these techniques in various situations and found that useful information can be gleaned and ideas generated which can be responded to through the design process. We have found that people living with dementia are keen to talk, to share their experiences and to respond to resource material in the right context and with the right formats and mediums.

DOI: 10.1201/9781003306054-5

Designers can engage with individuals with dementia to design residential facilities in a number of ways:

- Involving individuals with dementia in the design process – this can be done by inviting them to participate in design workshops, focus groups or user testing. This allows designers to gain a deeper understanding of the needs and preferences of individuals with dementia and to incorporate this information into the design of the facility.
- Conducting research – designers can conduct research, such as interviews, surveys or observational studies, to gain a better understanding of the experiences and needs of individuals with dementia. This research can be used to inform the design of facilities.
- Collaborating with dementia experts – designers can work closely with professionals who have expertise in dementia care, such as geriatricians, nurses or social workers. These professionals can provide valuable insights and perspectives on the specific needs of individuals with dementia.
- Using existing guidelines and standards – there are a number of guidelines and standards available for designing facilities for individuals living with dementia. Designers can use these guidelines to inform their design decisions and ensure that the facility meets the specific needs of individuals with dementia.
- Testing and prototyping – designers can create physical or virtual prototypes of the facility and test them with individuals with dementia to gather feedback and make any necessary adjustments.
- Involving family members – involving family members of individuals living with dementia can also provide important insights and perspectives on the design of residential facilities. They can provide valuable information on the day to day needs of individuals with dementia and their preferences for the design of the facility or home.

It is important to note that involving individuals with dementia in the design process can be challenging, and designers need to be sensitive to the specific needs and abilities of these individuals. Additionally, designers should also consider involving other stakeholders such as caregivers, staff and facility managers in the design process to get a holistic view of the needs and preferences of the people who will be using the facility.

Chris and Sally's House

A partnership between the Building Research Establishment, Loughborough University, Liverpool John Moores University and the Halsall Lloyd Partnership has taken the interactive design process to the next logical stage, the construction of a full size fully functioning dwelling as a demonstration project at the BRE's Innovation Park at Watford. This project is covered in detail in Chapter 7.

Living Well With Dementia

The Design Guide, which is presented in Chapter 10, is specifically addressed to the needs of people living with dementia. It is estimated that 70–80% of people diagnosed with dementia live at home. While a considerable amount of research and development has been directed at extra care, residential care homes and other specialist care communities which provide care tailored to the needs of people with dementia, in fact most people living with dementia continue living in their own homes and using the same spaces in their neighbourhoods and cities as everyone else.

Therefore, awareness of the issues associated with dementia should inform the design of all new dwellings and new neighbourhoods and the design of the public realm in general. Shops and other businesses serving the wider community should consider the specific needs of people living with dementia. Existing homes and neighbourhoods may be adapted to respond to this new awareness. In the longer term this approach (aging in place) will reduce pressure on health and social services and help prevent accidents, improving safety and security for all.

Only by trying to understand their experiences and by trying to perceive the world their way, can we begin to respond as designers working in the built environment.

Every three minutes someone develops dementia. The vast majority of these people will live in purpose designed care homes or in their own homes. There are currently 900,000 people in the UK living with dementia, a figure that is expected to dramatically increase in the coming years.

A definition of architectural design highlights the wide coverage and influence of design of interior and exterior spaces for people living with dementia. Design for people living with dementia can be broad and inclusive, from the small micro scale like the size of a chair to the larger macro city scale of the neighbourhood and the city. Good engaging design for people living in care homes, extra care schemes and specialist dementia care facilities can also involve music, dancing, art, painting and drawing, which can become therapeutic activities.

The principles of design engagement can be built around group and stakeholder joint working of people living with dementia, staff and their carers. The gentle development of face to face conversations in small groups is important as this enables a picture of the real requirements to emerge gradually, where all voices can be heard and form new creative relationships. All individual perspectives can be brought together so as to identify various tasks and common ground can be realised. Only then will external specialist expertise be brought into the process of engagement. This enables a bottom-up stage of engagement to develop.

Generally, design is an interactive process of planning or specification for the construction or assembly of a purpose made object. Design can be to make a functional object or a process or system. This could be anything from furniture, dwelling space, neighbourhood or part of a city. Traditionally (architectural) design might be described as firmness (structure), commodity (for the correct size) and delight (beauty or pleasure). This refers to Vitruvius (firmitas utilitas venustas) translated to English by Henry Woton in the 17th century (Wotton 1624). Design of homes for people living with dementia must take account of the needs of ageing people, and this will involve a two-way 'reflection in action' of the architect-designer and the user carers. This co-design is not just 'for' the users but 'with them' and cooperation with user/clients who may be living in the early stages of dementia with mood swings and conversation difficulties. They might have some difficulties of communication and making judgments. In response, design approaches and methods need to be clear and avoid being judgemental or confusing. Three-dimensional physical modelling and or computer-aided design can be useful and helpful in communication of complex spatial design issues. Physical models can also be used in the design of homes, and physical sand trays have been used as part of the living laboratory. Photo cue cards were used to enable understanding of the problems in public open spaces for people living with dementia.

The Role of Living Laboratories

The process of designing and engaging with people living with dementia can involve a number of ways of co-production which are at the basis of design collaboration. The living lab is a well-known European example and model of a well-worked process. MerseyCare is investigating the role of co-production in the delivery of their services, and co-production is central to the way that the MerseyCare Life Rooms are delivered. Figure 5.1 illustrates this process.

A living lab is a user-centric innovation milieu for everyday practice and research, with an approach that facilitates user influence in open and distributed innovation processes, engaging all relevant partners in real- life contexts, aiming to create sustainable value (Bergvall-Kåreborn and Ståhlbröst 2009).

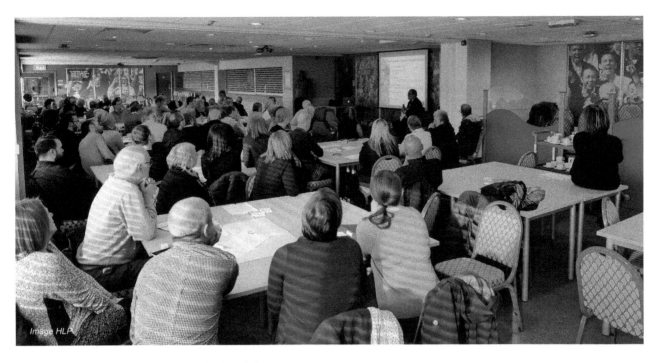

Figure 5.1 Innovate Dementia living laboratory

The active design engagement process of living laboratories can be the start of more detailed co-design production. Over an extended period of time, Innovate Dementia Europe held Living Laboratories involving about 150 people each week. Each lab included a presentation, group work and a shared lunch. At each stage of the living laboratory, it was important to get to know each other and break down the barriers between the professional experts and those living with dementia. The professionals learnt from those people living with dementia, who become the experts in this bottom-up approach.

A living lab is a pragmatic research environment which openly engages all relevant parties with an emphasis on improving the real-life care of people with dementia through the use of economically viable and sustainable innovations (Woods et al. 2013:13–14).

MerseyCare NHS Trust and Liverpool John Moores University were the UK partners for a European-funded project – Innovate Dementia, a 3-year INTERREG IVB-funded project working with partners in the Netherlands, Germany and Belgium to develop innovative solutions for people living with dementia. The project was part of a transnational cooperation programme to address the challenges that go beyond national borders. The ageing population means that there are increasing numbers of people living with dementia, and current methods of supporting people are economically unsustainable. There is a need to work collaboratively to develop innovative care solutions that enable people to live independently and well with dementia.

The project was built around four key themes which are:

- The use of intelligent lighting
- Exercise and nutrition
- Living environments
- Models of access.

The project used a living lab approach which brings together people living with dementia, health and social care professionals, academia and business to develop and test out innovative care solutions in real-life settings. Stakeholders met every 3 months to drive the project forward so people living with dementia were at the heart of innovation (Halsall et al. 2019).

Engagement Media and Techniques

There are various media and techniques for engaging and connecting with people living with dementia (Halsall et al. 2015).

A cue card is photographic record of an interior or an external public space that can be shared and discussed in a living lab. The participants can debate and identify good and bad aspects, from a lived experience perspective, of what the photographs illustrate. Critical comments can be written on the reverse of the photograph for group presentation in the living lab.

A sand tray is an informal and friendly way of creating fun and inspirational discussions amongst people living with dementia. A shallow wooden tray is filled with sand and various small tactile objects that provoke memories, such as an old coffee bottle, seashells, mint humbugs and flowers. Roses release fragrances, and birdsong plays in the background.

Music isn't just a nicety; it's a necessity for people living with dementia. Research proves that music reduces the need for anti-psychotic drugs and reduces the behavioural psychological symptoms of the condition such as anxiety, agitation and depression. Singing together in a choir is proven to be a therapeutic activity for people living with dementia. All kinds of dancing can be therapeutic and fun.

Taking a Labrador dog into a care home is a well proven way of engaging with people in a care home. Stroking a cat can bring back domestic memories. A yellow canary or a singing budgie in a cage can trigger recollections of childhood with grandparents or great aunts.

Good Environments and Living With Ageing

The whole environment needs to be considered a key mediating factor in supporting people to live well. We need to recognise that people ageing have a right to age in place in a safe place and secure environment, and we need to appreciate that an environment can be age friendly.

To design ageing-friendly dwellings and environments of the future, at different stages of ageing we need to work in collaboration with many people. We need multi-skilled professional teams to work with groups of people living in residential care homes, staff and their carers. This inclusive design process should set out to enable the voices of people and experts with lived experience of ageing to speak about their own environmental needs in their own terms.

Life and living in a care home or domestic environment need to be appreciated and communicated by people ageing themselves; we need to understand and expand on what it is like to live with a chronic illness or ageing disability. For example, some people living with ageing disabilities might take their own photographs (iPhone) of anything that they are unsure of, such as pavements, signage or steps and ramps. They can photograph their bedrooms, living spaces, kitchens and bathrooms and discuss their observations about whether the overall space can be well used.

The Participatory Approach

Three techniques have been used to facilitate participation:

Photo Cue Cards – Living Lab Format

Sets of cards with relevant photographic images on one side and space for comments on the other side were used to generate responses and discussion in a living lab format based on tables of six to ten people, as seen in Figures 5.2 and 5.3. The groups were mixed, including people living with dementia, carers and professionals. The results were recorded and analysed.

The photo cue cards have been used to explore responses to images of inside and outside spaces generically but also as an ongoing exploration – How Dementia Friendly Is Our City? This exercise has helped to highlight some of the difficulties experienced by people with dementia who use Liverpool city centre and to identify potential design responses.

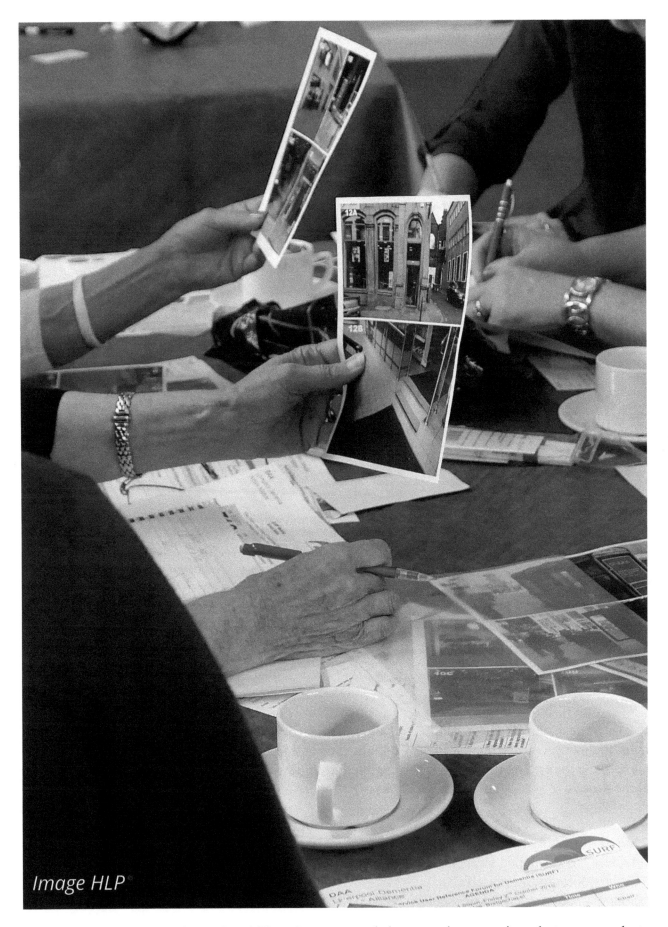

Figure 5.2 DAA (Dementia Action Alliance) group workshop members – using photo cue cards to respond to and comment on their experiences of Liverpool city centre

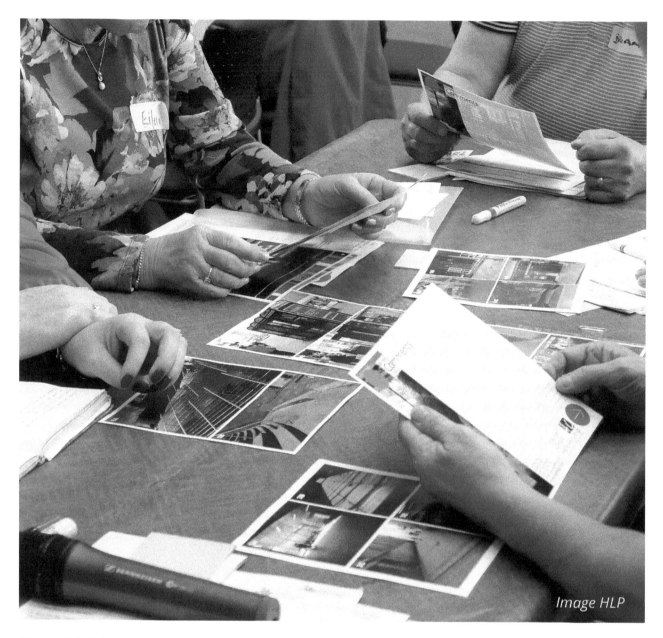

Figure 5.3 DAA meeting – group workshop

Connecting Minds Through Sandplay

The team have developed a hands-on method using a Jungian sand tray and a set of objects including stones, seashells, marbles, model houses and trees as well as moulds, sieves, spoons, buckets and rakes. The use of these is illustrated in Figures 5.4 and 5.5. The aim was to stimulate all the senses:

- Touch – sand, pebbles, objects
- Smell – 'sensory garden' of roses, herbs, spices
- Taste – old-fashioned sweets, ice cream
- Sight – coloured, shiny objects
- Sound – background music, shells.

In addition, memory was stimulated through postcards, newspapers and other items from the sixties.

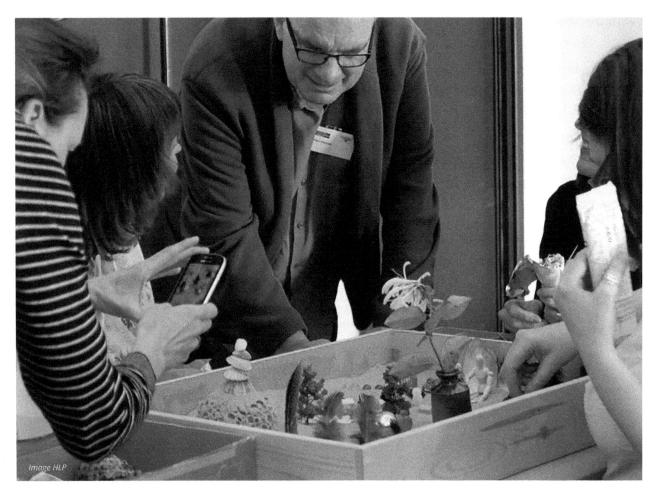

Figure 5.4 Sandplay workshop at the Albert Dock, Liverpool

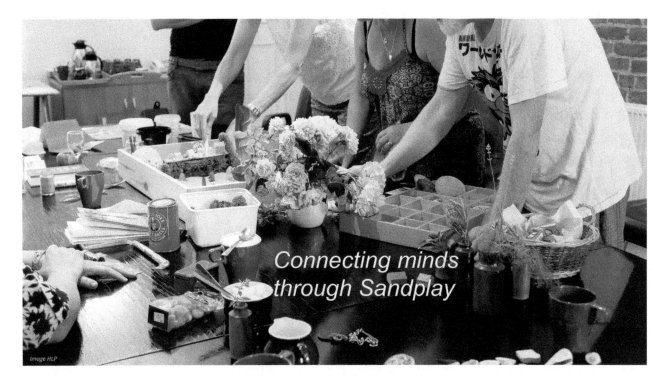

Figure 5.5 Sandplay workshop at Halsall Lloyd Partnership's offices

Hands-on Modelling – The Design *for* Dementia Bungalow

Figure 5.6 illustrates a foam board model being used to explore ideas for an ideal Design *for* Dementia Bungalow. The model is at a large scale to enable mixed groups to explore the concept and to envisage the spaces and connections between them. The model is demountable, including a full range of furniture and fittings. The garden is also fully modelled to the same scale so that the important interconnection between inside and outside environment can be demonstrated. Model human figures to the correct scale assist in understanding functional relationships and animate the model. This concept is being developed towards the implementation of a full-scale 'show bungalow' demonstrating design approaches which will assist living well with dementia.

This participatory approach has been implemented through a series of living labs which form an ongoing exploration of the issues and opportunities involved in responding to the challenge of dementia. These living labs and their outcomes are described in more detail.

Research Projects

This section provides an outline of some research initiatives which have grown up alongside the development of Design *for* Dementia and which have informed the concepts and ideas

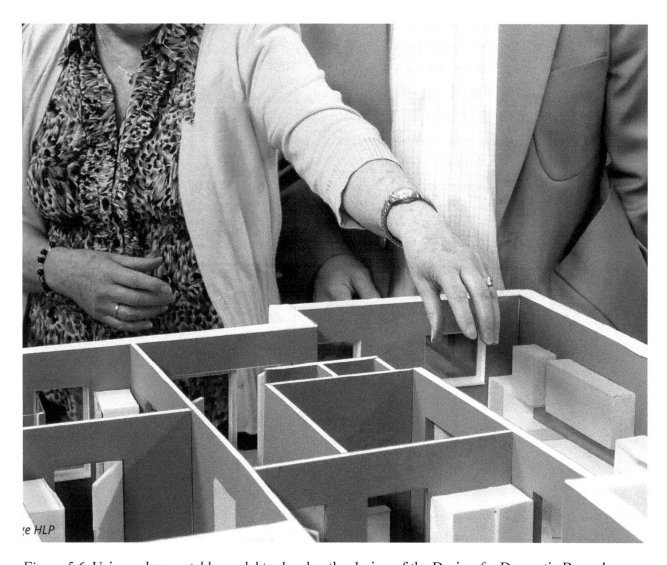

Figure 5.6 Using a demountable model to develop the design of the Design *for* Dementia Bungalow

included in this guide (Chapter 10). The outputs described are the result of activities by the team during 2015. All of the projects are based on the participatory design philosophy and techniques described and focus on the needs, frustrations and aspirations of those living with dementia.

Only by trying to understand their experiences and by trying to perceive the world their way, can we begin to respond as designers working in the built environment.

A brief outline of the projects is set out in the following with a summary of each contained within the following sections.

Project 1: The Dementia-Friendly Neighbourhood

Based on the premise that 70–80% of people living with dementia live in their own homes and use the same local environment and facilities as everyone else, how can the design of neighbourhoods be shaped to respond better to the needs of people living with dementia? And how can neighbourhoods and communities help people to live well with dementia?

Project 2: How Dementia Friendly Is Our City?

This exercise extends the lessons learnt from the dementia-friendly neighbourhood to a city scale, exploring responses to images of Liverpool City Centre. Its conclusions begin to point the way towards the aspiration of dementia friendly cities.

Project 3: Connecting Minds Through Sandplay

Explore Jungian sandplay to stimulate engagement by promoting play and relaxation and evoking memories.

Project 4: The Design *for* Dementia Bungalow

The Design *for* Dementia Bungalow is a design exercise which explores the design of an ideal model bungalow with all the features to live well with dementia. It includes an integrated Design *for* Dementia garden.

Research Project Summaries

Project Summary 1: The Dementia-Friendly Neighbourhood

Figures 5.7 to 5.10 illustrate features of this project.

Objectives

- Explore how neighbourhoods could be more responsive to the needs of people living with dementia
- Gain insight from people living with dementia about their environment.

Method

- Living lab including a mixed group of people, including carers, professionals and people living with dementia

- Photo cue cards were used to assist in stimulating a response to an assortment of images
- Results were collated and analysed.

What Can We Do to Make Neighbourhoods More Friendly and Useable by People Suffering From Dementia?

Neighbourhoods can and should be designed to fulfil the needs of *all* groups in the community. This means being not only accessible, safe, and secure but stimulating, with the conviviality of a mutually supportive community environment.

The benefits of this approach are:

- Tackling loneliness and isolation – promoting community inclusion
- Looking after people in their own neighbourhoods
- Reducing risk of accidents
- Reducing long-term cost to the health service and social services.

The Dementia Friendly Neighbourhood project explores this question through participation with the user groups involved in the Innovate Dementia Europe Project.

Event Format

The participatory methodology was living lab–based, asking mixed groups of people living with dementia, carers and professionals to explore their responses to a series of photo cue cards. The photo cue cards comprised a set of images showing interior and exterior environments. Participants listed their responses on the reverse.

Comments were collated and summarised, and conclusions were drawn from the exercise. Some examples are shown on the following pages.

Evaluation of the Living Lab

The workshop following the presentation generated a good level of discussion from a mixed group of people.

- The visual imagery stimulated a good response, with some significant results for the design of the built environment
- In both interiors and exteriors there were significant design features which, with more understanding of the issues of dementia, could have been approached differently to create a better environment for people with dementia in particular but also for everyone using these spaces
- Design guidance which recognises the issues of dementia and proposes practical approaches to design would assist in transmitting the message to those involved in design, construction, management and maintenance of neighbourhoods
- A joined-up approach is needed across all aspects of the built environment, not just in purpose-designed extra care or residential care schemes
- The involvement of people diagnosed with dementia in the design process is essential in developing a true understanding of what is needed
- The shared objective should be for an environment which caters for all on an equal footing, mitigating reliance on support services, which will generate a sustainable environment for the future.

Key Points Arising From the Living Lab

SAFETY AND SECURITY

- The visuo-perceptual issues experienced by people living with dementia demand special consideration in the design of internal and external environments. Hazards can arise from arbitrary changes in surface tonal value or from steps which may be invisible because of lack of contrast creating a trip hazard.

OPEN SPACE AREAS

- A green view and access to space for walking, socialising and enjoying the sunshine have particular therapeutic benefits for people with dementia.

USE OF COLOUR AND CONTRAST

- Colour, particularly at the red/yellow end of the spectrum, is valued. Contrast in tonal values can be used to distinguish a directional route or to identify the difference between horizontal and vertical surfaces or forms
- Colour could also help to identify, for example, an individual front door in a uniform row of properties.

PATTERNS

- Prominent patterns can cause disturbance – for example, herringbone paving with pronounced joints or large patterned curtains or wallpaper
- An uneven appearance of ground surface or patches of darker tone or colour can be confusing and potentially cause hesitation and perhaps accidents. A dark patch could be interpreted as a hole.

RECOGNITION OF FAMILIAR PLACES

- Images of older recognisable buildings or places were liked. Orientation through familiarity assists legibility.

PROBLEMS OF OBSTRUCTION

- Obstructions and clutter in the environment cause confusion and disruption, making it harder for people with dementia to move around. The needs of people with dementia and the visually impaired are similar in this respect.

SOCIABILITY

- Environments should encourage people to socialise. Institutional environments, such as chairs in rows or round the edge of a room discourage social mixing.

DISTINCTIVENESS IN DESIGN

- Sense of place can be developed by creating identity at a large or small scale, for example, chairs in a range of colours or designs or streets with distinctive features rather than repetitive uniformity.

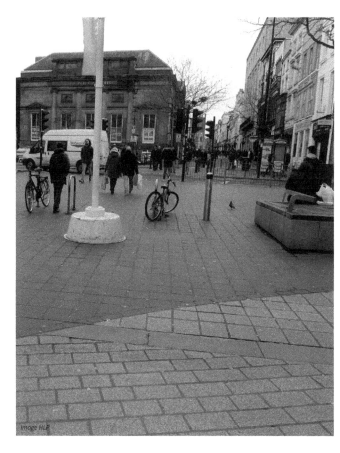

Summary
· People liked recognisable old buildings and open space.

Concerns
· Obstruction caused by cycle racks and flagpoles
· Random colour change of surface
· Uninviting seating
· Unclear signage
· Gloomy looking.

Design could be improved by:
· Being clutter free with clear routes for pedestrians
· Paving patterns that reflect movement routes
· Seats that are comfortable and look like seats
· Clear signage
· More colour - planting design.

Figure 5.7 The dementia-friendly neighbourhood – cue cards exercise – responses

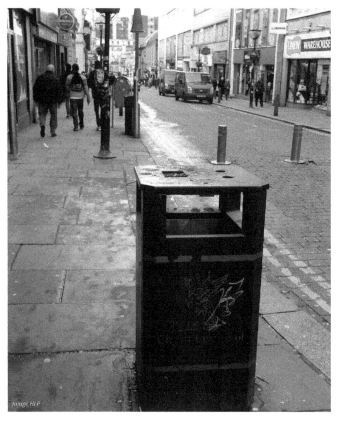

Summary
· People liked the busy local community shops.

Concerns
· Obstruction of the pavement by street furniture
· Dirty, slippy pavements
· Trip hazards
· Pavement too narrow
· Not people friendly.

Design could be improved by:
· Removing obstructions from the pedestrian areas
· Clearer visual distinction between road and pavement
· Better, more pedestrian friendly design
· More colour/planting.

Figure 5.8 The dementia-friendly neighbourhood – cue cards exercise – responses

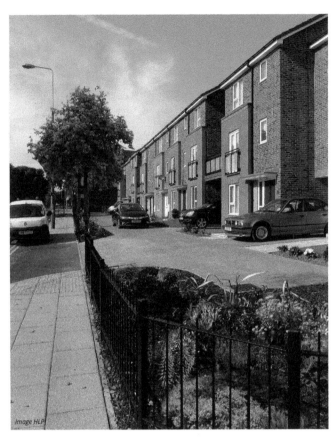

Summary

This image was liked by some people, particularly as an environment for young people or professionals.

Concerns

· Parked cars restricting access

· Steps to front doors

· Uniformity

· Balconies (although good safety rails).

Design could be improved by:

· Designing out the steps to achieve disabled access

· Features to distinguish between each house e.g. door colours

· More organised car parking.

Figure 5.9 The dementia-friendly neighbourhood – cue cards exercise – responses

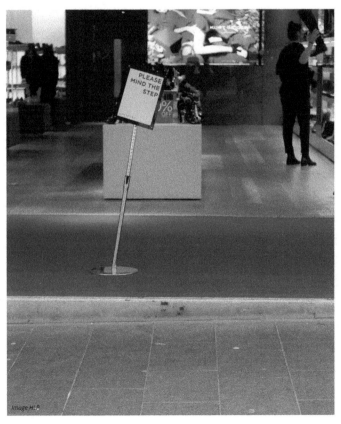

Summary

Shop thresholds are a particular area of concern. Perceptual problems can create risk hazards.

Concerns

· Concerns were regarding the trip hazard of the step. Clearly even the sign is an obstruction and potential trip hazard itself

· The red carpet could appear as a hole

· The step is indistinguishable from the pavement

· If the sign is perceived to be necessary it should be clear.

Design could be improved by:

· A distinctive colour on the tread and riser so that people going in or out can clearly see the step.

Figure 5.10 The dementia-friendly neighbourhood – cue cards exercise – responses

Project Summary 2: How Dementia Friendly Is Our City?

Figures 5.11 to 5.18 illustrate this project.

Objectives

- To see how dementia friendly Liverpool city centre is
- To explore the problems that people living with dementia may have in navigating and using the facilities of the city centre.

Method

- Living lab including a mix of people, including carers, professionals and people living with dementia
- Photo cue cards were used to assist in stimulating a response to an assortment of images
- Results were collated and analysed
- An independent equality act mini-audit was carried out on each image.

Understandably, most dementia-friendly design focuses on the inside private worlds of extra care housing, residential care projects, nursing homes or medical buildings and their surroundings.

However, the challenge of this project is finding a way to make our city centre and its buildings, streets, pavements and spaces more user friendly and accessible so that people living with dementia can live well with dementia.

People with dementia experience changes in perception and sight. If the designers get it wrong in terms of materials, texture, pattern or use of colour, then design can raise stress levels and increase the risk of falls amongst vulnerable user groups. People with dementia may have problems judging distances (visuospatial skills) and have difficulty with steps or seeing things in

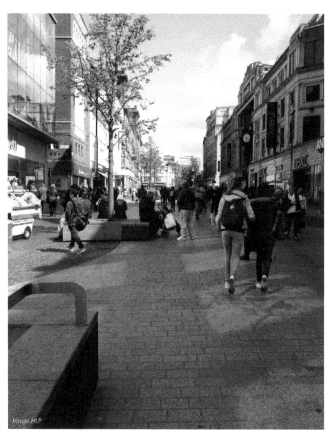

Comments from Workshop Participants

- Seats are uncomfortable, don't look like seats.
- Arbitrary paving patterns
- Grey bins blend in with grey floor
- Noise of buskers
- Cacophony of noise - buskers etc
- 'An awful place'
- Lively, busy, active, the centre of 'town' and it is important that this space is welcoming to all
- Seating is same colour as floor - would be better if seating was a different colour.

Figure 5.11 How Dementia Friendly Is Our City? Cue cards exercise – responses

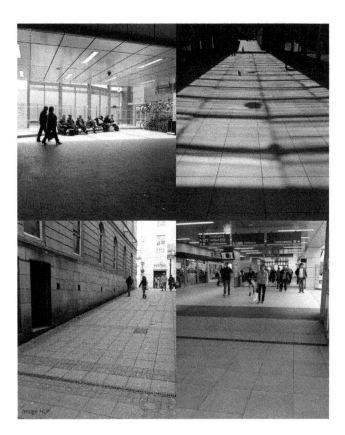

Comments from Workshop Participants

- Good use of natural light
- Good sitting space
- Handy for bikes
- Shadows on paving could cause a disturbing pattern
- The shadows make it difficult to judge the surface
- The ramp is too steep, difficult in high heels or when wet
- Handrails on the ramp?
- No steps as an alternative?
- The gradient of the ramp is too steep
- Black mat could read as a hole and cause someone with dementia to hesitate - potential accident.

Figure 5.12 How Dementia Friendly Is Our City? Cue cards exercise – responses

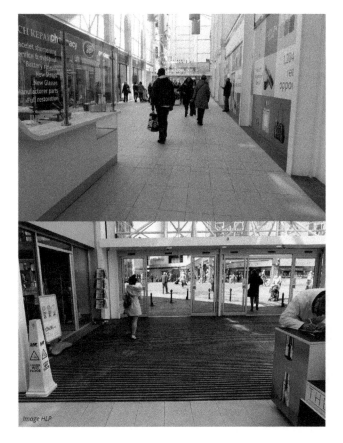

Comments from Workshop Participants

- Signs written on glass are very hard to read and seem very unclear.
- Should there be a tapping edge to assist visually impaired people?
- Black mat with shiny metal strips is disturbing
- Bollards are too low and distracting
- Black mat looks like a hole, or a step up
- The glass door needs clearer signs.

Figure 5.13 How Dementia Friendly Is Our City? Cue cards exercise – responses

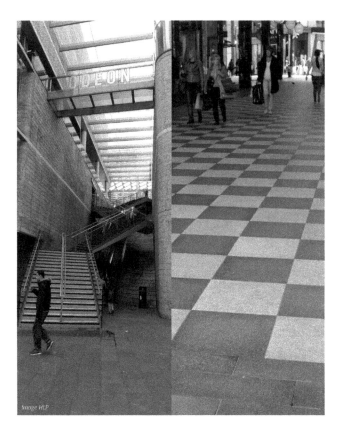

Comments from Workshop Participants

- 'Jazzy' paving pattern could be disturbing for people with dementia
- Checks on the floor design are very confusing and look very disorientating
- Hidden dark escalators
- Glass balustrades are disturbing
- Could bang your head on the stairs
- No clear signs - need a sign at eye level to say 'Odeon'.

Figure 5.14 How Dementia Friendly Is Our City? Cue cards exercise – responses

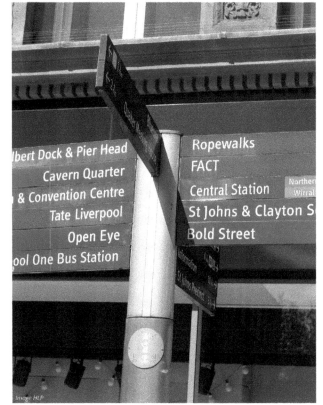

Comments from Workshop Participants

- Too high - not visible to people in wheelchairs or buggies
- White on blue is ok because of contrast
- Walking times are a good indication of distance
- Contrasting colours are good
- Too busy, too much information
- Needs more space between the individual signs
- Maybe have white lines between each sign to break them up
- Too much information - should be more selective
- Too close together - spacing between destinations should be increased
- Nothing stands out - colour could be selective to more important destinations.

Figure 5.15 How Dementia Friendly Is Our City? Cue cards exercise – responses

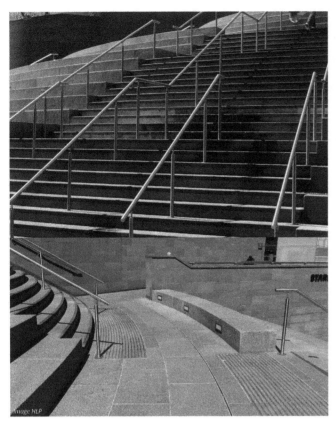

Comments from Workshop Participants

· Too steep, vertiginous, uncomfortable

· You could walk down expecting the steps to continue and fall over the stone plinth

· Dark strips could appear as holes but tactile paving is good for partially sighted

· Two different kinds of step is very confusing. Would be better if they were all the same depth

· Easily disorientated by different heights of step

· Curved edge to step can be hazardous

· Too many steps

· No signage to where the steps lead

· Confusing use - seating or steps?

· Too much of a travel distance

· Hand rail isn't continuous

· Takes too long to get up or down

Figure 5.16 How Dementia Friendly Is Our City? Cue cards exercise – responses

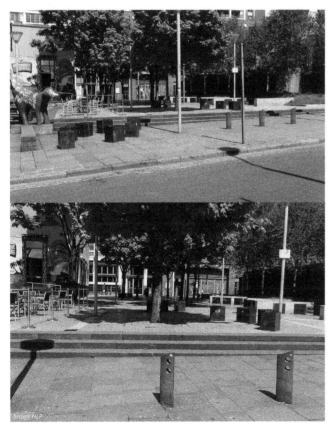

Comments from Workshop Participants

· Narrowing steps with tapered riser

· Obstructions - dark shadows

· But a pleasant active space in the summer

· Liked by skateboarders

· Handrails on steps?

· Is there an alternative ramped route?

· Not obvious or clear

· Step not clearly marked

· Bollards too low, so may not be seen and may be easy to walk into/trip over

· Steps and bollards appeared to be a bench

· Underneath appears very dark

· No handrail for steps.

Figure 5.17 How Dementia Friendly Is Our City? Cue cards exercise – responses

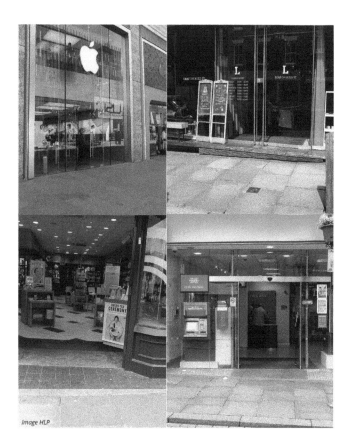

Comments from Workshop Participants

· Glass frontages cause confusing reflections
· Logo appears to be floating
· Tapering step with no hand rail - no disabled access
· Glass entrance makes it hard to distinguish which is the door
· Step appears as a slope, unsafe and hidden
· Black band/mat could appear as a hole - patterned flooring ditto
· Too many different floor surfaces
· All entrances are too dark.

Figure 5.18 How Dementia Friendly Is Our City? Cue cards exercise – responses

three dimensions. Visuospatial difficulties might lead to distortions and misperceptions of reality – a dark patch on a road can be mistaken for a hole, or a glossy surface might be perceived as being wet.

This exercise was carried out using Liverpool city centre as an exemplar and in order to benefit from the direct experience and participation of the user groups. There is no imputation that Liverpool city centre is any worse than other cities. Most cities present a poor pedestrian environment from a dementia accessibility perspective.

The city centre should not exclude anyone. This is the public realm, and our ambition is to make all of the public realm dementia friendly. People living with dementia may become confused about where they are, become disoriented or lose track of the day or time. Designers can help by creating clear legible routes through the city centre which are easy and comfortable to use. The environment should also provide a stimulus. The city should be a place to be enjoyed by all.

The How Dementia Friendly Is Our City? project was facilitated using photo cue cards: images taken on a lunchtime stroll through the city. In a living lab we asked a mixed group of people to comment on a range of themed photographs of different locations and to record their views on the back of the cards. The exercise asked for responses from a user viewpoint, including the viewpoint of those living with dementia and using the shared public realm of our city centre. An equality act 'mini-audit' provided a parallel commentary to the photo cues.

While this exercise was only a snapshot, it provides some insight for designers, businesses and managers about the issues being faced and perhaps shows the way towards improvements which could be made to assist Liverpool in becoming a dementia friendly city.

Some of the Lessons Learnt

The cue card exercise was a simple methodology aimed at stimulating responses from the group. It was not intended as a comprehensive design audit of the public realm of the city. However, there are some lessons that can be learned about the design of the pedestrian environment from the perspective of someone living with dementia.

The Pedestrian Environment

Design consideration is needed in response to the experience of people living with dementia. The pavement experience may be inhospitable:

- If it is obstructed by the bollards, bins, seats or equipment boxes. Clear unobstructed routes are essential
- Shiny, slippery or black tarmac patches may be misinterpreted as holes. Consistent surfaces in texture and tone are recommended
- Kerbs which are virtually invisible form trip hazards. Kerbs should contrast in tonal value
- Strong paving patterns such as chequerboard may cause disturbance – consistent light reflectance values are required
- Paving patterns or changes in colour which are arbitrary can cause confusion. Paving should be directional, assisting movement in a logical direction
- Lighting designed for traffic safety may not be right for pedestrians. Street lighting should indicate the direction of travel
- Pavement users include visually impaired people, people living with dementia as well as wheelchairs, mobility scooters and prams
- Pavements should have unobstructed zones wide enough to cater for all users
- Seats, which are an integral part of street furniture, may be confusing. Seats should look like seats
- Steps at changes in level should be avoided as far as possible. Where there are changes in level, there should be a clear choice between staircases, ramps or lifts
- Vertical objects such as litter bins or seating areas should contrast with paving so that they are clearly visible
- The city centre environment can be noisy and disturbing to people with dementia
- Noise can be absorbed or masked by trees or water features
- Signage should be clearly visible from a wheelchair position. Symbols and pictograms may be included. Too many signs on finger posts can confuse
- The pattern of shadows can be disturbing and make it difficult to judge the surface. They may be read as steps or obstacles
- Partially sighted people may use a white stick and can be assisted by the provision of a 'tapping edge'
- Small groups of steps can be difficult to judge. Handrails are needed. If there are handrails, they should be continuous. If there are steps, there should be a clearly visible ramp nearby
- Manhole covers can appear as a hole and should be recessed with matching paving infill.

Thresholds and Entrances

- Black rubber mats seem to be ubiquitous at entrances and thresholds. These may appear as holes to people with dementia and may cause them to hesitate in a busy thoroughfare and cause an accident. Some black mats have shiny metal strips which add to the confusion and

THE DEMENTIA INCLUSIVE PAVEMENT CONCEPT

A clear unobstructed pavement with directional paving orientation - wide enough for all categories of users to move confidently and freely, including white stick users and mobility scooters.

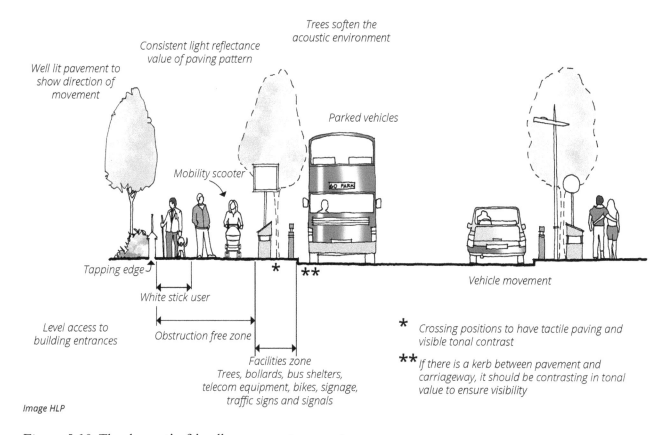

Image HLP

Figure 5.19 The dementia-friendly pavement concept

disturbance. Thresholds which have a consistent tonal value and light reflectance value (LRV) are safer. However, if there is a step, there should be a clear contrast, so that it is clearly visible

- Glass screens can be problematic. How can the fixed screen be distinguished from the door? Reflections in glass screens or balustrades also cause disturbance. 'Manifestations' (clearly visible patterns on glass) as required by regulation, must always be incorporated and clearly visible
- Contrasting door surrounds can assist in identifying the door position
- In the context of existing shop frontages, the design of thresholds suitable for use by those with dementia is a particular challenge. There is invariably a change in level. Pavements may slope across the entrance
- Entrances present a design challenge which must be tackled on a case-by-case basis in response to the principles outlined.

Conclusion

- *A more comprehensive design audit should be used to promote the dementia-friendly city concept*
- *This would involve the participation of the city council, businesses and city centre managers as well as user groups and other stakeholders.*

Project Summary 3: Connecting Minds Through Sandplay

Figures 5.20 and 5.21 illustrate this project.

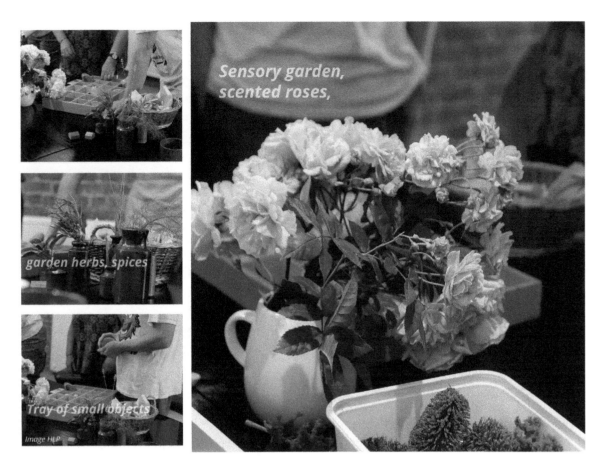

Figure 5.20 Connecting minds through sandplay

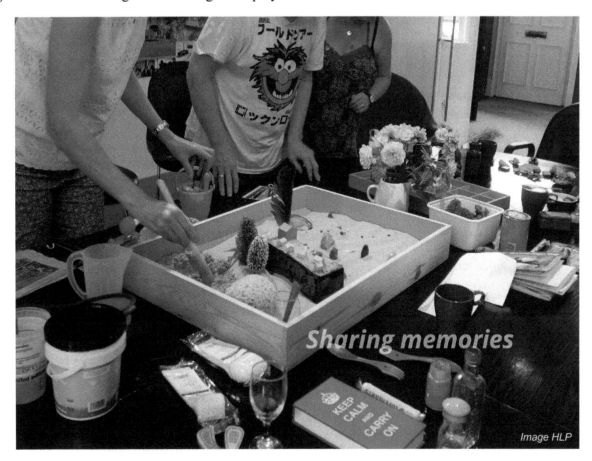

Figure 5.21 Connecting minds through sandplay

Objectives

- Explore the use of Jungian sandplay as a method for stimulating engagement, communication and participation involving people living with dementia.

Method

- Stimulate all the senses
- Promote play and relaxation
- Evoke memory.

Jungian Creative Play, Memory and the Senses

Jung was able to heal himself during a period of disorientation through the use of symbolic play, constructing a village using stones, mud and water on the banks of a lake, just as he had done as a child. In his building games, the creation of 'concrete' spontaneous imagery helped clarify his thoughts and released streams of fantasies.

Sandplay is a playful game that lasts about an hour and is aimed at encouraging creative lateral thinking, sensory awareness and memory recall. The game could apply to all people with or without dementia.

> I recall many times on beaches as a child in West Kirby, Scotland, Cornwall or Devon; long periods when time passed just playing in the sand and rock pools. As a child we hold sea shells to our ears on the sea shore, in the dry and wet sand. These memories are the building blocks of our sensory mind. We all have our own memories held within different objects, we can rediscover them in play. Jungian Sandplay can become art therapy for tactile and visual image making.
>
> (Dr Robert G MacDonald)

Sandplay uses a shallow tray painted blue inside to represent water or sky, filled with sand, measuring approximately 50 × 70 × 7 cm. Nearby is a collection of different small objects with which to play in the sand. The play can be photographed and recorded during the game and after sandplay is finished, when feedback is discussed and recorded.

Doing sandplay requires no special skill. The players are encouraged to play with the objects in the sand and out of the sand, to touch, smell, taste, listen, look and recall. What memories do the objects bring about? Jung used sandplay as a technique of 'active imagination' to provide a creative base for the expressive use of the arts as therapy.

Storr describes how Jung 'encouraged his patients to enter a state of reverie and fun in which judgement was suspended but consciousness preserved' (Storr 1983). What does the object feel like? Does the object have a distinctive taste? Can you hear the object? What do you see in the object? Does the object remind you of a person or place? When was the last time you remember seeing the object? Does the object provoke an emotion?

> 'I remember that day (wedding day) as clear as it can be . . . . but it's a struggle to recall what I did this morning.' It's happened to all of us at some time or another. You can't put a name to a face. You forget where you put your keys. You can't remember where you parked the car. Most of the time such slips are a nuisance, rather than a sign of something more serious. Dementia affects everyone in different ways. As well as problems with memory, other signs can include feeling confused even when in a familiar environment, problems thinking things through, and finding it hard to follow conversations.
>
> (Alzheimer's Society 2015)

Sandplay is part verbal, non-rational and unsophisticated; it encourages creative memory regression and stimulates the mind. Sandplay can be compared with artistic free painting, free drawing, free-form sculpture or free jazz. Therapies started their history with artists working with people in psychiatric and medical institutions. Perhaps there is a role for them in the 21st century?

Sandplay is a shared activity that integrates play and choice with small hand-sized objects. It involves an unplanned dialogue with individual's inner thoughts and memories. It's fun and joyful, and control is to be relaxed. Sandplay mirrors the eternal child in us all.

As a child I was always involved in drawing. I had a need to make marks and explore different materials. I drew on all surfaces; even the kitchen table! As a child, Daniel Libeskind drew on a large sheet of paper on his family dining table until his mother said, Daniel it's time for bed! I enjoyed making marks in snow, dust, chalk, earth, bird seeds and in my father's pet shop. I have always been taken by the real qualities of a blackboard and chalk. Geology was my subject of choice and fossils and rocks appealed. Later I experienced the sand and the primitive cave paintings of the Sahara Desert. Of all the environments that I know, the beach is the most special and wonderful. Now Crosby beach and Anthony Gormley's Iron Men are special and therapeutic. I love to collect objects to the north of Crosby beach and my fascination is with the original 'Cast Iron Shore' in Liverpool.

(Dr Robert G MacDonald)

Project Summary 4: The Design for Dementia Bungalow

Figures 5.22 to 5.28 illustrate this project.

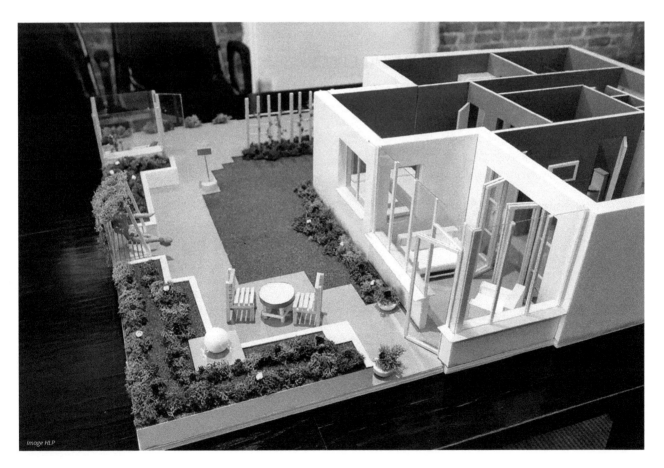

Figure 5.22 Design for Dementia bungalow model

DESIGN *for* DEMENTIA BUNGALOW

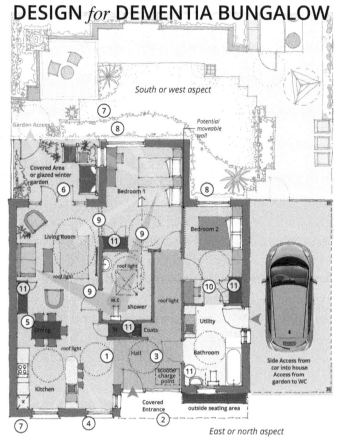

1. Open plan living from hall - kitchen dining - living room allows visual connection of spaces and reduces stress of multiple doors

2. Covered entrance and glazed screen promotes improved security and observation of outside - *'who is coming to the door?'*

3. Large entrance hall with easily accessible storage and scooter charge point. Easy to orientate from entrance

4. Kitchen and dining areas have natural daylight and views to the outside

5. Open plan living and dining promotes easy observation and inclusiveness

6. Sheltered rear space/winter garden allows outdoor enjoyment and activity for a longer period of the year, maximising sunlight and vitamin D manufacture in the skin

7. All rooms offer views to the front garden or rear garden areas. Gardens planted with interesting shrubs and flowers. *'Sensory'* garden providing stimulus to smell and taste as well as sight, sound and touch

8. Both bedrooms offer clear, interesting views to the rear garden even if a member of the family is bed bound. A direct connection is also created between living room and bedroom to facilitate inclusion of all family members and promote easy supervision

9. Visual links between living and bedroom areas are created including views of the toilet/wc

10. Additional visitor wc has direct access to bedroom 2. This wc also has a direct external link from the garden and parking area. This bathroom has been linked with a separate utility space to remove the washing machine, possible smells and noise from the open plan kitchen - living space

11. Functional storage - related to room functions

Image HLP

Figure 5.23 The Design *for* Dementia bungalow

DESIGN *for* DEMENTIA BUNGALOW

Conservatory outdoor space connected to the garden

Main bathroom with top light

Open plan living space connected to bathroom

Kitchen/dining area - views out to the entrance

Entrance hall - minimum number of doors and good views out

Main bedroom with views to the garden, living room and wc

Carer's bedroom with potential knock through panel within the wall to the main bedroom and ensuite connection to the shower room

Shower/utility room accessible from the garden and car port

Front entrance - covered and highly visible

Image HLP

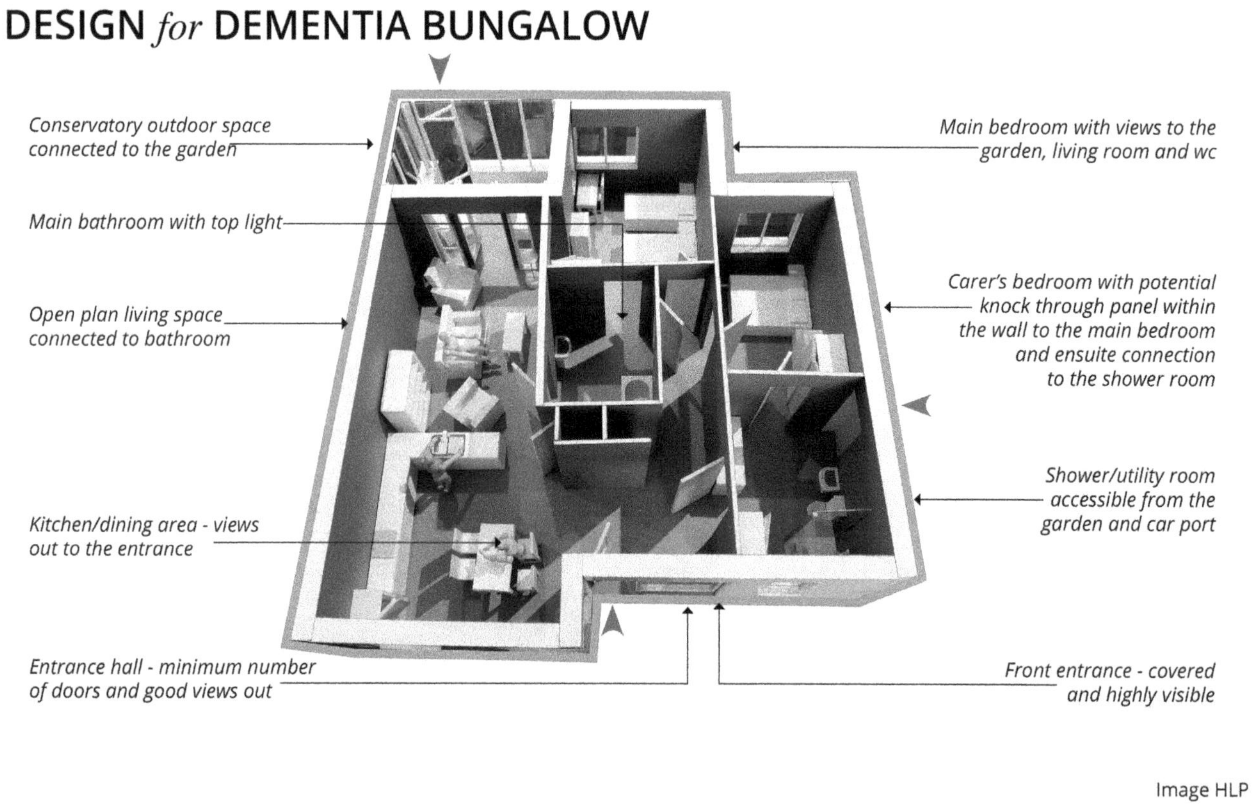

Figure 5.24 The Design *for* Dementia bungalow

DESIGN *for* DEMENTIA GARDEN

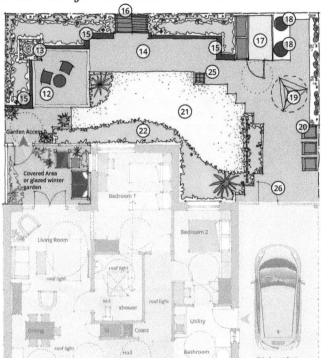

(12) Patio terrace with table set for eating or activities

(13) Visual focus - water feature; sound, movement, reflection

(14) Clear wide paths

(15) Raised beds, with areas of wider coping for sitting

(16) Visual focus - seating arbour

(17) Greenhouse or shed

(18) Compost bin/water butt

(19) Washing line

(20) Bins/recycling, screened from garden by timber trellis

(21) Lawn

(22) Low, fragrant planting next to windows

(23) Boundary fence softened by climbers

(24) Lighting to enable the garden to be enjoyed in the evening

(25) Bird table or bird bath to encourage visiting birds.

(26) Security gate and fence

Image HLP

Figure 5.25 The Design *for* Dementia garden

DESIGN *for* DEMENTIA GARDEN

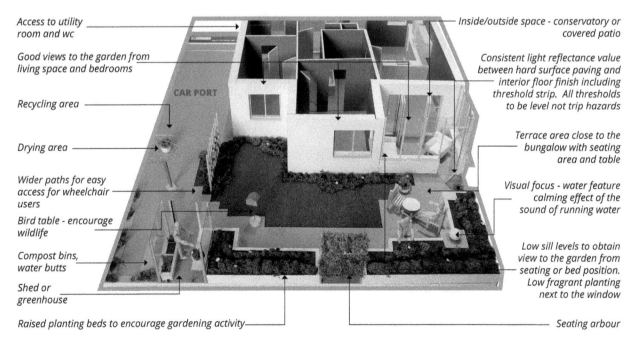

Access to utility room and wc

Good views to the garden from living space and bedrooms

Recycling area

Drying area

Wider paths for easy access for wheelchair users

Bird table - encourage wildlife

Compost bins, water butts

Shed or greenhouse

Raised planting beds to encourage gardening activity

Inside/outside space - conservatory or covered patio

Consistent light reflectance value between hard surface paving and interior floor finish including threshold strip. All thresholds to be level not trip hazards

Terrace area close to the bungalow with seating area and table

Visual focus - water feature calming effect of the sound of running water

Low sill levels to obtain view to the garden from seating or bed position. Low fragrant planting next to the window

Seating arbour

Image HLP

Figure 5.26 The Design *for* Dementia garden

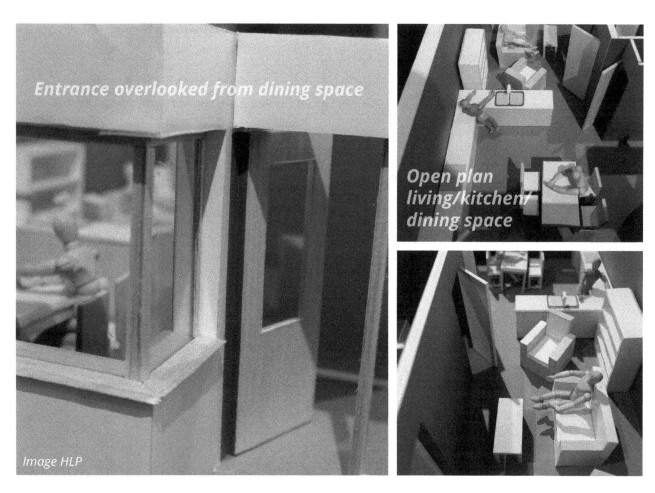

Figure 5.27 The Design *for* Dementia bungalow model

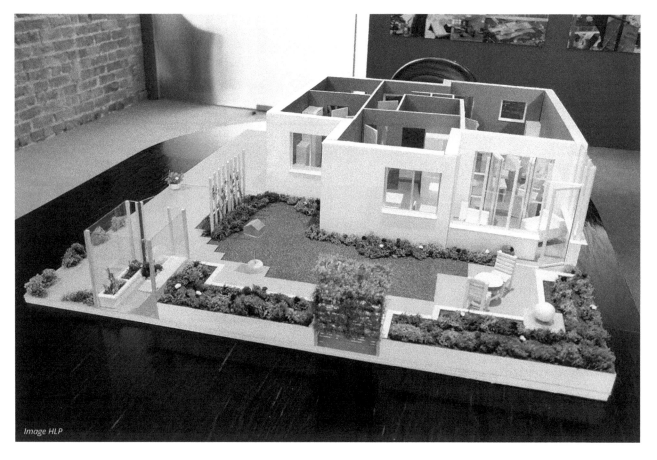

Figure 5.28 The Design *for* Dementia bungalow model

Concept

The Design *for* Dementia Bungalow was a research project carried out by HLP as an offshoot from the Innovation Dementia Europe, Living Lab engagement. It was based on a design participation process with the Service Users Reference Forum (SURF) and Dementia Action Alliance (DAA) members.

The concept was to design an ideal dwelling for someone living with dementia. It is a theoretical design for a potentially new archetype which could be incorporated into new housing layouts. From the outset the ideal was to design a dwelling which could be lived in by anyone rather than a special needs unit which could potentially stigmatize supported housing or housing for the elderly in a way which could isolate the users or make them more vulnerable by identifying them as different.

The Design *for* Dementia Bungalow would be aspirational as well as functional for someone living with dementia and their family or carer. Its design features would be beneficial to anyone living in it and attractive as a place to live. The design features focused on the needs of someone living with dementia should be discrete. Other features could be provided as built-in potential for future provision such as hoists and grab handles. Design should be non-institutional as far as possible.

Most importantly, it is hoped that the design principles developed in the model design can be adapted to other dwelling types and housing designs so that the Design *for* Dementia approach becomes written in to development briefs and that the ideal of being able to live comfortably at home as part of the community with dementia becomes a wider aspiration adopted by developers and designers. In the same way that 'Lifetime Homes' has become an adopted standard within the housing industry, Design *for* Dementia can become best practice. Lifetime Homes standards focus on design for disability and the incorporation of the needs of people who use a wheelchair, that is, those with physical disability. Design *for* Dementia demonstrates that cognitive disability can also be designed for, creating interior and exterior environments conducive for all impairments.

Objectives

- Tackle the main issues of living well with dementia through the development and refinement of the design of a single archetype. It is envisaged that the Design *for* Dementia Bungalow could be designed into mixed housing schemes or could form key components of specialist elderly care schemes. However, the design philosophy is 'long life, loose fit' – a dwelling which could be aspired to, and lived in, through life by anyone.

Methods

- Use the design principles established by the 'Design *for* Dementia' guide and other guidance. Design a model for a dementia-friendly dwelling
- Incorporate statutory standards and voluntary codes for design
- Participatory design process involving hands-on modelling to explore the design with the SURF group
- Evolutionary design process to demonstrate adaptability.

The Brief

- Satisfy a range of standards, including Lifetime Homes, Secured by Design and so on
- Simple layout, easily navigable
- Visual cues to assist orientation

- Visual connection and easy access between living room, bedroom and w.c.
- Low-level windowsills – view out from a low position
- Hoist route from bedroom to bathroom
- Option between shower or bath
- Separate w.c./utility area
- Natural light into the middle of the plan
- Car port with direct access to the bungalow
- Garden with patio area and raised planting beds for easy gardening
- Bedroom for carer – potential moveable wall
- Interior finishes appropriate for dementia
- Open plan kitchen/dining/living area with easy access to the garden
- Easy access between garden and w.c.
- Workable within mixed housing layouts
- Energy efficient low-carbon design and specification – affordable and comfortable
- Smart technology
- Level access throughout including thresholds
- Spaces large enough to provide good ease of movement
- Natural ventilation
- Clearly visible front entrance
- Easy natural flow between rooms
- Higher levels of artificial light (twice normal)
- Task-focused lighting
- Reduce the number of doors (or removable doors)
- Good views from seated position to front and rear
- Views to green and communal activity
- Tonal contrast between floors, walls and doors
- For the carer – balance privacy and access
- Views of the approach to the front entrance
- Viewable kitchen/bedroom/bathroom storage – easy to find things
- Easy to maintain.

Design Description

Spatial Organisation

The bungalow is designed around the bathroom as the central point of this plan to enable quick and easy access to the w.c. from all points of the plan. The movement pattern circulates the core in an open plan arrangement to ensure ease of navigation between the open plan spaces of the design. Doors are minimised to reduce confusion and assist visual permeability between spaces. The rear of the plan opens out into the garden.

The main spaces comprise a kitchen/diner/living room linked to a winter garden or conservatory at the rear. There are two bedrooms. The main bedroom is spacious and connected to the living room and the bath/shower room. The second bedroom is envisaged as being for a carer, for a visitor or as respite for a partner and is connected to a smaller second bathroom/utility area. This space has access to the carport/garden so that there is access to the w.c. from the garden.

Entrance

The front of the bungalow overlooks the street, and in this arrangement an east or north aspect is preferred, allowing the garden at the rear to orient to the south or west. The entrance is well overlooked from the kitchen and the entrance hall so that the residents can see who is approaching the front door. Windowsills of these spaces should be low enough to see out from seated position. An outside seat is also provided so that the resident can watch the world go by. The entrance is covered to provide protection from the elements while opening the door.

Once inside, movement is to the left for the more public areas and kitchen/diner/living and right for the more private areas. Good exterior lighting would be provided.

Opposite the main entrance is a wall which provides opportunities for expressing identity, (reminiscence wall) or a clock. Perhaps a small table for keys or other things, and behind the wall is storage and a space for coats and hats.

Communal Areas

At the front of the space is the kitchen with good views to the street. The kitchen could be equipped with a rise and fall worktop if required and is shown with a peninsular unit with a bar top for easy sociability and inclusiveness. The dining space adjoins the kitchen. A table for five or six people is shown so that visitors can be received. The main living space is grouped around a wall-mounted TV but also offers the potential for a view to the w.c. if needed.

The bathroom has a door for privacy. All internal doors would be capable of being easily removed in case this was required by the resident. All spaces and doorways are wide enough for wheelchair use, and wheelchair charging points would be provided in key rooms. If necessary, two wheelchair charging positions could be provided in the hall.

Private Areas

The main bedroom is shown connected to the living room by an open doorway to give easy movement between the bedroom and the living space.

If necessary, a hospital bed could be wheeled between these spaces. If required, a door on lift-off hinges could be installed or a pocket door which could be pushed back into a concealed position in the wall.

The bathroom in this arrangement ensures ease of access and generates confidence. Some of the user groups commented that two doors might cause confusion to someone living with dementia. In the plan, the entrance to the bathroom from the living room is shown with a door, while the entrance to the bathroom from the bedroom is shown as an opening. Alternatively, the door from the living room could be sealed off and a door from the bedroom installed. In either case, there would be provision for a hoist to be fitted to the ceiling between the bedroom and the bathroom to ease transfer of the resident from the bedroom to the w.c./shower.

Another debate was bath or shower. Some favoured a shower for accessibility reasons (it might be hard to get in and out of a bath). Others preferred a bath because the hissing sound of a shower caused them distress. In either arrangement the floor would be 'wash down' and fitted with a floor gulley, and all necessary grab rails and handles would be fitted.

Between the two bedrooms, a demountable panel is shown. This is a provision against the eventuality that the person living with dementia might need support and supervision through the night.

The second bedroom is smaller although fully wheelchair accessible and could be used by a carer, family member or visitor. It has its own bathroom, which in this iteration included a utility space. The noise from a washing machine or dryer can be disturbing to someone living with dementia, so this is positioned away from the main bedroom or living areas.

Some participants thought that the second bedroom should have its own bathroom and that the utility area should be separated off. This is an option and may be preferred by some people.

Car Port

Adjacent to the house is a car port to disabled access standards with space for wheelchair access. There is undercover access to the house through the utility area; it also provides a convenient connection to the garden and the outside clothes dryer.

Winter Garden/Conservatory

At the rear of the bungalow there is a small covered or glazed space providing a connection to the garden. This encourages the residents to sit out in the sun, experiencing sunlight, generating Vitamin D, and daylight assists in reinforcing circadian rhythms.

The Design for Dementia Garden

The garden is small but designed to provide space for relaxation and activities such as eating out, socialising and gardening. Raised beds and a shed or greenhouse are provided to assist gardening activities and appreciation of plants.

A small seating area encourages al fresco dining.

The garden is designed to stimulate the senses (a small sensory garden); colour and scent are promoted through the medium of plants. Sound and visual stimulus may be provided, a water feature, for example. Sight is stimulated by seasonal planting, form, foliage, flower, seed heads and so on to generate a garden scene all year round. Tactile experience is also provided through the materials used and the texture of leaves through the seasons.

The path through the garden is rotational and connects with the movement patterns through the bungalow.

The garden should also be designed to the bio-diverse, encouraging wildlife, including garden birds, to visit, providing additional year-round interest.

The Design for Dementia Bungalow

Most of all, it is safe and secure so that the residents can enjoy their peace and tranquillity.

The Design *for* Dementia Bungalow is not a paradigm or 'one size fits all'. Dementia comes in many different forms, and it is experienced in different ways by different individuals who may live in different circumstances with different types of support. It demonstrates a set of design principles which can be utilised in various contexts to suit the need of the individual concerned.

The design which emerged through participation of the SURF and DAA groups is quite large (approximately 110 m² including the covered external area) and would occupy a significant length of street frontage including its in-curtilage parking space. It would therefore be an expensive dwelling. The Design *for* Dementia Garden is relatively shallow so that the interface distances could be 'tightened up', reducing the site area requirements.

Design Participation Evaluation – 'Hands-on Modelling'

The chosen medium for communication and dialogue was a foam board model, open topped so that the interiors could easily be manipulated, at a scale of 1:25. Wooden mannequin figures were used to animate the spaces and to assist understanding of the ergonomic aspects of the design. The furniture was moveable, as were the garden features. The SURF group responded well to this format.

Points of Discussion

• The bungalow was liked as an ideal model but also as a way of explaining to housing providers – the council, housing associations or builders – what was needed by people living with dementia

- A degree of customisation is needed. Therefore, the design should be flexible, with alternative layouts, in particular, a choice between bath and shower. Some people felt that they couldn't use a bath; others found the sound of a shower annoying. Plans have been amended to show a wet room en-suite to the main bedroom and a bath in place of a shower in the combined utility area
- However, plan variants should show a range of options. In the same way, the kitchen layout should have design variants to cope with different needs and aspirations. Choice of appliances is an important consideration. There is concern about gas in particular – that someone could forget to turn it off and cause a fire. Induction hobs with safety cut-outs are a potential solution to this problem
- The 'Design *for* Dementia Bungalow' needs to be able to easily respond to the different stages or types of condition involved. Potential solutions are: removable doors, ceiling mounted hoist positions or removable wall panels. This 'evolutionary' plan concept enables a responsive design which can be customised to suit individual needs
- Maintaining the garden was another concern, although the greenery and convivial surroundings were appreciated. Suggestions included artificial turf – to save grass cutting while maintaining a green view. Many people living with dementia gain great enjoyment and relaxation from their gardens but are concerned about future maintenance
- The carer's needs and lifestyle must also be considered. A degree of privacy and respite is necessary.

Summary

Good, appropriate design of the built environment can help people living with dementia to sustain their capacity for longer and promote their independent living. The design of both the interior domain and the external environment can assist in creating a better living environment for all. In order to achieve this design engagement with people living with dementia and their carers, health care professionals should form part of the design process to ensure that designers have understood the needs, requirements and aspirations of people living with dementia. A range of techniques is available to facilitate this process, and formats such as living laboratories and hands-on design techniques such as cue cards, sand trays and physical modelling can help generate a creative interaction. In this regard the significance of the Design *for* Dementia bungalow should be noted; the Design *for* Dementia bungalow project was used by Bill Halsall and Robert G MacDonald in presentations at many dementia-focused conferences and exhibitions, feeding back the lessons learnt and gathering further responses to the features of design. It became a precursor to the Design *for* Dementia Demonstration Project at the Building Research Establishments Innovation Park.

The dementia demonstrator Chris and Sally's House has taken design research to the logical next step on a full-scale, fully functional house which functions both as an experimental platform and resource and an educative tool.

References

Alzheimers Society, 2015. *Dementia 2015: Aiming Higher to Transform Lives*. Alzheimers Society: London.

Bergvall-Kåreborn, B., and Ståhlbröst, A., 2009. Living lab: An open and citizen-centric approach for innovation. *International Journal of Innovation and Regional Development*, 1, 356–370. https://doi.org/10.1504/IJIRD.2009.022727.

Halsall, W., and MacDonald, R., 2015. Volume 2 – Design *for* Dementia – research projects, outlines the research projects and describes the participatory approach. ISBN 978-0-9929231-2-9.

Halsall, W., MacDonald, R., and Landi, D., 2015. Volume 1 – Design *for* Dementia – a guide with helpful guidance in the design of exterior and interior environments. *Halsall Lloyd Partnership Liverpool.* ISBN 978-0-9929231-1-2.

Halsall, W., MacDonald, R., and Landi, D., 2019. Volume 3 Design *for* Dementia – the international dimension. ISBN 978-0-9929231-1-2.

Storr, A., 1983. Individuation and the creative process. *The Journal of Analytical Psychology*, 28 (4), 329–343. https://doi.org/10.1111/j.1465-5922.1983.00329.x.

Woods, L., Pendleton, J., Smith, G., and Parker, D., 2013. *Innovative Dementia Baseline Report: Shaping the Future for People with Dementia*. Liverpool John Moores University Press: Liverpool, England.

Wootton, H., 1624. *The Elements of Architecture*. John Bill: London.

6 Personas and the Evidence Base of Dementia-Inclusive Design

Sue Hignett and Eef Hogervorst

Introduction

The guidance for both housing and care facilities has mostly been based on professional consensus rather than robust research evidence. Despite best design intentions, the inclusion of people living with dementia has been limited depending on the stage and progression of the disease. To address this challenge, Dr Charlotte Jais (PhD at Loughborough University), supported by Prof Hignett and Prof Hogervorst, her supervisors, developed a building design tool to support the voice of people living with dementia in the design process, which will be discussed in this chapter (for more details, see Jais 2019).

Personas

One approach to inclusive design is the use of personas to explore interactions by representing the needs and abilities of a user group. Personas are often in the form of a short profile of an archetypal (typical) member of a specific group and can be evidence-based or assumption-based. Evidence-based personas are more reliable, as they use scientific research rather than individual opinions and/or preconceptions about a user group (Adlin and Pruitt 2010).

A qualitative methodological approach was taken with iterative development and review process to:

- Establish what is already known through a literature review and scoping survey
- Develop the personas and the design tool (three formats).

The literature review and scoping study results were combined to create the first version (V1) of the personas focusing on eating, toileting, physical activity and social interactions. The literature review identified 4,124 papers, of which 57 were retained. These data were combined with the scoping study ($n = 113$ respondents) which considered which activities (ADLS and iADLs) were felt to be specifically relevant to, or important for, people with dementia, with ideas for design solutions to support these activities. This produced very lengthy descriptions, so a higher-level approach was taken to combine social interaction with eating (at communal mealtimes) and toileting with physical activity to support residents using the toilet independently.

The World Health Organisation (WHO 2012) suggested that problems linked to dementia can be understood in three stages: (i) early stage (1–2 years), (ii) middle stage (2–4/5 years) and (iii) later stage (5+ years). The initial personas focused on the two most common types of dementia, Alzheimer's disease and vascular dementia. Generic symptoms and care needs were taken from a range of sources (to allow combinations across all forms of dementia and integration of specific characteristics (Prince et al. 2015; WHO 2012). It was decided that a four-stage

DOI: 10.1201/9781003306054-6

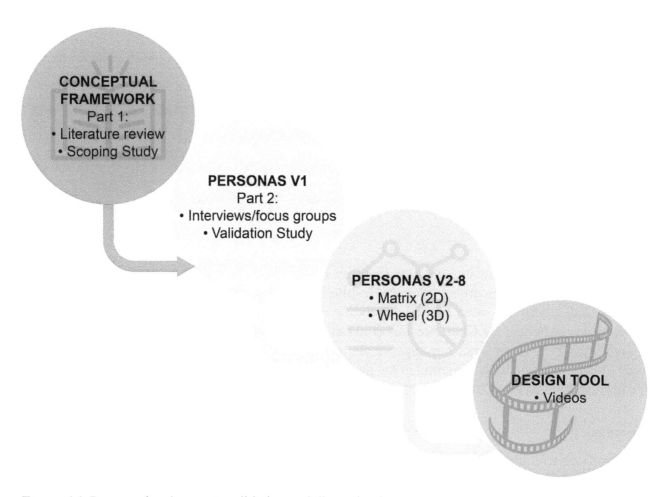

Figure 6.1 Persona development, validation and dissemination

framework (A, B, C, D) would be most effective for the design tool, with two personas for the middle stage (B and C):

A.   Alison: early stage with short-term memory problems
B.   Barry: early middle stage
C.   Chris(tine): late middle stage
D.   David: later stage of vascular dementia (through to end of life), with severe communication difficulties

The personal information included a demographic outline for age, sex, previous employment and marital status. The clinical information (diagnosis and symptoms) had six sections for clinical condition (stage and type of dementia); current living situation; and physical, cognitive, perceptual and communication abilities. The built environment section linked symptoms to design recommendations. For example, the Alison persona recommends clear signage in bathrooms (Namazi and Johnson 1991), contrasting toilet seats (Lord and Dayhew 2001), familiar fixtures in bathrooms (Boger et al. 2013) and domestic-style dining rooms (Van Hoof and Kort 2009). The David persona recommends hoists to assist with toileting (Garg and Kapellusch 2012), ensuring that bathrooms could accommodate specialist equipment and multiple carers (Day et al. 2000), and providing an adjustable table for use with a wheelchair at mealtimes (Chaudhury et al. 2013).

Development of Personas

Data were collected with architects, care home developers and care home workers using semi-structured interviews. To better illustrate the large variation in symptoms and needs within persons living with dementia, the persona design was further modified to illustrate a wider range of symptoms, design and care needs on a good day (green section), an average (orange) day and a bad (red) day. These are illustrated in Figures 6.2–6.5. Changes related to ageing were also added: Alison included visual changes (wearing glasses), Chris(tine) included hearing aids and David included mobility challenges (using a walking frame for 5 years). Additional information was added to support communication between clinicians and designers with clinical assessment scores.

Finally, the personas were applied and validated at five care environments ($n = 13$; managers, nurses, and care team leaders).

Alison, illustrated in Figure 6.2, represents someone with early dementia (70 years old) who is widowed and used to work in a shop. On a good day, her needs and symptoms are minimal, closely reflecting those of a healthy older adult. On an average day she experiences minor difficulties, and on a bad day she is likely to need more support.

Barry, illustrated in Figure 6.3, is a 74-year-old retired postman who has been diagnosed with dementia and is currently living in his own home. He has difficulty with word finding, planning and organising and has a small risk of falls (physical changes). On an average day he sometimes forgets recent events (including personal information about himself) and may need support for numerical tasks. On a bad day he may have communication difficulties and be confused, particularly in new environments (navigation information processing).

Christine, shown in Figure 6.4, illustrates the third stage of living with dementia. The persona includes a generic 'ageing' characteristic of hearing loss, where since the age of 70 years she managed with bilateral hearing aids. These aspects may present dementia-related challenges in remembering to wear the hearing aids and the physical dexterity (usability) for operation and

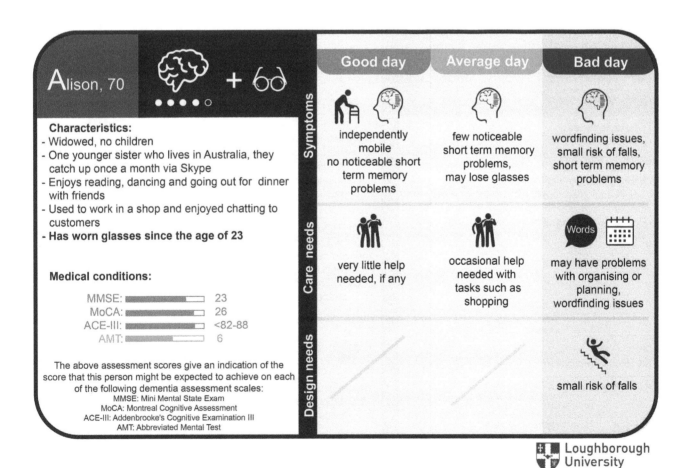

Figure 6.2 Alison: early stage with short-term memory problems

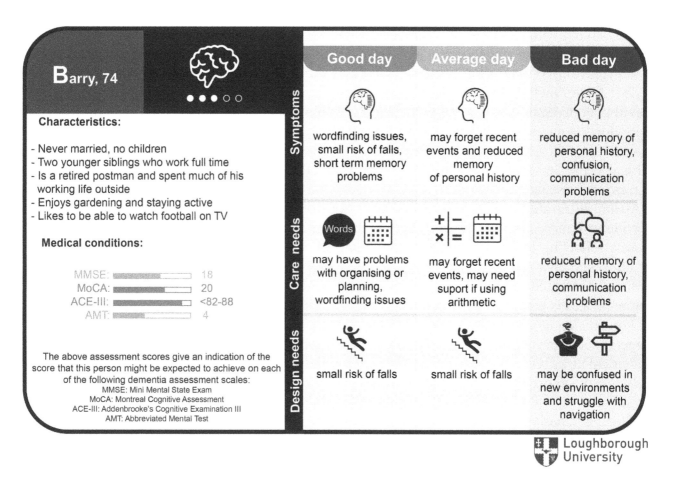

Figure 6.3 Barry: early middle stage

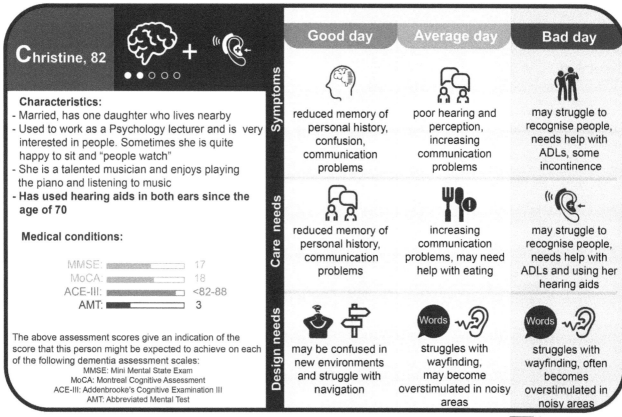

Figure 6.4 Christine: late middle stage

maintenance (battery changes). As Christine is a talented musician, the hearing challenges can contribute to frustration with her changing capabilities and limitations.

The couple persona (Chris and Sally) represents that, in many settings, the primary caregiver will be the marriage partner (with more women), including couples moving into care homes together.

Chris and Sally, illustrated in Figure 6.5, have been married for over 50 years and love to spend time with their three grandchildren. Sally is starting to find it harder to care for Chris as his dementia progresses. They both have good, average and bad days; Chris has the same symptoms, care and design needs as Christine. If their bad days coincide, Sally needs considerable help and may have to stay awake to care for him throughout the night.

David, illustrated in Figure 6.6, represents the later stages of dementia. David was an office manager and enjoyed painting. On a good day his symptoms, care needs and design needs are the same as Christine on a bad day. On an average day, he is likely to have problems with incontinence and will need support with ADLs, such as toileting and eating. On a bad day, he is likely to have severe mobility problems and communication difficulties and may be completely dependent on carers for all ADLs.

Following the final validation study, the personas were given 'voices' as short films with patient actors. For example, Christine's daughter explains her care needs, and David's carer explains his care needs in the nursing home. The five films were installed in the demonstrator house as dissemination to both professional (building design and clinical care) and public visitors. These films were shown to Loughborough alumni who had selected the dementia-inclusive home as their primary interest for funding. Feedback was overwhelmingly positive, with many older people recognising the persona and their worth for improving design features and guiding designers and architects.

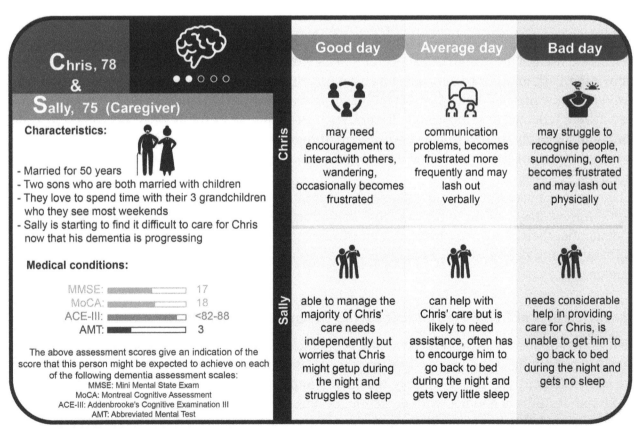

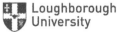

Figure 6.5 Chris and Sally (couple)

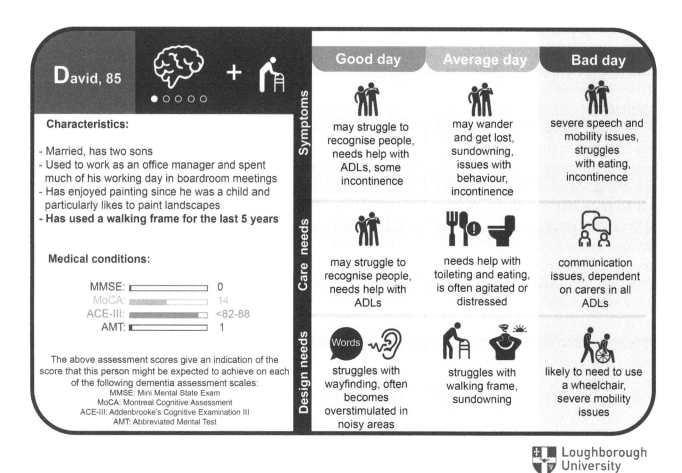

Figure 6.6 David: later stage of vascular dementia through to end of life

The personas developed through this research represent a fundamental component of the evidence base used in the design of Chris and Sally's House, the demonstration project at the BRE's Innovation Park in Watford, and acted as a resource through the design process. The design was based around Chris and Sally's perceived needs and aspirations. Elements of other personas like David were reflected in some design drivers, such as the potential future provision of a day room downstairs, closely related to the downstairs bathroom/w.c., designed with a possible future use of assisting end-of-life care. In the absence of real clients, the personas became substitute end users.

The persona make designers and architects aware of changes within and between people living with different stages of dementia and how that affects design needs. The general characteristics of dementia, their influence on the design of Chris and Sally's House and how these could be addressed using design and technology in people's homes are described in the next part of this chapter.

Characteristics of Dementia Influencing the Design of Chris and Sally's House

As outlined in previous chapters, dementia is characterised by gradual and progressive (or stepwise and sudden in VD) cognitive impairment of which forgetfulness; loss of organisation skills and contrast sensitivity are often early features to impact activities of daily life.

The risk for falls is doubled with dementia, because of changes in gait and contrast perception (Fernando et al. 2017). Once older people have falls resulting in fractures, their risk for reduced mobility, prolonged hospitalisation, institutionalisation and mortality increases significantly. Preventing falls in older people, particularly in those with dementia, is essential.

Fall risk is increased by thresholds, loose rugs and thick carpets; slippery and shiny floors in the kitchen and bathrooms; and ill-lit patterned steep and uneven stairs. Risk for injury can occur due to sharp corners on appliances and surfaces, exposure to scalding hot water and hot hobs, which might be forgotten to be turned off after use.

Patterns on soft furnishings such as rugs, carpets, walls and curtains and clutter on surfaces and noise from appliances can contribute to confusion, possible hallucinations, delusions, restlessness and other behavioural issues, as described in Chapter 3. To deal with forgetfulness and disorientation (e.g., losing keys and missing appointments), technology can be used effectively. The Alzheimer's Society has a range of products which can help mitigate these issues.

Part M of UK Building Regulations was introduced to ensure that future houses built would have fewer challenging features and would take an inclusive design approach. Wheelchair access, slip-resistant floors in the bathrooms with no patterns and sockets at wheelchair height, for instance, are included.

Hence, many of the issues mentioned previously could be solved by adhering to part M by implementing sockets at wheelchair height, using slip-resistant flooring without patterns, including railings where needed (bathrooms, stairs, beds, etc.), improving stair access (light, height of steps with contrasting strips), not including thresholds and widening access to allow improved access by creating an open plan living/dining/kitchen space. Many guidelines exist for designing for dementia but are often not rooted in evidence-based findings. In Chris and Sally's house, suggestions through patient and public involvement (PPI) were implemented and combined with features proven to work in research to improve the life of people with dementia and their partners or carers.

Dementia symptoms and needs are related to (i) cognitive, (ii) sensorimotor and (iii) behavioural changes which respond to different design and digital technology solutions. These solutions in Chris and Sally's House are outlined for individual rooms and living spaces.

Understanding Symptoms and Needs Related to Cognitive Issues Affecting Daily Life

Loss of memory is a hallmark in dementia, and both subjective as well as objective loss of memory can be an early marker, particularly in Alzheimer's disease, the most common dementia. These memory issues can start from forgetting shopping lists and appointments to not being able to remember family members. Linked to this is a lack of orientation in time, place and person.

Language issues can present with word finding problems but also in the inability to produce understandable language or to understand written/spoken language, making communication and understanding instructions difficult.

Planning disturbances are initially more common in people with vascular dementia but, as dementia progresses, usually become an issue for all dementia types and can result in problems cooking, dressing, banking, planning and executing trips and other instrumental activities of daily life. Loss of weight is often seen very early in dementia and can lead to loss of muscle mass, leading to falls and immobility. It is probably related to forgetting to eat, cook and/or shop.

Design Solutions to Mitigate Cognitive Change Affecting Activities of Daily Life

Cooking requires all cognitive functions and is a complex activity of daily living. To aid with memory loss, the kitchen should have glass fronted cabinets to allow easy identification of material needed. The fridge needs to be energy efficient and have a self-closing door. The hobs and kettle need to turn off automatically when not occupied or used, and taps are programmed to not scald the skin (part M). Taps need to be colour coded (red and blue) to help identify the hot and cold taps.

One of the most important and best evaluated elements, suggested by US-based research and patient and public involvement, is a downstairs wet room, where bits of the porcelain are visible from all angles downstairs (see subsequently; Caspi 2014; Day et al. 2000; Fleming et al. 2014; Hyde 1989; Marquardt et al. 2014; Namazi and Johnson 1991; Torrington 2009; van Hoof et al. 2013). This wet room is installed in the middle of the downstairs area, with glimpses of the toilet acting as reminders of where to find to it, which helps reduce anxiety and agitation. Incontinence is a problem in the later stages of dementia, and this central wet room feature helps maintain independence in toileting.

Digital Technology to Aid With Cognitive Loss in Dementia Affecting Activities of Daily Life

A tablet or large-font calendar with dates and time for orientation in time supplemented with reminders for appointments and planning activities could be placed on the wall, requiring wiring. This can be as simple as a digital clock supplied by the Alzheimer's Society and a whiteboard for appointments or an advanced remote programmable tablet. There could also be a computer tablet on the wall, which could be activated at mealtimes, with pictures of personalised meal choices, which when touched could be connected via Wi-Fi to producing online shopping lists for delivery and pictures how to prepare and cook the food. Food storage boxes need to be labelled with pictures for easy identification.

Medicine cabinets in the bathroom could be fitted with sensors to remind people with a voiceover to take their medicine if the cabinet doors have not been used at the expected time and to brush their teeth. A loss of teeth doubles the risk for dementia and is linked to loss of

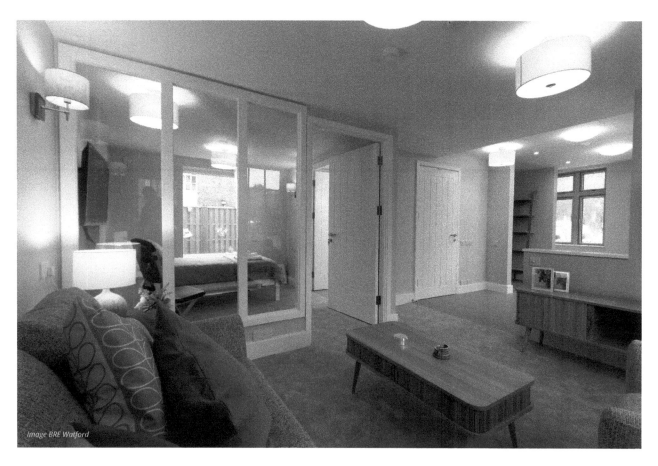

Figure 6.7 Completed lounge, Chris and Sally's House
Source: image BRE

weight and not eating. Dental hygiene is very important as a preventative factor in the development of frailty.

Clothes wardrobes in the bedrooms could also have sensors in the doors with voiceovers to remind people to get dressed and washed in the morning once the bed sensors were be activated.

Understanding Symptoms and Needs Related to Sensorimotor Changes in Dementia

There are several sensorimotor changes in dementia, and these can present early. First, best known are changes in contrast sensitivity, which make navigation and getting around more difficult. Especially in conditions of poor light (stairs, dusk), this can contribute to falls.

Second, there is a known loss of blue/green colour perception, which has stimulated a debate about the provision of red toilet seats or cutlery, for example. However, this may not be the best approach, provided there is sufficient contrast between surfaces. In addition, more recent studies have shown general colour discrimination issues, which is not limited to the blue–yellow axis (Javaid et al. 2016; Kim et al. 2022). To help with loss of contrast sensitivity, a 30% light reflectance value between floors, skirting boards, walls and furniture was suggested by previous research to be optimal for navigation in space and identification of objects (Bright et al. 2000).

The risk for falls can be compounded by changes in gait. Toes tend to touch the surface before the heel in dementia, which can lead to trips and falls. Loss of balance can also occur in dementia (often due to orthostatic hypotension), leading to falls.

Grip strength reduces with age and can predict dementia onset and affect activities of daily living (opening cans, taps, doors, etc.).

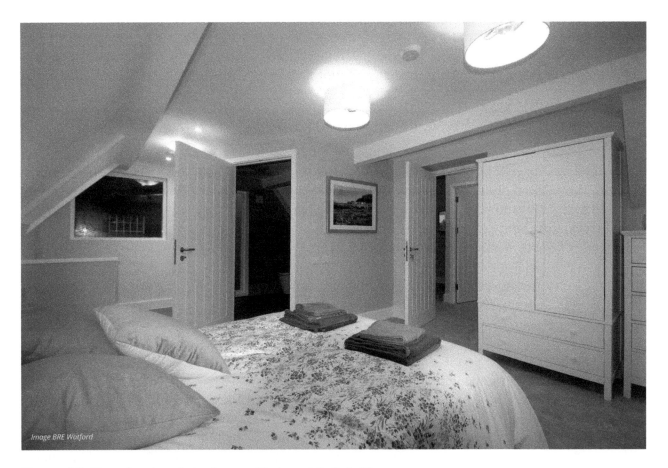

Figure 6.8 Completed main bedroom, Chris and Sally's House
Source: image BRE

Design Solutions to Mitigate Sensorimotor Changes in Dementia

Floors could have underfloor heating with slip-resistant, neutral-coloured fabrics, which are easy to clean, but can look and feel like carpet, with adequate contrast between skirting boards, walls and floor (30% difference in LRV).

Light bulbs are installed with double the intensity throughout the house. Windows need to be large to let in natural light. To further allow easy access and reduce injury, the path throughout the space needs to be clear; rugs, mats, thresholds and walls in traditional houses need to be removed or avoided to render an open plan kitchen/dining area/lounge.

A lift could be installed close to the entrance to allow easy access to the upstairs areas for later stages of dementia. Stairlifts for frailty are often not practical and may be hard to navigate in dementia.

To stimulate activity and independence as long as possible, stairs and bathrooms need to have grab rails to help independence and reduce falls.

All surfaces, cupboards and tables need to be rounded to remove the risk of injury in case of a loss of balance.

For grip strength loss, handles, taps and locks (using fingerprint ID) need to be easy to use.

To reduce noise disturbance, the washing machine should be situated in a separate utility store insulated to be soundproof. This could be adjacent to the ground floor bathroom for ease of plumbing installation.

Digital Technology to Mitigate Sensorimotor Changes in Dementia

In hospital settings, most falls occur around the bed and in the bathroom (Hignett, Sands, Fray et al. 2013; Hignett, Sands and Griffiths 2013). Sensors could be placed in the bathroom to alert third parties if someone spent longer than 30 minutes in this room, indicating a possible fall. An activated voiceover could ask people if they were okay and contact emergency services. The visible wet room is also downstairs, to be reached more easily.

Understanding Symptoms and Needs Associated With Behavioural and Psychiatric Symptoms in Dementia

Behavioural and psychiatric symptoms of dementia, including aggression, depression, apathy, agitation, drowsiness, sundowning, nightwandering, hallucinations and delusions, are difficult to deal with and are the most likely reasons for carers reaching burn-out and for patients requiring residential/nursing home care (see Chapter 4).

Many BPSD are probably related to anxiety and disorientation and/or frustration in the inability to communicate, plan or remember effectively. Issues with auditory and visual perception and a lack of reality testing can lead to hallucinations, agitation and delusions but can be reduced through design features. Especially in the common but often not diagnosed Lewy body dementia, the following perceptual issues can be prominent:

- Shiny floors can be perceived as 'wet' and need to be matt and non-slip;
- Dark rugs and mats can be perceived as holes in the floor;
- Extreme contrast in flooring materials can be perceived as having different heights and lead to trips and falls;
- Noise of the washing machine can be misinterpreted, and lead to agitation, fear and restlessness;
- Many older people's homes are stuffy, badly ventilated and overheated. This can affect alertness and induce drowsiness. In addition, poor ventilation can increase eye discomfort and dryness, further reducing vision and wellbeing;

- Patterns in curtains/on floors can be perceived as moving ('snakes') and create anxiety;
- People do not recognise themselves in the mirror, leading to anxiety.

Design Solutions to Mitigate Behavioural and Psychiatric Symptoms in Dementia

Calming colours developed via mood boards include greens (lounge, kitchen), purples (bedroom) and blues (dayroom), while the kitchen wall has an uplifting colour, yellow. Large windows with low windowsills were installed for optimal natural light to aid circadian rhythm. These windows should ideally provide views to green, which have been found to lift mood and reduce stress, as does access to safe gardens outside (but beware of slippery or uneven garden paths or ponds). Exposure to daylight with regular walks *outside* in green areas is important for circadian rhythm maintenance, sleep, mood and well-being and should be encouraged by doors leading to outside areas with no thresholds or steps.

Gardening has shown benefits in dementia. Raised beds in limited outside space or plant boxes inside or outside on balconies could be installed for people to garden and tend to vegetables and flowers for sensory stimulation, activity and reminiscence.

Digital Technology to Reduce and Mitigate Behavioural and Psychiatric Symptoms in Dementia

Insulation and underfloor heating could be installed with sun-energy panels on the roof for efficient heating and provision of energy.

An automated ventilation system could be installed with sensors to allow circulation of air through automatically opening and closing windows (using buoyancy driven natural ventilation).

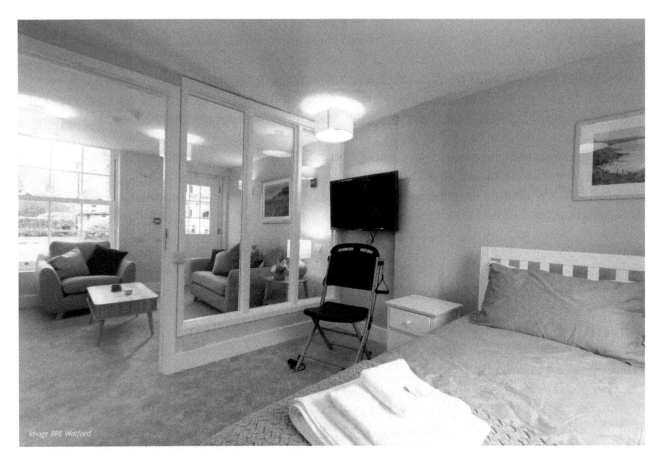

Figure 6.9 Completed dayroom view to lounge in Chris and Sally's House showing Acti-chair
Source: image BRE

To reduce overheating in the summer, solar analysis can be conducted using computer modelling and used to design automated external solar shading to protect the rooms inside from direct sunshine and glare.

Phone or other GPS-based locators, such as My-SOS tracker (https://peoplesafe.co.uk/products/mysos/) can allow carers to locate people with dementia without hindering them in their freedom to wander. Some bus and train companies recognise bracelets with programmed chips to help bring people to their destination. Shopping trips to the local market and trips to activity centres with dementia groups can also be highly beneficial. However, research has shown that older people spend most of their time at home, being sedentary.

For this purpose, the Acti-chair was developed (Ma et al. 2018) people with dementia. The Acti-chair has resistance bands with electronic feedback to allow people to do resistance band exercises safely at home. These exercises were shown to improve memory in middle-aged and older people with and without dementia and can also improve leg strength, which helps reduce falls and increases mobility. (Elliott-King et al. 2019; Hogervorst et al. 2012) Feedback on the correct use of the resistance bands (speed, orientation, strength) is given through colour changing of the handlebars of the bands. People can use the TV screen to communicate with friends and family using adapted Skype and Facetime and engage in the evidence-based cognitive stimulation therapy programme (Spector et al. 2003).

Sensors in the floors and bed and on doors linked to timers could identify night wandering and sundowning. If people get up and try to leave the house at night, a gentle voice could remind them of the time and ask them to get back to bed.

The Later Stages of Dementia, Design Solutions and Feedback by Patient and Public Involvement

As dementia progresses, basic activities of life cannot be carried out independently any longer, and people need constant care.

A overhead tracking hoist to allow access to the wet room upstairs was considered a good but expensive feature to aid washing and toileting by a non-trained and often older carer. A mobile (floor-based) hoist could offer a cheaper option, to be made available if needed.

A lift for access to the second floor was considered highly desirable in PPI and allowed easy access to the upstairs. Cheaper versions should be explored, as this desirable feature could be very expensive to install (in excess of £25,000).

We had initially included a small kitchenette upstairs to prepare small meals/drinks and support an overnight carer, but this feature was considered superfluous by some individuals, with a sense to keep the house as 'normal' as possible. The lift allowed easy transfer of meals, rendering the kitchenette upstairs obsolete.

In the later stages of dementia, most people will be bedridden and no longer mobile. Separate rooms for carer and patient were considered desirable for better sleep and rest.

A dayroom could be installed downstairs for people to take a nap. The opaque and decorated glass wall to the lounge still allows visual contact with carers. However, this feature was not considered desirable by several of the patients, carers and service provider contributors who evaluated the house. Daytime naps can affect nighttime sleep and should perhaps be avoided, but many older people do report daytime napping needs. Personalisation here is key; a separate room off the lounge should be provided which could be used as a dining area, study, library, storage or for a daybed/guest bed or a quiet room.

In conclusion, Chris and Sally's House meets the needs for symptoms seen in people with moderate dementia and also gave guidance for people with mild (kitchen) and severe stages (upstairs). In the next part of the chapter we present the evidence base for the key design features advised, design rationale and how these integrate with characteristics of people with dementia.

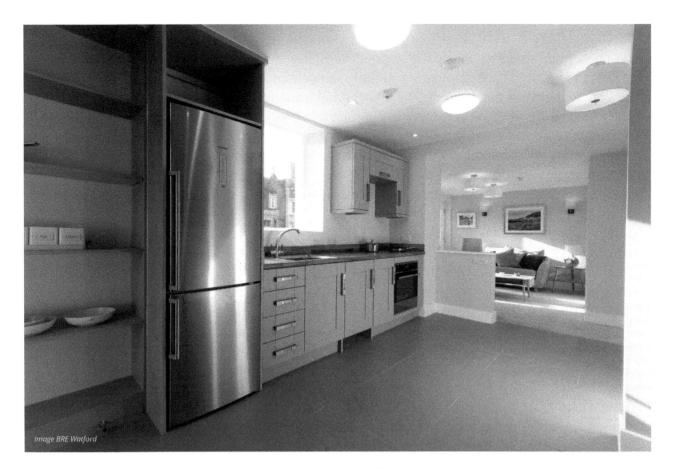

Figure 6.10 Completed kitchen/dining, Chris and Sally's House
Source: image BRE

Evidence Base – Review

The design features of Chris and Sally's House have been independently reviewed, room by room. References for each design feature demonstrate a robust evidence base for the design rationale. The design evolution and development of Chris and Sally's House are described in full in Chapter 7.

Kitchen/Dining

Key Design Features

- Open plan arrangement
- Legibility between rooms
- Easy access to w.c. and shower room with good visibility for orientation
- Lift access to first floor to accommodate wheelchair plus carer
- Minimising doors
- Walkability as well as wheelchair access
- Kitchen with glass doors and drawers for visibility of kitchen equipment
- High- and low-level work surfaces
- Rounded corners to minimise risks from falls
- View to green – good aspect
- Good natural and artificial light
- Tonal contrast between floor, walls, door, kitchen unit fronts and worktops based on approximately 30% difference in light reflectance values
- Personalisation and memories to make it feel like a home

Design Rationale

- The open plan arrangement provides good visibility between the kitchen/dining and living areas of the house. This helps Chris and Sally to negotiate the spaces and facilitates visual and oral contact between them, producing a social environment. The design objective of legibility is satisfied by this open arrangement in contrast to a more conventional approach of a corridor with multiple doors of similar appearance. People living with dementia can be confused by too many choices, so keeping choices simple and obvious is recommended
- For similar reasons, doors have been minimised
- The space is designed to accommodate wheelchair access but also walkability. Chris and Sally can move through their house, holding onto furniture, worktops and so on. Possible additional handles strategically positioned to aid workability
- The worktops and table have rounded corners to minimise risk of harm through falls
- A lift was designed in, potentially as a future provision. The lift is big enough to take a person in a wheelchair as well as a carer on the basis that people living with dementia may not be happy on their own
- There is easy access to the w.c. and shower room with a door wide enough to take a wheelchair. There is good visibility from the kitchen/diner as well as the lounge
- Visibility of the w.c. in particular is seen as providing reassurance and reducing problems of incontinence
- A new window has been introduced to the south elevation to achieve a view to green. Research by Edinburgh University has indicated that a view to green has a beneficial effects in reducing stress
- The increase in natural light is also beneficial for Chris and Sally, as the ageing eye deteriorates
- Good artificial light has also been provided to approximately twice normal, and a mix of ambience, feature and task lighting has been designed in to help visibility of the space and objects in it. All light fittings are fitted with LED light sources for increased visibility and reduced electricity consumption
- The kitchen layout has been designed within the restricted space available to provide a compact easily useable ergonomic modern kitchen; a lower-level worktop provides a food prep area for someone sitting in a wheelchair
- The kitchen units have glass-fronted doors and drawers to make it easier to find things. Cooker, fridge and dishwasher have stainless steel fronts, contrasting with the kitchen units to self-identify their function, as opposed to an integrated design where they appear as kitchen units
- Light-reflectance values have been calculated to provide approximately 30% difference in value between adjoining surfaces – floors, walls, doors, kitchen fronts and surfaces. These calculations have included furniture and timber elements such as furniture legs and the tonal contrasts produced by skirtings to enable Chris and Sally to interpret space and form within their house and to negotiate their space in comfort and security. The following section provides the literature references for the evidence base used in the design features of the Chris and Sally House.

Evidence Base

Open plan arrangement:

- Open plan spaces support a more homely environment (Chaudhury and Cooke 2014; Nordin et al. 2015)

  Legibility between rooms:

- Legibility can be enhanced through the use of visual contrast (Day et al. 2000)
- Clear sight lines, even lighting, matt finishes and lack of clutter aid legibility (Waller and Masterson 2015)

- Legibility can be supported through furniture, fixtures and fittings and logical room layouts (Charras et al. 2016; Marquardt and Schmieg 2009)
- Using colour as a cue significantly improves reaction time and day to day functioning for Alzheimer's sufferers (Bosch et al. 2012)
- Colour can influence how a space performs and is experienced, creating an illusion of space and assisting with wayfinding (Dalke 2008)
- Easy access to w.c. and shower room with good visibility for orientation:

  - Visibility of toilets is linked to increased use (Day et al. 2000; Fleming et al. 2014; Hyde 1989; Marquardt et al. 2014; Namazi and Johnson 1991; Torrington 2009; van Hoof et al. 2013)
  - Not being able to locate the toilet can be distressing and may lead to incontinence (Caspi 2014).

Lift access to first floor, to accommodate wheelchair plus carer:

- Issues with mobility may prevent older people from using rooms on the first floor (Renaut et al. 2014)
- Stairs are hazardous for some people with dementia (Gross et al. 2015).

Minimising doors:

- Open plan spaces support a more homely environment (Chaudhury and Cooke 2014; Nordin et al. 2015)
- Locked doors can create frustration (Mooney and Nicell 1992).

Walkability as well as wheelchair access:

- Room layout can be used to support 'furniture walking' (McMurdo 2001)
- A good floor space for older people, particularly those with dementia, allows and encourages activity, involvement, comfort and ultimately identity in a positive way. People with dementia need to feel that every detail is designed to generate well-being. The floor is key to this environment (Dalke et al. 2004).

Kitchen with glass doors and drawers for visibility of kitchen equipment:

- Lack of visibility of items in the kitchen may prevent people with dementia from accessing them (Wherton and Monk 2010)
- Kitchen cupboards with clear panels may support cooking activities by ensuring that relevant equipment is easily visible and therefore accessible (Grey et al. 2015).

High- and low-level work surfaces:

- Older adults may get tired more easily from standing and may find it useful to have a lower work surface at which they can sit (Maguire et al. 2014)
- Worktops with different heights may be useful for different tasks (Steinfeld et al. 1979).

Rounded corners to minimise risks from falls:

- Rounded corners on kitchen units are recommended (Marsden et al. 2001)
- Rounded corners and smooth edges on furniture are recommended (Pinto et al. 2000)
- Ergonomics and functionality cannot be separated from emotional appeal. Natural materials and realistic textured woods with delicate contrasts offer authentic feelings of comfort and wellbeing (Dalke et al. 2004).

View to green – good aspect:

- Visual access to a garden may reduce agitation (Edwards et al. 2013)
- Visual access to a garden may stimulate conversation and social interaction (Hernandez 2008)
- Visual access to a garden can support health and wellbeing (Hartig et al. 1991; Leather et al. 1998)
- Visual access to the outdoors helps to maintain circadian rhythms, stimulate serotonin production, lift mood and increase alertness (Digby and Bloomer 2014)
- Views of nature and positive distractions improve patient comfort.

Good natural and artificial light:

- Even lighting aids visibility and mobility (Torrington and Tregenza 2007)
- High lighting levels are recommended for kitchens (Marsden et al. 2001)
- Increased lighting can contribute to improved nutritional intake (McDaniel et al. 2001).

Tonal contrast between floor, walls, door, kitchen unit fronts and worktops based on approximately 30% difference in light reflectance values

- Contrast sensitivity is reduced in people with dementia (Lakshminarayanan et al. 1996)
- Reduced contrast sensitivity is linked to fall risk (Lord 2006)
- Contrasting colours can be used to support orientation and accessibility (Andersson et al. 2011; Caspi 2014)
- Using colour as a cue significantly improves reaction time and day-to-day functioning for Alzheimer's sufferers (Bosch et al. 2012)
- Equality Act guidelines on colour and contrast to differentiate between critical surfaces (wall and floor, walls and doors) (Bright et al. 2000)
- A colour scheme can add interest and variety to the patient environment – the absence of variety can cause sensory deprivation. Patients in care homes need variety in colour, lighting and artwork for their well-being (Mahnke and Mahnke 1987)
- Solid-coloured flooring has less of an ability to hide dirt, stains and dents over time. Debris and dust are two of the worst culprits; however, flecks and wood grains in the flooring pattern are more forgiving. Maintenance draws advantages from flecked flooring because it disguises bits of debris that can accumulate between cleanings. It also decreases the length of time before a floor needs to be replaced. (Dalke et al. 2004).
- Very white, shiny or dark flooring should be avoided because the reflected light can disturb or dazzle patients with Alzheimer's according to the stage of their condition (Goodman and Watson 2010).

Personalisation and memories to make it feel like a home:

- Personalisation is a key component of creating a suitable environment for people with dementia (Chaudhury and Cooke 2014; Grey et al. 2015)
- Personalisation supports the creation of a homely environment (Day et al. 2000; Falk et al. 2009)
- Personalisation can support feelings of control and autonomy (Schwarz et al. 2004)
- Personalisation can be used to support links with the past (Passini et al. 2000)
- Personalised environments can support continuation of self and normality (Edvardsson et al. 2010; Grey et al. 2015).

Lounge

Key Design Features

Walkability

- View to green
- Visibility to the w.c.
- Open plan with visibility to kitchen and entrances
- Tonal contrast between walls, floor and furniture
- Curtains with highlighted edge for ease of use
- High level of ambient and task lighting
- Accessible and visible storage
- Rounded corners to reduce risk of falls

Design Rationale

- The lounge area is continuous with the kitchen/living room in an open plan arrangement enabling Chris and Sally to negotiate their home. The spatial interconnectivity generates a high level of legibility within the dwelling
- Within the lounge area, the themes of walkability, rounded corners and visible accessible storage are continued from the kitchen
- There is a transition in floor finish between the kitchen and lounge from floor tile to carpet. LRVs have been calculated to achieve a close LRV between the two surfaces to avoid a visual trip
- Tonal contrasts have also been achieved between floors, walls and furniture of approximately 30% LRV to enhance spatial perception
- Fabrics have been selected to comply with these design principles, including contrasting leading edges on curtains and contrasting arms on seating
- Curtains draw back, clearing window opening to allow as much natural light as possible into the room
- A high level of ambient and task lighting has been achieved through both natural and artificial lighting
- Paint colours have been selected from AzkoNobel's range of dementia-inclusive colours, producing a pastel colour scheme
- The windows and doors are glazed to maximise view to green and sunlight from the south elevation, maximising exposure to UV radiation and promoting vitamin D production in the skin. The lounge door is the garden door, giving level access to the garden. LRVs at thresholds are co-ordinated to avoid a visual trip hazard
- The doorway to the w.c. has been carefully situated to enable views to the w.c. when open. This is considered an aim to comfort and security and to reducing problems of incontinence
- The lounge area is connected to the day room, with a glazed screen to enable a visual connection.

Evidence Base

Walkability:

- Room layout can be used to support 'furniture walking' (McMurdo 2001)
- A good floor space for older people, particularly those with dementia, allows and encourages activity, involvement, comfort and ultimately identity in a positive way. People with dementia need to feel that every detail is designed to generate well-being. The floor is key to this environment (Dalke et al. 2004).

View to green:

- Visual access to a garden may reduce agitation (Edwards et al. 2013)
- Visual access to a garden may stimulate conversation and social interaction (Hernandez 2008)
- Visual access to a garden can support health and wellbeing (Hartig et al. 1991; Leather et al. 1998)
- Visual access to the outdoors helps to maintain circadian rhythms, stimulate serotonin production, lift mood and increase alertness (Digby and Bloomer 2014)
- Views of nature and positive distractions improve patient comfort (Ulrich et al. 2008).

Visibility to the w.c.:

- Visibility of toilets is linked to increased use (Day et al. 2000; Fleming et al. 2014; Gross et al. 2015; Hyde 1989; Marquardt et al. 2014; Namazi and Johnson 1991; Torrington 2009; van Hoof et al. 2013)
- Not being able to locate the toilet can be distressing and may lead to incontinence (Caspi 2014).

Open plan with visibility to kitchen and entrances:

- Open plan spaces support a more homely environment (Chaudhury and Cooke 2014; Nordin et al. 2015)
- Visual access is important (Fleming et al. 2008; Fleming et al. 2014; Fleming and Purandare 2010; Marquardt et al. 2014; Marquardt and Schmieg 2009)
- Visual access to important spaces can support wayfinding and can increase use of these spaces (Passini et al. 2000)
- Using colour as a cue significantly improves reaction time and day to day functioning for Alzheimer's sufferers (Bosch et al. 2012).

Tonal contrast between walls, floor and furniture:

- Contrast sensitivity is reduced in people with dementia (Lakshminarayanan et al. 1996)
- Reduced contrast sensitivity is linked to fall risk (Lord 2006)
- Contrasting colours can be used to support orientation and accessibility (Andersson et al. 2011; Caspi 2014)
- A colour scheme can add interest and variety to the patient environment – the absence of variety can cause sensory deprivation. Patients in care homes need variety in colour, lighting and artwork for their well-being (Mahnke and Mahnke 1987)
- Using colour as a cue significantly improves reaction time and day-to-day functioning for Alzheimer's sufferers (Bosch et al. 2012)
- Insomnia is one of the most frequent psycho-behavioural problems to affect Alzheimer's patients, often caused by the inversion of the wake/sleep pattern called the circadian rhythm. Preference should therefore be given to light, clear flooring colours that offer better light reflective properties. (Bright et al. 2000)
- Colour can influence how a space performs and is experienced, creating an illusion of space and assisting with wayfinding (Dalke 2004).

Curtains with highlighted edge for ease of use:

- Contrasting colours can be used to support orientation and accessibility (Andersson et al. 2011; Caspi 2014).

High level of ambient and task lighting:

- High levels of lighting can assist with task visibility (Falk et al. 2009; Grey et al. 2015).

Accessible and visible storage:

- Open shelves increase visibility (Grey et al. 2015)
- Adequate storage space is important (Marsden et al. 2001).

Rounded corners to reduce risk of falls:

- Rounded corners and smooth edges on furniture are recommended (Pinto et al. 2000)
- Ergonomics and functionality cannot be separated from emotional appeal. Natural materials and realistic textured woods with delicate contrasts offer authentic feelings of comfort and wellbeing (Dalke et al. 2004).

Day Room

Key Design Features

- Alternative uses: dining room, quiet room or day room for end-of-life care
- View to green with blackout blinds
- Hoist to shower room
- Pocket door between day room and shower room for flexibility between alternative uses
- Multiple wheelchair charging positions

Design Rationale

The day room is planned as a flexible space which can be used for:
- Dining room
- Quiet room
- Hobby room
- End-of-life care
- It has a glazed screen to the living room so that visual contact can be maintained compatible with these uses
- Like the other rooms, it has an external window for a view to green. The window is fitted with a blackout blind to assist daytime sleeping and control over natural light conditions
- Curtains draw back, clearing window opening to allow as much natural light as possible into the room
- It has a wheelchair position and charging point to assist carers in end-of-life care mode
- A pocket door to the adjoining shower room can be kept closed during its normal function and is painted to match the wall colour to be virtually invisible in dining room, quiet room or hobby room mode. This avoids confusion of doors and lack of privacy in the bathroom in these uses
- In end-of-life care or case of serious illness when one of the occupants maybe confined to bed, the pocket door can be kept in the open position, enabling convenient access to the shower room
- The ceiling is pre-adapted to take a hoist system so that the occupant can be managed from the bed to the w.c. and shower
- The w.c. is visible from the bed position
- The colour scheme reflects the principle of achieving 30% LRV difference between walls, floors and furnishing.

Evidence Base

Alternative uses: dining room, quiet room or day room for end-of-life care:

- Flexible spaces are useful for adapting to changing needs (Grey et al. 2015; Maguire et al. 2014; Pynoos et al. 1989; Simmons 2011)
- Day rooms should reflect their purpose and should have warm welcoming colours to encourage use (Goodman and Watson 2010).

View to green with blackout blinds:

- Visual access to a garden may reduce agitation (Edwards et al. 2013)
- Visual access to a garden may stimulate conversation and social interaction (Hernandez 2008)
- Visual access to a garden can support health and wellbeing (Hartig et al. 1991; Leather et al. 1998)
- Visual access to the outdoors helps to maintain circadian rhythms, stimulate serotonin production, lift mood and increase alertness (Digby and Bloomer 2014)
- Views of nature and positive distractions improve patient comfort (Ulrich et al. 2008).

Hoist to shower room:

- Changes in mobility occur as dementia progresses (World Health Organisation 2012)
- Hoists may be required as needs change (Grey et al. 2015).

Pocket door between day room and shower room for flexibility between alternative uses:

- Flexible spaces are useful for adapting to changing needs (Grey et al. 2015; Maguire et al. 2014; Pynoos et al. 1989; Simmons 2011).

Multiple wheelchair charging positions:

- Flexible spaces are useful for adapting to changing needs (Grey et al. 2015; Maguire et al. 2014; Pynoos et al. 1989; Simmons 2011)
- Changes in mobility occur as dementia progresses (World Health Organisation 2012).

Shower Room

Key Design Features

- Wheelchair accessible
- Wet area for shower
- Non-slip floor
- Hoist to shower and toilet
- Tonal contrasts between floor, walls, grabrails, seat
- Storage with washer/drier
- Pocket door to the dining/day room
- Shower curtains with magnetic closing
- Retractable seat in shower enclosure.

Design Rationale

- The room is designed as a fully wheelchair-accessible room fully equipped with grab rails and other aids in compliance with Part M4(3) of the Building Regulations. (The kitchen units have a fixed worktop at the usual height rather than a rise and fall worktop, to accommodate appliances but also to fulfil the brief for a house anyone would be happy to live in (if needed, a rise and fall worktop could be retrofitted)

- The store/airing cupboard accommodates the washing machine as well as shelving for linen. The washing machine is situated outside of the kitchen to reduce noise disturbance to Chris and Sally, and easy access to clean linen is an advantage in the context of assisted bathing
- The room is a wet room – all surfaces are washable for easy cleaning
- The ceiling is pre-fitted with supports for future provision of a hoist from the day room to aid assisted bathing
- The pocket door is lockable from the inside to ensure privacy
- The window is openable manually, and the room is fitted with an extract fan
- Tiling colours are carefully selected to ensure LRV contrasts between floor and walls. A darker band provides sufficient contrast with the white grab rails (Stirling recommends 45–55% difference)
- The handwash basin has rounded edges to minimise the risks of falls and has two cross-head taps marked H&C for familiarity and ease of use for someone living with dementia
- The colour of the toilet seat will be of an LRV to provide 30% contrast with floor and walls.

Upstairs Shower Room

- The upstairs shower room is designed for full wheelchair accessibility per Building Regs Part M
- It is fully equipped with necessary grab handles, drop down seat and so on in accordance with recommendations
- Floor and wall tiles have been selected to achieve LRVs with tonal contrast between floors, walls, sanitary ware and bathroom aids
- The w.c. is visible from the bed position
- A ceiling-mounted hoist system enables Chris or Sally to be easily moved from bed to shower/w.c. to facilitate assisted bathing.

Evidence Base

Wheelchair accessible:

- Flexible spaces are useful for adapting to changing needs (Grey et al. 2015; Maguire et al. 2014; Pynoos et al. 1989; Simmons 2011)
- Changes in mobility occur as dementia progresses (World Health Organisation 2012).

Wet area for shower:

- Wet rooms avoid the need to cross a threshold or step into a shower tray (Grey et al. 2015)
- Wet areas allow more space and freedom of movement for carers (Van Hoof and Kort 2009)
- Step-in shower trays are considered hazardous (Lowery et al. 2000).

Non-slip floor:

- Non-slip flooring is recommended for people with dementia (Grey et al. 2015; Wong et al. 2014)
- Urinary and faecal incontinence are a feature of Alzheimer's disease, so it is essential to choose flooring that is practical and easy to maintain, particularly in patient rooms and bathrooms (Goodman and Watson 2010).

Hoist to shower and toilet:

- Changes in mobility occur as dementia progresses (World Health Organisation 2012)
- Hoists may be required as needs change (Grey et al. 2015).

Tonal contrasts between floor, walls, grabrails, seat:

- Contrast sensitivity is reduced in people with dementia (Lakshminarayanan et al. 1996)
- Reduced contrast sensitivity is linked to fall risk (Lord 2006)
- Contrasting colours can be used to support orientation and accessibility (Andersson et al. 2011; Caspi 2014)
- Equality Act guidelines on colour and contrast to differentiate between critical surfaces (wall and floor, walls and doors) (Bright et al. 2000).

Wash-down surfaces for ease of cleaning:

- Ease of cleaning is an important design consideration (Boger et al. 2013)
- Storage with washer/drier:

  - Reduced noise in dining areas contributes to improved nutritional intake (Thomas and Smith 2009)
  - High noise levels can be problematic for people with dementia (Van Hoof and Kort 2009; Wong et al. 2014).

Pocket door to the dining/day room:

- Visibility of toilets is linked to increased use (Day et al. 2000; Fleming et al. 2014; Gross et al. 2004; Hyde 1989; Marquardt et al. 2014; Namazi and Johnson 1991; Torrington 2009; van Hoof et al. 2013)
- Not being able to locate the toilet can be distressing and may lead to incontinence (Caspi 2014)
- Visual access is important (Fleming et al. 2008, 2014; Fleming and Purandare 2010; Marquardt et al. 2014; Marquardt and Schmieg 2009)
- Visual access to important spaces can support wayfinding and can increase use of these spaces (Passini et al. 2000).

Shower curtains with magnetic closing:

- Used previously in dwellings for people with dementia (van Hoof et al. 2013).

Retractable seat in shower enclosure:

- Flexible spaces are useful for adapting to changing needs (Grey et al. 2015; Maguire et al. 2014; Pynoos et al. 1989; Simmons 2011)
- Shower seat is one example of an adaptation that can be made to meet changing needs (Grey et al. 2015).

Main Bedroom

Key Design Features

- Fully wheelchair accessible
- View to green

- Hoist to shower room
- Curtains and blackout blinds
- Wheelchair charging position
- Ambient and task lighting
- Adjoining kitchenette area – for preparation of light meals and drinks and storage of medication.

Design Rationale

- The main bedroom is designed to full wheelchair standards per Building Reg Part M4(3), allowing full accessibility around the bed and other furniture
- There is a wheelchair charging point adjacent to the bed to allow a wheelchair to be charged in a convenient position
- A hoist runs across the ceiling to facilitate moving Chris or Sally from the bed to the shower or w.c.
- The room has a view to green from the bed position
- Curtains draw back, clearing window opening to allow as much natural light as possible into the room
- The w.c. is visible from the bed when the door is open for comfort and security and to reduce incontinence at nighttime
- Adjoining the bedroom is a small kitchenette or tea room area. This area may be used for the preparation of drinks and light meals if Chris or Sally were confined to bed. It could also function for the storage and preparation of medication
- There is good provision for both ambient and task lighting to twice normal levels. The room is naturally lit from each side
- Windows are provided with black-out blinds to help sleep patterns
- LRVs have been calculated for walls and floor furniture/furnishings to achieve a 30-point approximate difference.

Evidence Base

Fully wheelchair accessible:

- Flexible spaces are useful for adapting to changing needs (Grey et al. 2015; Maguire et al. 2014; Pynoos et al. 1989; Simmons 2011)
- Changes in mobility occur as dementia progresses (World Health Organisation 2012).

View to green:

- Visual access to a garden may reduce agitation (Edwards et al. 2013)
- Visual access to a garden may stimulate conversation and social interaction (Hernandez 2008)
- Visual access to a garden can support health and wellbeing (Hartig et al. 1991; Leather et al. 1998)
- Visual access to the outdoors helps to maintain circadian rhythms, stimulate serotonin production, lift mood and increase alertness (Digby and Bloomer 2014)
- Views of nature and positive distractions improve patient comfort (Ulrich et al. 2008).

Hoist to shower room:

- Changes in mobility occur as dementia progresses (World Health Organisation 2012)
- Hoists may be required as needs change (Grey et al. 2015).

Curtains and blackout blinds:

- Reduced exposure to light at nighttime promotes melatonin production (Nioi et al. 2017)
- Blackout blinds can be used to reduce light exposure (Nioi et al. 2017).

Wheelchair charging position:

- Flexible spaces are useful for adapting to changing needs (Grey et al. 2015; Maguire et al. 2014; Pynoos et al. 1989; Simmons 2011)
- Changes in mobility occur as dementia progresses (World Health Organisation 2012).

Ambient and task lighting:

- High levels of lighting can assist with task visibility (Falk et al. 2009; Grey et al. 2015).

Adjoining kitchenette area – for preparation of light meals and drinks and storage of medication:

- Flexible spaces are useful for adapting to changing needs (Grey et al. 2015; Maguire et al. 2014; Pynoos et al. 1989; Simmons 2011).

Bedroom 2

Key Design Features

- Respite for carer
- View to green
- Blackout blinds
- Tonal contrasts for easy visibility
- Wheelchair adaptable.

Design Rationale

- Bedroom 2 has been considered a respite room for the carer and has wheelchair adaptability
- An additional window has been installed to provide a view to green and good natural light
- Curtains draw back, clearing window opening to allow as much natural light as possible into the room
- Both the new window and the existing high-level windows are equipped with blackout blinds. The high-level blinds are remotely operated
- LRVs have been calculated for walls, floor coverings and furniture/furnishings
- Curtains have contrasting edges.

Evidence Base

Respite for carer:

- Carer strain is common amongst carers of people with dementia (Prince et al. 2015).

View to green:

- Visual access to a garden may reduce agitation (Edwards et al. 2013)
- Visual access to a garden may stimulate conversation and social interaction (Hernandez 2008)

- Visual access to a garden can support health and wellbeing (Hartig et al. 1991; Leather et al. 1998)
- Visual access to the outdoors helps to maintain circadian rhythms, stimulate serotonin production, lift mood and increase alertness (Digby and Bloomer 2014)
- Views of nature and positive distractions improve patient comfort (Ulrich et al. 2008).

Blackout blinds:

- Reduced exposure to light at nighttime promotes melatonin production (Nioi et al. 2017)
- Blackout blinds can be used to reduce light exposure (Nioi et al. 2017).

Tonal contrasts for easy visibility:

- Contrast sensitivity is reduced in people with dementia (Lakshminarayanan et al. 1996)
- Reduced contrast sensitivity is linked to fall risk (Lord 2006)
- Contrasting colours can be used to support orientation and accessibility (Andersson et al. 2011; Caspi 2014)
- Equality Act guidelines on colour and contrast to differentiate between critical surfaces (wall and floor, walls and doors) (Bright et al. 2000)
- Using colour as a cue significantly improves reaction time and day-to-day functioning for Alzheimer's sufferers (Bosch et al. 2012)
- Colour can influence how a space performs and is experienced, creating an illusion of space and assisting with wayfinding (Dalke et al. 2004).

Wheelchair adaptable:

- Flexible spaces are useful for adapting to changing needs (Grey et al. 2015; Maguire et al. 2014; Pynoos et al. 1989; Simmons 2011)
- Changes in mobility occur as dementia progresses (World Health Organisation 2012).

Key Design Feature:

Acoustic insulation installed on the building walls and roof, within the internal walls and between the floors.

Design Rationale:

To manage internal and external noise to create an optimal indoor acoustic environment.

Evidence base:

High noise levels can be problematic for people with dementia, causing poor sleep, agitation, confusion and fear (Garre- Van Hoof and Kort 2009; Wong et al. 2014).

Summary

The personas are useful for creating an environment that is suitable for people at different stages of dementia. The different stages (Alison to David on good/average/bad days) are useful to consider how the design of the house needs to be flexible and adaptable for future changes, such as mobility, with installation of a hoist, for instance.

Each persona shows how symptoms, care needs and design needs differ on good, average and bad days. We suggest that the use of evidence-based personas may provide a more accessible way to design for people living with dementia. The use of the personas throughout the design process can help to maintain the focus on the needs of people living with dementia during design discussions.

Acknowledgements

This work was supported by the Design Star Centre for Doctoral Training, Arts & Humanities Council (AHRC) www.designstar.org.uk/; Martin Habell, Adonika Brown, Rushcliffe Care Group, Halsall Lloyd Partnership, Building Research Establishment.

Graphic design by Charlotte Jais and Zuli Galindo Estupiñan.

References

Adlin, T., and Pruitt, J., 2010. *The Essential Persona Lifecycle – Your Guide to Building and Using Personas.* Morgan Kaugman: Burlington, MA.

Alzheimer's Society, www.alzheimers.org.uk/get-support/staying-independent/memory-aids-and-tools [Accessed 10 Jun 2023].

Andersson, M., Lindahl, G., and Malmqvist, I., 2011. Use and usability of assisted living facilities for the elderly: An observation study in Gothenburg Sweden. *Journal of Housing for the Elderly*, 25 (4), 380–400.

Boger, J., Craig, T., and Mihailidis, A., 2013. Examining the impact of familiarity on faucet usability for older adults with dementia. *BMC Geriatrics*, 13 (1), 63.

Bosch, B., Arenaza-Urquijo, E.M., Rami, L., Sala-Llonch, R., Junqué, C., Solé-Padullés, C., Peña-Gómez, C., Bargalló, N., Molinuevo, J.L., and Bartrés-Faz, D., 2012. Multiple DTI index analysis in normal aging, amnestic MCI and AD. Relationship with neuropsychological performance. *Neurobiology of Aging*, 33 (1), 61–74.

Bright, K., Cook, G., and Luck, R., 2000. Deafness, design and communication in the built environment. *COBRA 2000, 30 Aug–1 Sept 2000*. University of Greenwich: London.

Caspi E., 2014. Wayfinding difficulties among elders with dementia in an assisted living residence. *Dementia*, 13 (4), 429–450.

Charras, K., Eynard, C., and Viatour, G., 2016. Use of space and human rights: Planning dementia friendly settings. *Journal of Gerontological Social Work*, 59 (3), 181–204.

Chaudhury, H., and Cooke, H., 2014. Design matters in dementia care: The role of the physical environment in dementia care settings. M. Downs, and B. Bowers (Eds.), *Excellence in Dementia Care*. 2nd ed. Open University Press: UK, 144–158.

Chaudhury, H., Hung, L., and Badger, M., 2013. The role of physical environment in supporting person-centered dining in long-term care: A review of the literature. *American Journal of Alzheimer's Disease and Other Dementias*, 28 (5), 491–500.

Dalke, H., 2008. Sensory design & healthcare: Colour design and lighting. *Design, Health and Community Colloquium*. Newcastle-upon-Tyne, UK (Unpublished).

Dalke, H., Littlefair, P.J., Loe, D.L., and Camgöz, N., 2004. *Lighting and Colour for Hospital Design*. The Stationery Office: London.

Day, K., Carreon, D., and Stump, C., 2000. The therapeutic design of environments for people with dementia. A review of the empirical research. *The Gerontologist*, 40 (4), 397–416.

Digby, R., and Bloomer, M.J., 2014. People with dementia and the hospital environment: The view of patients and family carers. *International Journal of Older People Nursing*, 9 (1), 34–43.

Edvardsson, D., Fetherstonhaugh, D., and Nay, R., 2010. Promoting a continuation of self and normality: Person-centred care as described by people with dementia, their family members and aged care staff. *Journal of Clinical Nursing*, 19 (17–18), 2611–2618.

Edwards, C.A., McDonnell, C., and Merl, H., 2013. An evaluation of a therapeutic garden's influence on the quality of life of aged care residents with dementia. *Dementia* (London, England), 12 (4), 494–510.

Elliott-King, J., Peel, E., and Hogervorst, E., 2019. Acute cognitive effects of physical activity for people who have Dementia. *International Journal of Neurodegenerative Disorders*, 2, 9.

Falk, H., Wijk, H., and Persson, L.-O., 2009. The effects of refurbishment on residents' quality of life and wellbeing in two Swedish residential care 259 facilities. *Health & Place*, 15 (3), 687–694.

Fernando, E., Fraser, M., Hendriksen, J., Kim, C.H., and Muir-Hunter, S.W., 2017. Risk factors associated with falls in older adults with dementia: A systematic review. *Physiotherapy Canada. Physiotherapie Canada*, 69 (2), 161–170.

Fleming, R., Crookes, P.A., and Sum, S., 2008. A review of the empirical literature on the design of physical environments for people with dementia. https://api.semanticscholar.org/CorpusID:12700893 [Accessed 23 Jan 2022].

Fleming, R., Goodenough, B., Low, L.-F., Chenoweth, L., and Brodaty, H., 2014. *The Relationship Between the Quality of the Built Environment and the Quality of Life of People with Dementia in Residential Care*. Dementia: London, 1–8.

Fleming, R., and Purandare, N., 2010. Long-term care for people with dementia: Environmental design guidelines. *International Psychogeriatrics/IPA*, 22 (7), 1084–1096.

Garg, A., and Kapellusch, J.M., 2012. Long-term efficacy of an ergonomics program that includes patient-handling devices on reducing musculoskeletal injuries to nursing personnel. *Human Factors: The Journal of the Human Factors and Ergonomics Society*, 54 (4), 608–625.

Goodman, C., and Watson, L., 2010. Design guidance for people with dementia and for people with sight loss. *Thomas Pocklington Trust Research Findings Number*, 35 (Dec).

Grey, T., Pierce, M., Cahill, S., and Dyer, M., 2015. *Universal Design Guidelines Dementia Friendly Dwellings for People with Dementia, Their Families and Carers*. National Disability Authority: Dublin, Ireland.

Gross, J., Harmon, M.E., Myers, R.A., Evans, R.L., Kay, N.R., Rodriguez Charbonier, S., and Hadjri, K., Rooney, C., and Faith, V., 2015. Housing choices and care home design for people with dementia. *HERD: Health Environments Research & Design Journal*, 8 (3), 80–95.

Hartig, T., Mang, M., and Evans, G.W., 1991. Restorative effects of natural environment experiences. *Environment and Behavior*, 23 (1), 3–26.

Hernandez, R.O., 2008. Effects of therapeutic gardens in special care units for people with dementia. *Journal of Housing for the Elderly*, 21 (1–2), 117–152.

Hignett, S., Sands, G., Fray, M., Xanthopoulou, D., Healey, F., Griffiths, P., 2013. Which bed designs and patient characteristics increase bed rail use? *Age & Ageing*, 42, 531–535.

Hignett, S., Sands, G., and Griffiths, P., 2013. In-patient falls: What can we learn from incident reports? *Age & Ageing*, 42, 527–531.

Hogervorst, E., Clifford, A., Stock, J., Xin, X., and Bandelow S., 2012. Exercise to prevent cognitive decline and Alzheimer's disease. *JADPD* 2, e117.

Hyde, J., 1989. The physical environment and the care of Alzheimer's patients: An experiential survey of Massachusetts' Alzheimer's units. *The American Journal of Alzheimer's Care and Related Disorders & Research*, 4 (3), 36–44.

Jais, C., 2019. Designing for dementia: Personas to aid communication between professionals developing built environments for people with dementia. PhD. Loughborough University.

Javaid, F.Z., Brenton, J., Guo, L., and Cordeiro, M.F., 2016. Visual and ocular manifestations of Alzheimer's disease and their use as biomarkers for diagnosis and progression. *Frontiers in Neurology*, 7, 55.

Kim, H.J., Ryou, J.H., Choi, K.T., Kim, S.M., Kim, J.T., and Han, D.H., 2022. Deficits in color detection in patients with Alzheimer disease. *PloS One*, 17 (1), e0262226.

Lakshminarayanan, V., Lagrave, J., Kean, M.L., Dick, M., and Shankle, R., 1996. Vision in dementia: Contrast effects. *Neurological Research*, 18, 9–15.

Leather, P., Pyrgas, M., Beale, D., and Lawrence, C., 1998. Windows in the workplace sunlight, view, and occupational stress. *Environment and Behavior*, 30, 739–762. doi: 10.1177/001391659803000601.

Lord, S.R., 2006. Visual risk factors for falls in older people. *Age and Ageing*, 35 (Supplement 2), ii42–ii45. Loughborough University (2018): Loughborough, UK.

Lord, S.R., and Dayhew, J., 2001. Visual risk factors for falls in older people. *Journal of the American Geriatrics Society*, 49, 508–515.

Lowery, K., Buri, H., and Ballard, C.G., 2000. What is the prevalence of environmental hazards in the homes of dementia sufferers and are they associated with falls. *International Journal of Geriatric Psychiatry*, 15, 883–886.

Ma, J., Hogervorst, E., Magistro, D., Chouliaras, V., and Zecca, M., 2018. Development of sensorised resistance band for objective exercise measurement: Activities classification trial. *Annual International Conference of the IEEE Engineering in Medicine and Biology Society*, 3942–3945.

Maguire, M., Peace, S., Nicolle, C., Marshall, R., Sims, R., Percival, J., and Lawton, C., 2014. Kitchen living in later life: Exploring ergonomic problems, coping strategies and design solutions. *International Journal of Design*, 8 (1), 73–91.

Mahnke, F., and Mahnke, R., 1987. *Color and Light in Man-Made Environments*. New York: Van Nostrand Reinhold Co.

Marquardt, G., Bueter, K., and Motzek, T., 2014. Impact of the design of the built environment on people with dementia: An evidence-based review. *Health Environments Research & Design Journal*, 8, 127–157.

Marquardt, G., and Schmieg, P., 2009. Dementia-friendly architecture: Environments that facilitate wayfinding in nursing homes. *American Journal of Alzheimer's Disease and Other Dementias*, 24 (4), 333–340.

Marsden, J.P., Meehan, R.A., and Calkins, M.P., 2001. Therapeutic kitchens for residents with dementia. *American Journal of Alzheimer's Disease and Other Dementias*, 16 (5), 303–311.

McDaniel, J.H., Hunt, A., Hackes, B., and Pope, J.F., 2001. Impact of dining room environment on nutritional intake of Alzheimer's residents: A case study. *American Journal of Alzheimer's Disease and Other Dementias*, 16 (5): 297–302. http://doi.org/10.1177/153331750101600508. PMID: 11603166.

McMurdo, M.E., 2001. Falls prevention. *Age and Ageing*, 30, 4–6.

Mooney, P., and Nicell, P.L., 1992. The importance of exterior environment for Alzheimer residents: Effective care and risk management. *Healthcare Management Forum*, 5 (2), 23–29.

Namazi, K.H., and Johnson, B.D., 1991b. Physical environmental cues to reduce the problems of incontinence in Alzheimer's disease units. *The American Journal of Alzheimer's Care and Related Disorders & Research*, 6 (6), 22–28.

Nioi, A., Roe, J., Gow, A., McNair, D., and Aspinall, P., 2017. Evaluating blue spectral irradiance, illuminance level and the associations with health and wellbeing in older adults: OPENspace View project. L. Brotas, S. Roaf, and F. Nicol (Eds.), *Design to Thrive Proceedings Volume II: PLEA 2017*. NCEUB: Edinburgh.

Nordin, S., Elf, M., McKee, K., and Wijk, H., 2015. Assessing the physical environment of older people's residential care facilities: Development of the Swedish version of the Sheffield Care Environment Assessment Matrix (S-SCEAM). *BMC Geriatrics*, 15 (1), 3.

Passini, R., Pigot, H., Rainville, C., and Tetreault, M.-H., 2000. Wayfinding in a nursing home for advanced dementia of the Alzheimer's type. *Environment and Behavior*, 32 (5), 684–710.

Pinto, M., De Medici, S., Van Sant, C., Bianchi, A., Zlotnicki, A., Napoli, C., 2000. Technical note: Ergonomics, gerontechnology, and design for the home-environment. *Applied Ergonomics*, 31 (3), 317–322. ISSN 0003–6870.

Prince, M., Wimo, A., Guerchet, M., Ali, G.-C., Wu, Y.-T., Prina, M., . . . Xia, Z., 2015. *World Alzheimer Report 2015 the Global Impact of Dementia. An Analysis of Prevalence, Incidence, Cost and Trends*. Alzheimer's Disease International (ADI): London.

Pynoos, J., Cohen, E., and Lucas, C., 1989. Environmental coping strategies for Alzheimer's caregivers. *American Journal of Alzheimer's Care and Related Disorders & Research*, 4 (6), 4–8.

Renaut, S., Ogg, J., Petite, S., and Chamahian, A., 2014. Home environments and adaptations in the context of ageing. *Ageing and Society*, 1–26.

Schwarz, B., Chaudhury, H., and Tofle, R.B., 2004. Effect of design interventions on a dementia care setting. *American Journal of Alzheimer's Disease and Other Dementias*, 19 (3), 172–176.

Simmons, D., 2011. Sustainable living in long-term care: For people with dementia/Alzheimer's. *Educational Gerontology*, 37 (6), 526–547.

Spector, A., Thorgrimsen, L., Woods, B., Royan, L., Davies, S., Butterworth, M., and Orrell, M., 2003. Efficacy of an evidence-based cognitive stimulation therapy programme for people with dementia: Randomised controlled trial. *The British Journal of Psychiatry: The Journal of Mental Science*, 183, 248–254. https://doi.org/10.1192/bjp.183.3.248.

Steinfeld, E., Schroeder, S., and Bishop, M., 1979. *Accessible Buildings for People with Walking and Reaching Limitations*. U.S. Department of Housing and Urban Development, U.S. Government Printing Office: Washington, DC.

Thomas, D.W., and Smith, M., 2009. The effect of music on caloric consumption among nursing home residents with dementia of the Alzheimer's type. *Activities, Adaptation & Aging*, 33 (1), 1–16.

Torrington, J.M., 2009. The design of technology and environments to support enjoyable activity for people with dementia. *ALTER – European Journal of Disability Research/Revue Européenne de Recherche Sur Le Handicap*, 3 (2), 123–137.

Torrington, J.M., and Tregenza, P.R., 2007. Lighting for people with dementia. *Lighting Research and Technology*, 39 (1), 81–97. http://doi.org/10.1177/1365782806074484.

Ulrich, R.S., Zimring, C., Zhu, X., DuBose, J., Seo, H.-B., Choi, Y.-S., . . . Joseph, A., 2008. A review of the research literature on evidence based healthcare design. *Health Environments Research & Design Journal*, 1 (3), 61–125.

van Hoof, J., Blom, M.M., Post, H.N.A., and Bastein, W.L., 2013. Designing 278 a "think-along dwelling" for people with dementia: A co-creation project between health care and the building services sector. *Journal of Housing for the Elderly*, 27 (3), 299–332.

Van Hoof, J., and Kort, H.S.M., 2009. Supportive living environments: A first concept of a dwelling designed for older adults with dementia. *Dementia*, 8 (2), 293–316.

Waller, S., and Masterson, A., 2015. Designing dementia-friendly hospital environments. *Future Hospital Journal*, 2 (1), 63.

Wherton, J.P., and Monk, A.F., 2010. Problems people with dementia have with kitchen tasks: The challenge for pervasive computing. *Interacting with Computers*, 22 (4), 253–266.

WHO, 2012. *Dementia: A Public Health Priority.* World Health Organization: Geneva.

Wong, J.K.-W., Skitmore, M., Buys, L., and Wang, K., 2014. The effects of the indoor environment of residential care homes on dementia suffers in 280 Hong Kong: A critical incident technique approach. *Building and Environment*, 73, 32–39.

7 Case Study – Chris and Sally's House

Bill Halsall and Eef Hogervorst

Introduction

The evidence base outlined in Chapter 6 provided a secure, grounded foundation for the design of the Dementia Demonstration Project at the BRE's Innovation Park at Watford. In particular, Loughborough University's work on personas provided a very accessible way of designing for people living with dementia.

For over a year, the HLP design team worked with the academic team at Loughborough to develop theory into practice and to interpret the needs and requirements of the personas into the alternative design scenarios which are outlined in this chapter.

This process involved taking into account the various constraints imposed by the existing building as well as matters of the supply chain and availability of materials and products. The team were on a journey tackling the real life issues involved in converting an existing house into a dementia-resilient home.

Living With Dementia

Chris and Sally's House is a demonstration project which forms part of the Building Research Establishment's Innovation Park in Watford. Completed in 2018, the demonstration project represents the culmination of several years' research into design for dementia.

The Design for Dementia home is a design paradigm which responds to the growing issues of dementia in society. The concept has evolved into a more broadly based concept – a home for life.

Design for Dementia

The demonstration project is based on the design principles described in *Design for Dementia – A Guide* co-authored by Bill Halsall and Dr Robert G MacDonald of Liverpool John Moores University (2015). A distinguishing feature of this work has been the participatory nature of the approach, involving health professionals, academics and carers, along with people with dementia. Innovative participatory techniques have been evolved to generate a user-responsive design process and research outputs. A key element in the development of the design principles has been a participative design approach in partnership with the Liverpool-based Dementia Action Alliance and the Service Reference User's Forum. Bill Halsall with Dr Robert G MacDonald of Liverpool John Moores University developed participatory methods to facilitate direct co-design with people living with dementia. This process is referred to in Chapter 5. The main premise of *Design for Dementia – A Guide* is that approximately 70% of people living with dementia live in their own homes and use the same facilities and centres as everybody else. Design for dementia can help people living in their own homes to sustain their capacity for longer and maintain their quality of life as members of the community. This principle extends to the design of the public realm and to publicly accessible buildings as well as the domestic environment. Responding to this issue

DOI: 10.1201/9781003306054-7

SITE LOCATION - AERIAL

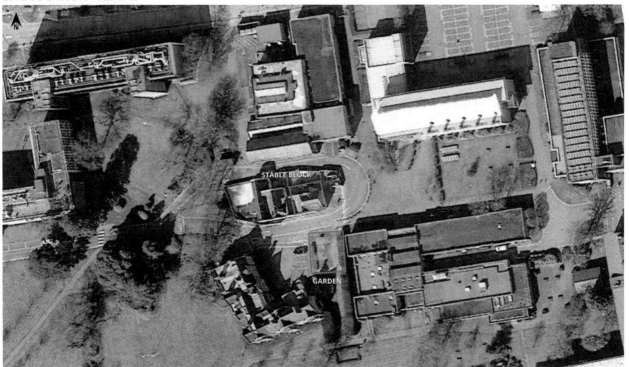

Image HLP

Figure 7.1 Site location of Chris and Sally's House – demonstration project BRE

as designers, we should envisage a future where housing, neighbourhoods, local facilities and centres must all respond to the needs and aspirations of those living with dementia and to enable them as far as possible to live well with dementia.

The Demonstration Project

Chris and Sally's House demonstrates how a typical two-up two-down cottage could be converted and adapted to deliver the key objectives of helping people to age in place, sustaining their capacity and independence for longer through design in accordance with the principles described in *Design for Dementia*. The demonstration project has been delivered through a partnership including the BRE, HLP and Loughborough University, who have provided much of the research and evidence base which underpins the project. Many other stakeholders, suppliers and researchers have become involved in the venture.

It is a logical development of the Design for Dementia Bungalow design exercise described in Chapter 5. In the case of Chris and Sally's House, the opportunity was to carry out a full-scale working demonstration project as a conversion project. In this case it demonstrates how an existing building could be converted into a dementia-friendly dwelling. In contrast to the Design for Dementia Bungalow, the house conversion project introduces additional building-specific constraints. However, the advantage of a conversion project is that it may be more representative of the real situation of many people in having to adapt their home, now or in the future, to cater for the experience of living with dementia.

Chris and Sally are personas developed by Loughborough University based on their research into the experience of dementia and the support systems which can aid people living with dementia. The house has been designed through intense attention to detail covering every aspect of the needs of people living with dementia to respond to the needs and aspirations of Chris and Sally.

THE STABLE BLOCK

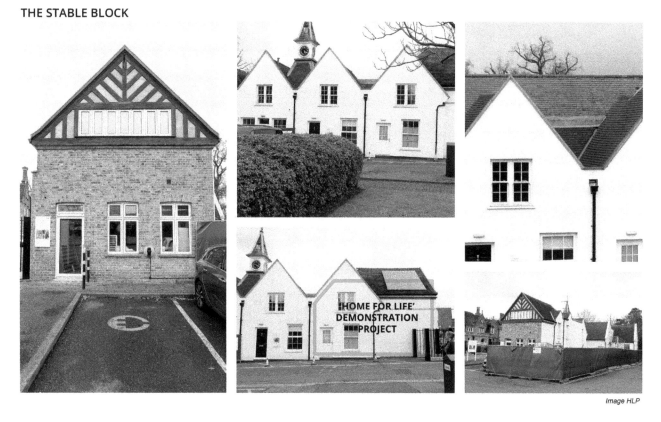

Image HLP

Figure 7.2 The stable block, Chris and Sally's House – demonstration project BRE

The Design for Dementia Home is a first step. Taking the simplest archetype and applying Design for Dementia principles, the project explores the issues and proposes design solutions which may then be applied to a wider range of archetypes, including existing dwellings and refurbishment projects. The lessons learnt can be more widely applied in a range of different contexts.

The Design for Dementia Home is not just designed for dementia. It envisages scenarios which cater for a range of abilities and disabilities and builds on well-established design standards, including Lifetime Homes and Secured by Design.

In this respect the design philosophy is 'long life, loose fit' – a comfortable aspirational home and a good place to live for anyone, but with dementia needs considered in every detail.

Importantly, the Design for Dementia Home comes with a Design for Dementia Garden reflecting the health benefits of a green view and the enjoyment and stimulus of linked outside space.

It aspires to be a comfortable home rather than an institution: a house in which anyone would be happy to live.

Collaborative Research

Chris and Sally's House, therefore, is a multi-disciplinary and multi-stranded collaborative project for which Halsall Lloyd Partnership (HLP), architects, landscape architects and interior designers, as well as key partners: Loughborough University, Liverpool John Moores University and the Building Research Establishment, have facilitated a bridge between academic research and practical implementation.

The design of Chris and Sally's House has responded to three briefs, as follows.

A Demonstration Project

How can design help people living with dementia retain their capacity, age in place and live safely and comfortably for longer?

3D MODEL VIEWS - STABLE BLOCK

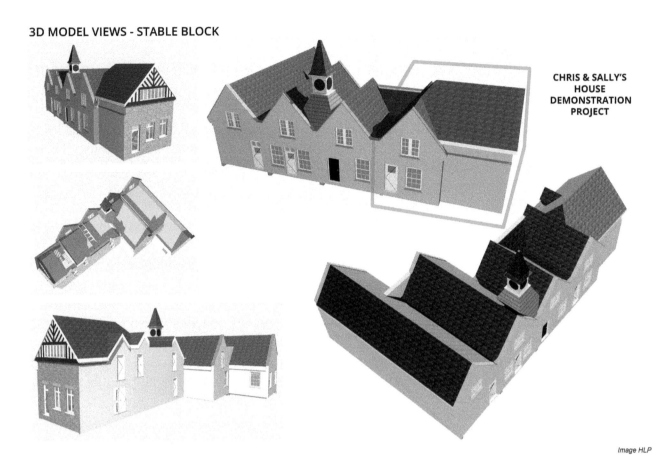

CHRIS & SALLY'S HOUSE DEMONSTRATION PROJECT

Image HLP

Figure 7.3 Chris and Sally's House – demonstration project BRE

A Research Platform

To carry out ongoing evidence-based research into living with dementia.

A Learning Tool

To assist people living with dementia and their carers, developers and institutions in the care, health and housing sectors to understand how new housing design and existing properties can be improved to cater for ageing in place.

The broad objective of the Chris and Sally's House project is to create the opportunity for a win-win-win outcome as a response to the impact of the dementia epidemic.

- A win for people living with dementia, living in their own homes safely and comfortably for longer
- A win for family, friends and carers, easing the burden of care and the stress of a move to an extra care or residential care facility
- A win for the health and care system, potentially reducing the pressures caused by the projected exponential increase in demand for dementia care services.

Housing, health and social care agencies are increasingly interested in the potential of the principles and practice demonstrated through Chris and Sally's House as one approach to easing the burden of care presented by an ageing society.

The Design Brief

- The brief has evolved to include a response to a range of impairments associated with ageing and to personas derived from Loughborough University research

- The brief, therefore, combines design for physical impairment as well as cognitive impairment in the context of adaptation of an existing dwelling
- The design principle is adaptive; that is, the plan can evolve to respond to progressively debilitating illness, enabling people to live sustainably and retain capacity for longer in their own homes
- The building which forms the basis for the demonstration project is the stable block at BRE Garston. Two units are to be designed into one adaptive home – Chris and Sally's House. These buildings are not in fact residential; one was part of a stable, and the other was formerly a bank. The most recent use is as a research facility
- The building has a complex form, including roof geometry and window design and position, which impose some limiting constraints both structurally and in design. Limitations include door positions as well as former modifications, openings and beams
- Although these constraints are restrictive compared to a new build option, the conversion scenario arguably represents a more realistic situation confronting people living in older property which may be unsuitable for their needs and aspirations
- The scenarios illustrated, therefore, demonstrates a range of practical design solutions to achieve the project objectives
- The brief and design have evolved through participation with Loughborough University and Liverpool John Moores University team. HLP have developed the concept and design through a range of iterations and scenarios.

Who Are Chris and Sally?

As discussed in Chapter 6, Chris and Sally are personas developed by Loughborough University. The personas represent a set of characteristics presented by people living with dementia at different stages.

Chris and Sally Personas

- Married for 50 years
- Two sons, who are both married with children
- They love to spend time with their three grandchildren, whom they see most weekends
- Sally is starting to find it difficult to care for Chris now that his dementia is progressing.

Chris – 78 Years Old

- Good day – may need encouragement to interact with others, wandering, occasionally becomes frustrated
- Average day – communication problems, becomes frustrated more frequently and may lash out verbally
- Bad day – may struggle to recognise people, sundowning, often becomes frustrated and may lash out physically.

Sally – 75 Years Old

- Good day – able to manage the majority of Chris' care needs independently but worries Chris might get up during the night and struggles to sleep
- Average day – can help with Chris' care but is likely to need assistance, often has to encourage him to go back to bed during the night and gets very little sleep
- Bad day – needs considerable help in providing care for Chris, is unable to get him to go back to bed during the night and gets no sleep.

The Scenario

The imagined scenario, illustrated in Figure 7.4, is that Chris and Sally are living in a two up–two down cottage. This archetype is a plan form which finds expression throughout the UK in many variations; whether manifested as a country cottage or an urban terrace, it is one of the simplest typologies and is widespread geographically. The layout of the stable block provides an approximation of the two up–two down with a similar floor area.

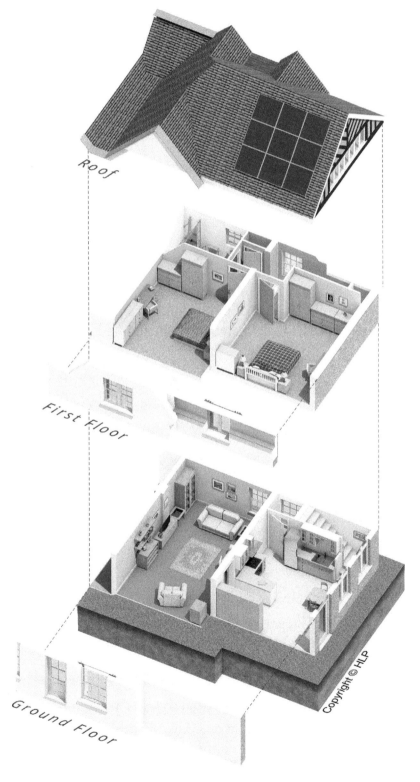

Roof

First Floor

Ground Floor

Image HLP

Figure 7.4 Reimagined property ready for conversion/refurbishment to suit Chris and Sally's requirements

Key Design Objectives of the Demonstration Project (Refer to Chapter 5)

These objectives were determined based on the requirements of the Chris and Sally personas and on available research carried out by Loughborough University. Design principles drew on *Design for Dementia – A Guide* published by HLP and co-authored by Bill Halsall with Dr Robert G MacDonald. The objectives evolved from a series of design meetings between HLP, BRE, Loughborough University and John Moores University.

A House in Which Anyone Would Be Happy to Live

The ambience of the house should feel like a home rather than an institution. While there will be of necessity design features which are a direct response to the condition of dementia, these should as far as possible be covert rather than overt. They should not stigmatise the house in any way or draw attention to the unusual nature of the design brief.

Layout

The layout should be simple and easy to navigate so that Chris and Sally can easily access all parts of the house with the aid of visual cues leading from one space to the next. An open-plan ground-floor linking living room, dining and kitchen is the main living space. A structural wall was removed to enable this flow of space.

Accessibility and Walkability

All parts of the house should be easily accessible by wheelchair. Also the room arrangements and furniture should provide walkability – ease of movement assisted by a network of objects to lean on for support. The house satisfies a range of standards, including Lifetime Homes and Part M of the Building Regulations.

Visual Connections Internally

Key visual connections are:

• Between kitchen/dining and living space
• Between the sitting space and the w.c. (when door open)
• Between the bed position and the w.c. (when door open).

In general, doors are avoided as far as possible to assist orientation and navigability. Visibility of the w.c. from the main sitting area provides comfort and a feeling of security, reducing anxiety and risks of incontinence.

Views out to the Garden

A view to green reduces stress significantly, and contact with nature provides daily visual interest in the changing seasons. Low-level window sills enable a view out from a seating position.

Maximising Natural Light and Artificial Light

The body's natural circadian rhythm (body clock) can become disoriented through the condition of dementia, creating confusion between night and day. Maximising natural light into the home helps to regulate the body clock and avoid confusion. The ageing eye requires better light – both natural and artificial (twice normal lighting levels are indicated). Good task lighting is needed.

Bathing Arrangements

Bathrooms are wet rooms, including accessible shower at each floor level. Disability aids are provided.

Separate Utility/Washing Area

The noise of a washing machine can disturb someone living with dementia. Therefore, this should be situated in a separate utility area rather than in the kitchen.

Carer's Bedroom

A separate bedroom for the carer is advised. People living with dementia may suffer broken sleep patterns, which may be disturbing and disruptive for the carer. There is a balance to be struck between privacy for the carer and access.

Ventilation

Good ventilation is a key requirement. People living with dementia and older people generally need a higher room temperature for comfort. This can lead to reluctance or, indeed, inability to open windows. If the house is efficiently sealed and weather stripped, there can be a build up of CO_2, leading to drowsiness and loss of capacity. A sophisticated ventilation system has been designed combining both natural and artificial ventilation using carbon dioxide monitoring and automatic actuators on windows to ensure good ventilation at all times (refer to Chapter 7).

Visual Perception

The use of colour and light reflectance values helps people living with dementia to navigate their world. The tonal value of walls, floors, kitchen units and other articles of furniture can be used to aid perception of space and visibility of objects in space.

Light-reflectance values can be measured using a light-reflectance meter. On a scale of 1 to 100, where 1 is black and 100 is white, the light-reflectance value of surfaces can be measured. The aim is to achieve a difference of at least 30 points between adjoining surfaces. This objective was tackled through a comprehensive interior design scheme including all surfaces, fixtures, fittings and furniture. The aim is to achieve sufficient contrast at every junction and interface.

Analysis of Chris and Sally's Original Home Scenario

In the reimagined two up–two down terraced house, illustrated in Figure 7.5, Chris and Sally have experienced a number of difficulties as they have got older.

The Immediate Issues

- The only bathroom and toilet are upstairs. Getting there quickly is an issue. This provision is inadequate to accommodate the problem of incontinence
- It has become hard to get into or out of the bath
- The stairs are a struggle, particularly long flights with no resting places/half landings, and too narrow for a stairlift. Although the couple can manage the stairs for the moment, in future they will need better provision and possibly the need for the use of a wheelchair
- The views of the garden are poor
- Access to the garden is difficult
- Thresholds are too high to be navigable in a wheelchair
- The lighting (natural and artificial) is inadequate to cater for the ageing eye

- The ventilation is poor, and windows are hard to open and to clean. The couple worry about their fuel bills and don't want to feel any draughts. Condensation and mould growth result on cold walls and ceilings
- On a sunny day, they can suffer from glare
- Their house is small, with restricted headroom at first floor
- The house is cluttered because of inadequate storage. As Chris' memory deteriorates, he prefers to have things out where he can see them.

THEIR HOME - *Hypothetical Home*

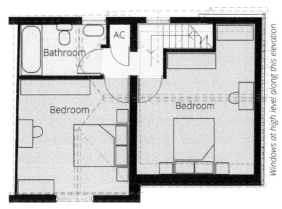

EXISTING FIRST FLOOR

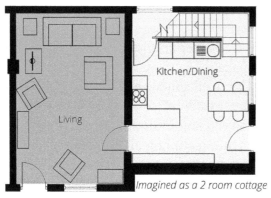

Imagined as a 2 room cottage

EXISTING GROUND FLOOR

IMMEDIATE ISSUES

- The only bathroom is upstairs
- Getting there quickly
- The upstairs bathroom is inadequate for incontinence issues.
- Bath is hard to get in and out
- Stairs are a struggle
- Although the couple can manage stairs at the moment, in the future they will need better provision for wheelchair use
- Views of the garden are poor
- Access to the garden is difficult
- Thresholds are not navigable in a wheelchair
- Lighting is not adequate for the ageing eye levels it needs to be raised
- More natural light needed
- Ventilation is poor - windows are hard to open and to clean
- On a sunny day there is glare
- The house is a small cottage with restricted headroom at first floor.

ISSUES FOR THE FUTURE

The first item that would need to be addressed would be access to the toilet. A shower room situated downstairs with a w.c. would help them greatly.

Creating an organised memory cabinet would help tackle the issue of clutter.   The unit would be easily accessible helping them to file all their paperwork and photographs and would display their knick-knacks. This would be designed in a way that would organise clutter and display memories too.

Currently Sally can't see Chris when he's in the garden, so if he had a fall she wouldn't be aware of it. The windows would need to be improved, creating views to the garden so that Sally can see Chris when he's outside.

Lighting levels need to be improved throughout the house. Opening windows and adding additional light sources would help.

It is important to retain familiar items which will reassure Chris & Sally's of their home. Simple changes could make a lot of difference and aid them now and in the future.

Image HLP

Figure 7.5 Original home scenario – Chris and Sally's House

What Will Happen in the Future?

The first issue that would need to be addressed would be access to the toilet. A shower room situated downstairs with a w.c. would be a great help.

Creating an organised memory cabinet would help to tackle the issue of clutter. The unit would be easily accessible, helping them to file all their paperwork and photographs. They could also display their knick-knacks. They should be able to organise their clutter and display their treasured items and memories.

Currently, Sally can't see Chris if he's in the garden, so if he had a fall, she would't be aware of it. The windows would need to be improved, creating views to the garden so that Sally can see Chris when he's outside.

Inside, the room separation could cause confusion for Chris. Too many doors cause disorientation.

Lighting levels need to be improved throughout the house; opening windows would improve light levels and ventilation. Additional light sources would help. Bulbs could be replaced with high-powered LED luminaires to achieve an instant improvement.

Familiar items should be retained to reassure Chris and Sally that this is still their home.

Simple changes could make a lot of difference and aid them now and in the future, but the major design problems they experience could be tackled by more serious changes to the house.

Adaptive Design Scenarios

A series of adaptive design scenarios were explored by HLP in conjunction with Loughborough University, Liverpool John Moore's University and the BRE. The intention was to investigate a range of design options which might be adopted to ameliorate the design issues of Chris and Sally's original house. Through this collaborative approach to the design issues identified, utilising experts in various fields, HLP aimed to evolve a design solution which would tackle both the problems presented to Chris and Sally by their home in the context of Chris' developing prognosis of dementia and the physical constraints imposed by the design and construction of their house.

Adaptive Design Scenario 1

This design proposed a fairly low level of intervention in the fabric of the house, as illustrated in Figure 7.6. A knock-through opening was created between the kitchen and the living room to allow ease of movement, better visual connection and navigability. A platform lift was installed between the kitchen and the bedroom. This provided disabled access throughout the house (a platform lift was preferred to a stairlift, because people living with dementia can experience disorientation caused by the movement pattern of the stairlift).

Internal finishes would be reviewed, including features such as rugs, which can form a trip hazard, or mirrors, which can cause disturbance to people living with dementia.

Adaptive Design Scenario 2

Adaptive Design Scenario 1 addressed some of Chris and Sally's problems, as illustrated in Figure 7.7. However, the design of the bathroom, although now accessible by lift, was still too far away from living areas to address issues such as incontinence. Equally, it did not fulfil modern requirements for wheelchair accessibility and was invisible from the lounge or kitchen. Adaptive Scenario 2 proposes a downstairs toilet and washbasin accessed from the dining room, shortening the travel distance and instilling greater confidence – the knowledge that it is there and reachable in emergency. The new w.c. would be designed to dementia-friendly principles and include features such as grab handles, a wheelchair turning circle and a lower washbasin.

ADAPTIVE DESIGN SCENARIO 1

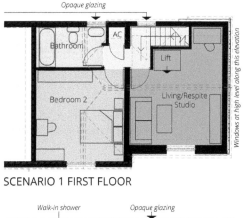

SCENARIO 1 FIRST FLOOR

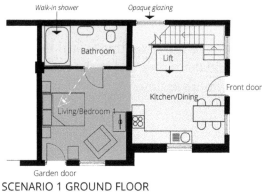

SCENARIO 1 GROUND FLOOR

ADAPTATIONS

- Install lift
- Living space upstairs
- Move bedroom downstairs
- Add bathroom with dementia friendly design
- Retain upstairs bathroom.

Image HLP

Figure 7.6 Adaptive Design Scenario 1

ADAPTIVE DESIGN SCENARIO 2

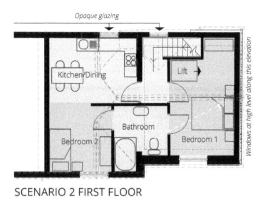

SCENARIO 2 FIRST FLOOR

ADAPTATIONS

- Install lift
- Retain 2 bedrooms upstairs
- Add kitchen/dining upstairs
- Add dementia friendly bathroom upstairs.

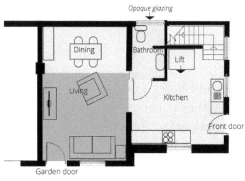

SCENARIO 2 GROUND FLOOR

Image HLP

Figure 7.7 Adaptive Design Scenario 2

The upstairs bathroom would also be re-provided to similar dementia-friendly and accessibility standards. Adaptive Design Scenario 2 shows a separate but visually connecting dining area forming part of what was the living room and a small kitchenette area adjoining a single bedroom upstairs. The design intention here is to provide space upstairs for longer-term care of Chris as his dementia progresses while still allowing a more normal environment for Sally downstairs.

Adaptive Design Scenario 3

The design shown in Figure 7.8 addresses the issues in a different way, providing a full bathroom at each level. Upstairs this follows a double entry system to provide direct accessibility from both bedrooms (this idea was rejected because the two doors could cause confusion). It also shows a downstairs bedroom, potentially a dayroom, so that Chris could rest while being in contact with Sally in the living room and kitchen/dining room. The lift is shown in a different position to allow space for the full bathroom downstairs, but this produces rather poor kitchen arrangements and the need to relocate the front door.

Adaptive Design Scenario 4

Figure 7.9 also shows two bathrooms/w.c.s upstairs and downstairs. The upstairs bathroom is to full wheelchair standard and is quite generous in size, while the downstairs w.c. is to minimum wheelchair accessibility standards. The lift is better positioned at ground floor but necessitates a rather long corridor upstairs. Adaptive Design Scenario 4 provides perhaps a better and more conventional balance between accommodation at the ground and first floors compared to some of the previous options.

ADAPTIVE DESIGN SCENARIO 3

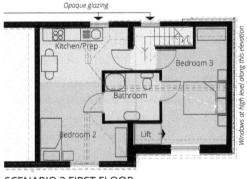

SCENARIO 3 FIRST FLOOR

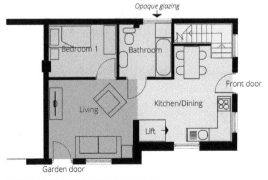

SCENARIO 3 GROUND FLOOR

Image HLP

ADAPTATIONS

- Install lift
- 2 bedrooms upstairs
- Add bedroom downstairs
- Add kitchen/dining upstairs
- Add dementia friendly bathroom downstairs and upstairs.

Figure 7.8 Adaptive Design Scenario 3

ADAPTIVE DESIGN SCENARIO 4

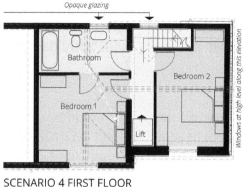

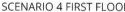

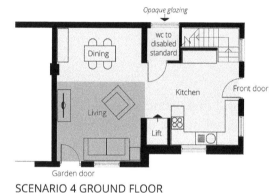

SCENARIO 4 FIRST FLOOR

SCENARIO 4 GROUND FLOOR

ADAPTATIONS

• Install lift

• 2 bedrooms upstairs

• Add bedroom downstairs

• Disabled w.c. downstairs

• Add dementia friendly bathroom upstairs.

Image HLP

Figure 7.9 Adaptive Design Scenario 4

Adaptive Design Scenario 5

Figure 7.10 shows Scenario 5, which is a development of Adaptive Design Scenario 4 but with more emphasis on sight lines between the living room and downstairs bathroom. Upstairs, the idea of a small kitchenette adjoining the bedroom developed in Adaptive Design Scenario 3 returns but in a smaller, less intrusive form. At ground floor, the concept of a small day room adjoining the lounge is retained but is in the form of a recess which can be closed off with a sliding door. The thinking behind this is that at some stage it is feasible that Chris will spend more of his days in bed, and the proximity of living room and kitchen and the day-to-day activities of Sally would assist in breaking down loneliness and isolation. Wheelchair charging points are also shown so that the wheelchair can be easily accessed from bed positions. The potential for a hoist system in the main bedroom has been provided. In view of the complex room/ceiling profile, this has determined a 45° door position to the upstairs bathroom, which also improves visibility and accessibility from the bed position. Both bathrooms now show a walk-in shower arrangement, but the upstairs bathroom has the flexibility to install a bath if required (some people living with dementia prefer a bath to a shower on the basis that the noise of a shower can be an irritation). Bedroom 2 now has a single bed and is perceived as a respite for Sally if Chris is restless at night.

Adaptive Design Scenario 6

In this scenario, illustrated in Figure 7.11, the lift is placed close to the stairs to shorten the length of the corridor on the first floor and to create a better kitchen at ground floor. The bathroom arrangements have been rationalised with a smaller w.c./shower room downstairs and a larger bathroom upstairs. The ground floor plan also shows a separated space for the washing machine in recognition of the fact that many people living with dementia may be disturbed by the noise

ADAPTIVE DESIGN SCENARIO 5

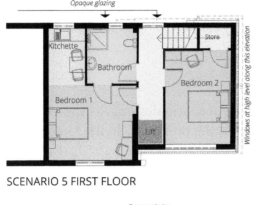

SCENARIO 5 FIRST FLOOR

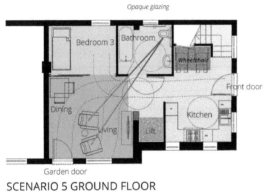

SCENARIO 5 GROUND FLOOR

Image HLP

ADAPTATIONS

- Install lift - wheelchair
- 2 bedrooms upstairs
- Add daybed recess downstairs
- Add kitchenette upstairs
- Add dementia friendly bathroom downstairs and upstairs.

Figure 7.10 Adaptive Design Scenario 5

ADAPTIVE DESIGN SCENARIO 6

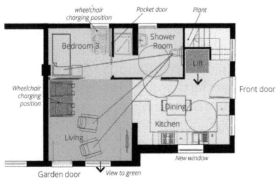

SCENARIO 6 FIRST FLOOR

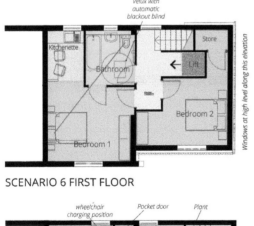

SCENARIO 6 GROUND FLOOR

Image HLP

ADAPTATIONS

- Install lift - wheelchair
- 2 bedrooms upstairs
- Add daybed recess downstairs
- Add kitchenette upstairs
- Add dementia friendly bathroom downstairs and upstairs.

Figure 7.11 Adaptive Design Scenario 6

nuisance of a washing machine and the acceptance that the washing machine is better situated in its own insulated storeroom.

Internal visual connections are further developed so that the downstairs toilet is visible from the dayroom as well as the living room. At the first floor, the visibility of the w.c. from the bed position is improved.

Adaptive Design Scenario 7

This design is a more detailed iteration of the previous scenario designs, as shown in Figure 7.12. More consideration has been given to wheelchair charging positions. In the kitchen, a lower area

ADAPTIVE DESIGN SCENARIO 7

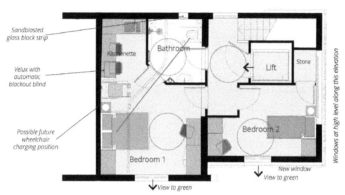

SCENARIO 7 FIRST FLOOR

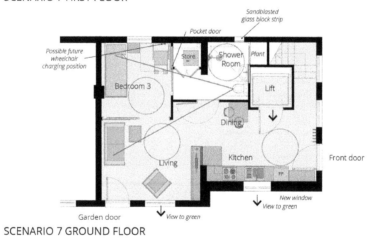

SCENARIO 7 GROUND FLOOR

ADAPTATIONS

- Install lift - wheelchair plus 1 person
- 2 bedrooms upstairs *(1 to M4 standard)*
- Daybed recess downstairs
- Kitchenette upstairs
- Dementia friendly bathroom downstairs and upstairs. *(M4 standard)*

REV C

- Dining table space added
- Washing machine space in store
- Wheelchair charging point on both floors
- Building regulations M4 standard apart from Bed 1, Bathrooms - M4
- 'Walkability'
- Simplify upstairs store

Image HLP

Figure 7.12 Adaptive Design Scenario 7

of worktop has been included to provide a range of different heights and the possibility to perform some tasks from a seated or wheelchair position. Consideration was given to an adjustable-height rise and fall kitchen to full wheelchair standards. Although this might be desirable in some situations, it was decided that it was not appropriate here because one of the key aspirations of the brief was for a house that anyone would want to live in rather than for a specialised solution.

Other provisions include access to both sides and the end of each bed by wheelchair and better space for storage and for appropriate furniture. The kitchenette upstairs was retained in a reduced and more integrated form. It was felt that this would be useful in a situation where Chris would need more intensive nursing care, providing space for administering medicines. Provision for making a cup of tea or a simple meal was envisaged as being potentially very useful in this scenario.

Equally the downstairs day room was envisaged as a feature which could flexibly fulfil a range of functions, such as:

- A day room for Chris close to the living room and kitchen
- End-of-life care
- A small dining room
- A quiet room to alleviate distress in some situations
- Space for hobbies or other activities.

Direct access from the day room to the shower room has been allowed for in this layout with a sliding pocket door so that this can be sealed off when required.

Conclusions

Through discussion among the design group (including HLP, BRE and Loughborough University), it was decided that Adaptive Design Scenario 7 would be proceeded with for detailed design and construction.

This was because, in the context of the requirement for a demonstration project, Adaptive Design Scenario 7 shows the most comprehensive range of adaptations while remaining a house that anyone would want to live in. It also provides the most intensive range of features to enable Chris and Sally to retain their capacity for longer and to live relatively independently with the assistance of design adaptations provided. Figures 6.2–6.6 in Chapter 6 show how the demonstration project also could adapt to other personas, Alison, Barry, Christine and David, achieving maximum benefits for the demonstration aspects of the project.

There have been some compromises arising out of the physical constraints of the existing building, reimagined as a two up–two down cottage, and by financial/sponsorship limitations.

Principally, the size of the kitchen and living room have been reduced as additional facilities; particularly, bathrooms and w.c.s have been introduced, and inevitably there is less space for other main rooms, including bedrooms. Similarly, intrusions of the roof geometry have affected the positioning of the hoist, wardrobes and so on because of the low eaves levels involved.

Through limitations on cost, some aspects remain as potential future provisions. In particular, the space for a lift was provided, but a platform lift was not installed at the time of writing. However, this does reflect real life, and the concept is that through a 'long life loose fit' design philosophy, the house can be designed to be dementia adaptable, compatible with progressive stages of adaptation as required.

For Chris and Sally, the process of remodelling their house would be very disruptive, and one of the less interventionist adaptive design scenarios may be more realistic. In the context of the design of a demonstration project, the most comprehensive adaptation package is more relevant. Dementia takes many forms and affects individuals differently. Therefore, there is no definitive answer to the question of how to adapt an existing dwelling to accommodate living with dementia to sustain capacity and independent living for longer. A range of measures may be appropriate to different people in different circumstances, so it is appropriate to show a range of iterations (1–7). Every house or apartment will also be different so that in terms of adaptation, there is no single 'one size fits all' solution. Designers should interpret the lessons learnt to suit the individual and the constraints of the property. In the context of a new build, there is more flexibility, of course, to build in future capacity to planned housing projects so that adaptations can be fitted when needed. This is particularly relevant to the use of space and space standards for new building projects so that there is designed-in flexibility.

The Interior Design of Chris and Sally's House

The interior layout, finishes, colours, furniture and lighting were carefully curated to respond to the needs of Chris and Sally as understood through the medium of the persona studies research by Loughborough University. This is illustrated in Figure 7.13. Particular attention was given to the spatial experiences of people living with dementia and the cognitive impairments associated with the various forms of dementia and their manifestations as experienced by the persona.

Key features of the design include an open plan layout to aid navigability and transparency of spaces to assist understanding of the functionality and relationships between spaces. The 'view to the loo' has been one of the main drivers of the design on both ground and first floors.

Although the design is fundamentally a refurbishment project, the interiors have been designed to fulfil Part M of the Building Regulations to full wheelchair accessibility standards. This has had a major impact on the detail design of spaces, including, for example, wider doors, well-positioned bathroom aids, provision for a hoist in the bedroom and wheelchair charging positions.

GROUND FLOOR SCENARIO 7

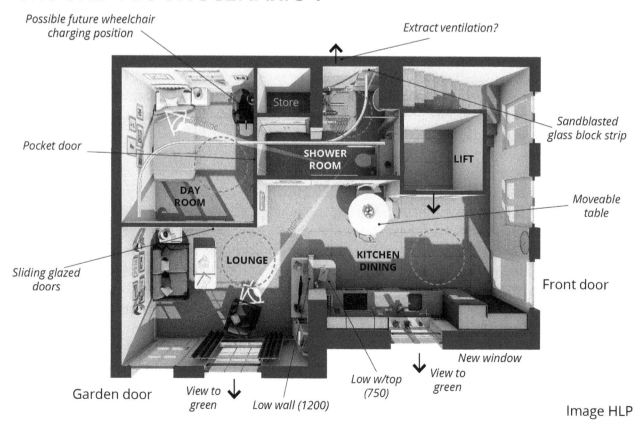

Figure 7.13 Ground floor Scenario 7

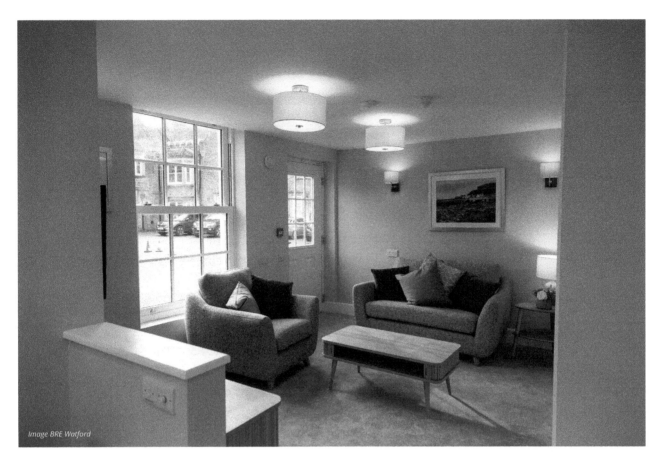

Figure 7.14 View of lounge near completion

Heating and ventilation strategies are described in detail in Chapter 8 but are based on maintaining comfortable temperatures and a good level of ventilation in all rooms. Electric underfloor heating was selected to avoid wall-mounted radiators and reduce carbon emissions through the use of fossil fuel–free green electricity. The ventilation system is partially automatic, with actuators operated by sensors to reduce the build-up of CO_2 in the house while maintaining comfortable temperatures. Older people may be more sensitive to drafts and nervous about fuel use. Windows may be kept closed to avoid drafts. This can result in a build-up of CO_2, producing drowsiness and exacerbating the effects of dementia. The heating and ventilation strategy tackles this issue (refer to Chapter 8).

Noise reduction is another design factor. Excessive noise can be very disturbing for people living with dementia. Acoustic installation is installed in the building's walls, floor and roof; within the external walls; and between floors.

To aid comprehension of spaces and objects in space, the design is based on the light reflectance values of all surfaces. To identify differences in colour/surface, the amount of light a surface/colour reflects is measured by its light reflectance value. A difference of 30% difference in LRV is targeted between all walls, floors and visible surfaces.

The light reflectance value of finishes is a useful method for designing and selecting materials to assist people living with dementia to perceive their environment more clearly. If the LRVs of adjacent materials are close in value, then their appearance to the ageing eye will be consistent and unthreatening. This is particularly relevant to floor finishes because a change in LRV at floor level could be misinterpreted as a step.

Alternatively, contrast can be used to give definition to different surfaces, such as between walls and floors. A minimum LRV of 30% is required to create this contrast.

FIRST FLOOR SCENARIO 7

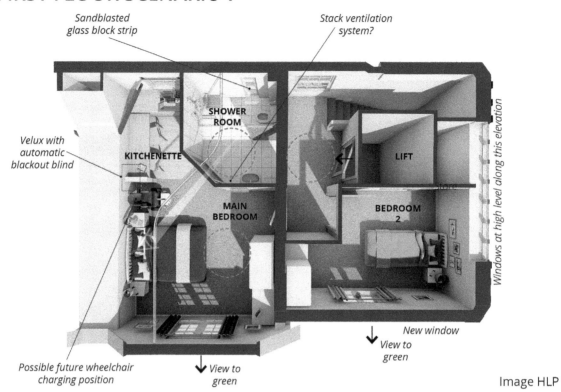

Figure 7.15 First floor Scenario 7

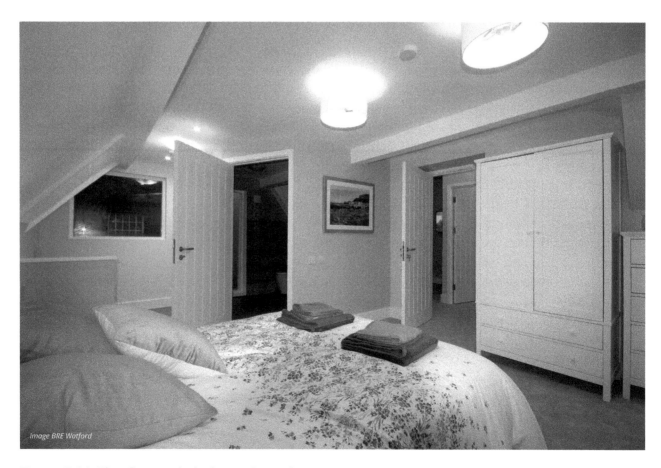

Figure 7.16 First floor main bedroom Scenario 7

Contrast between walls and floors, skirting boards, architraves and doors will help people living with dementia to perceive their environment more clearly and help them to negotiate it. Doors which are accessible can also be distinguished from doors which are non-accessible such as service rooms by the applied use of colour.

A Walkthrough of Chris and Sally's House

PROPOSED INTERVENTIONS

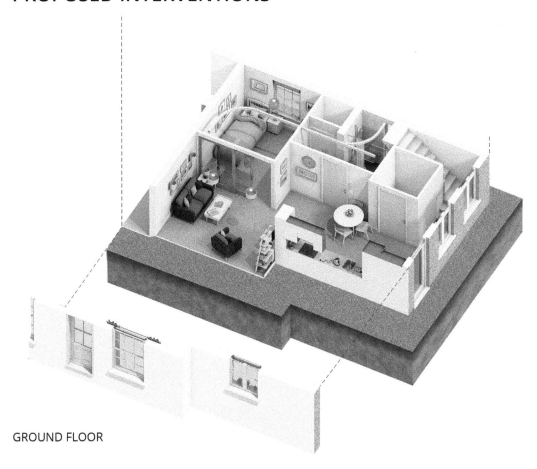

GROUND FLOOR

- Wheelchair accessible lift

- Kitchen with varied worktop heights glazed doors

- New manual and automatic opening windows

- Open plan living/kitchen dining space

- Dayroom/dining room/quiet room

- Shower room downstairs with hoist access from dayroom.

- Living room with view to w.c.

- Walkability as well as wheelchair access

- 'View to Green'

- Light reflectance values differentiate between walls/floors/furniture

- Floors finishes have consistent light reflectance values avoiding trip hazards

- Thresholds are wheelchair accessible

- Noise reduction features

Image HLP

Figure 7.17 Ground floor proposed intervention

PROPOSED INTERVENTIONS

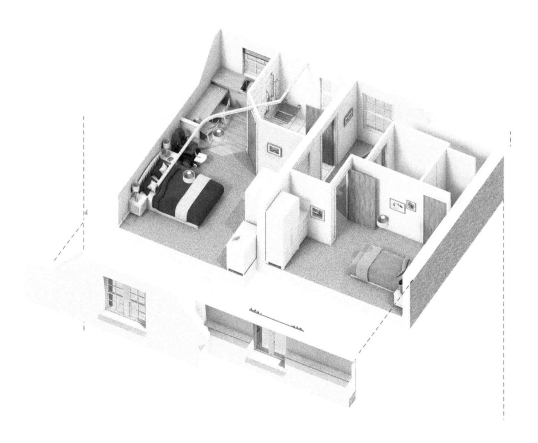

FIRST FLOOR

• Main bedroom and adjoining shower room to wheelchair standards with a hoist and view from bed to w.c.

• Wheelchair accessible lift

• Kitchenette for food and drink preparation/medication

• Carer's bedroom

• New manual and automatic opening windows

• Walkability as well as wheelchair access

• 'View to Green'

• Light reflectance values differentiate between walls/floors/furniture

• Floors finishes have consistent light reflectance values avoiding trip hazards

• Thresholds are wheelchair accessible

• Noise reduction features

Image HLP

Figure 7.18 First floor proposed intervention

A Tour of Chris and Sally's House

Kitchen/Dining Room (Figure 7.19)

- The kitchen/dining room and living room form an open plan arrangement with good visibility to aid navigation and legibility. There is ample space to negotiate a wheelchair through the spaces but also good walkability. Chris and Sally can make their way through the spaces, making use of kitchen units, tables, chairs and so on for additional support
- Doors are minimised to avoid confusion
- In the kitchen area, wall and floor units have glazed fronts to allow Chris and Sally to locate kitchen utensils and so on. This helps to declutter the kitchen. Otherwise, items could be left on the kitchen surfaces for ease of finding. Kitchen equipment is shown as what is it – stainless steel fronts to identify fridge freezer, dishwasher, cooker and extract fan, as opposed to, perhaps more fashionably, disguising them as kitchen cupboards
- The light reflectance values are calculated to provide a 30% difference between floor and base unit front, between fronts and worktop and between worktop and wall finish. There is a lower-level worktop next to the cooker so that Chris or Sally can use it from an alternative position such as seated or from a wheelchair
- Personalisation and familiarity are reinforced by pictures or photographs on the walls to make it feel like home and stimulate memories. A view to green is provided by the kitchen window overlooking the garden
- Corners of worktops, tables and chairs are rounded to minimise risk of falls, and the tabletop and chair seats have light-coloured surfaces to contrast with walls and floors
- Table and chair legs are conventional, avoiding pedestals or swivels, because they will be used for leaning on

KITCHEN/DINING

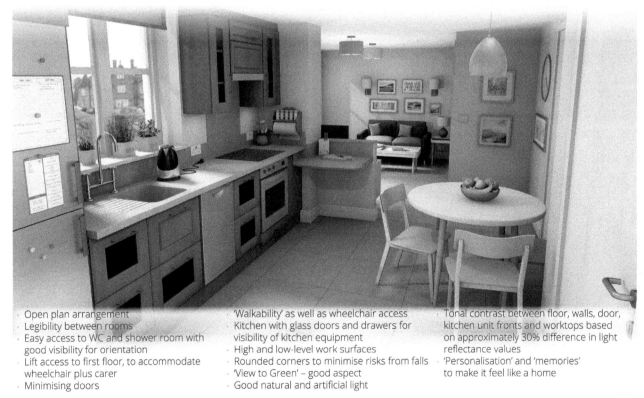

- Open plan arrangement
- Legibility between rooms
- Easy access to WC and shower room with good visibility for orientation
- Lift access to first floor, to accommodate wheelchair plus carer
- Minimising doors

- 'Walkability' as well as wheelchair access
- Kitchen with glass doors and drawers for visibility of kitchen equipment
- High and low-level work surfaces
- Rounded corners to minimise risks from falls
- 'View to Green' – good aspect
- Good natural and artificial light

- Tonal contrast between floor, walls, door, kitchen unit fronts and worktops based on approximately 30% difference in light reflectance values
- 'Personalisation' and 'memories' to make it feel like a home

Image HLP

Figure 7.19 Kitchen/dining, Chris and Sally's House

- Skirting boards and architraves also help to define form and assist cognition of the spaces
- Lighting is concentrated over usable surfaces – task lighting to help the occupants see what they are doing. Approximately twice the usual lighting levels are achieved
- There is a clock with a large face on the wall to assist in keeping track of time and help to reinforce the rhythms of the natural body clock
- The w.c. is visible both from the kitchen/living area and the lounge.

The Lounge

- The lounge (Figure 7.20) has good views towards the garden, providing a view to green. The windows sill is at a low height to provide views from a seated position. It has a good visual connection to the kitchen. The floor is carpeted but to similar LRV as the kitchen floor and detailed at the junction to avoid a trip hazard
- Again, the tonal contrast between floors, walls and furniture has been gauged to generate a 30% contrast at all junctions, aiding spatial perception. Curtains have a highlighted edge for ease of use, and there is a contrast between the arms and cushions of the sofa and armchair
- There is high-level ambient and task lighting from a variety of sources, including wall lights and table lights
- Open shelving can be used to display personal items, assisting in generating familiarity and personalisation with pictures and photographs on the wall
- The occasional tables have wooden frames and legs to provide good stability and tonal contrast with the floor finishes and are fitted with white tops for contrast with both the floor and the timber elements.

LOUNGE

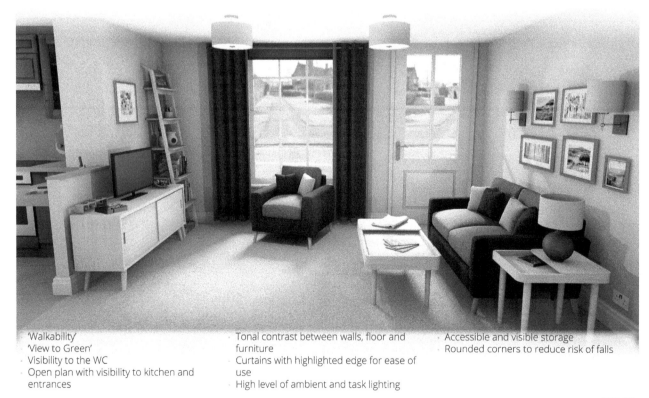

'Walkability'
'View to Green'
Visibility to the WC
Open plan with visibility to kitchen and entrances

Tonal contrast between walls, floor and furniture
Curtains with highlighted edge for ease of use
High level of ambient and task lighting

Accessible and visible storage
Rounded corners to reduce risk of falls

Image HLP

Figure 7.20 Lounge, Chris and Sally's House

DAYROOM

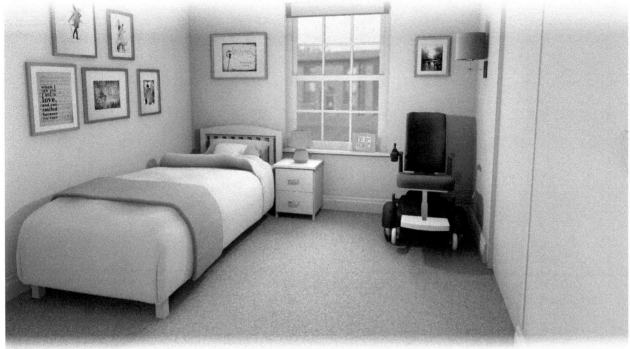

· Alternative uses: dining room, quiet room or   · Hoist to shower room   · Multiple wheelchair charging positions
  day room for end of life care   · Pocket door between day room and shower
· 'View to Green' with blackout blinds   room for flexibility between alternative uses

Image HLP

Figure 7.21 Dayroom, Chris and Sally's House

Dayroom

- As described earlier, the day room (Figure 7.21) has flexibility in use. It could be used as a quiet room or dining room as well as a room for end-of-life care. It is visually connected to the downstairs w.c. via a pocket door reflecting this range of potential uses. It has potential for a hoist to be fitted in future to transfer from the bed to the shower room
- The screen between the dayroom and the living room is glazed to allow two-way vision and connection between the two rooms, as well as some degree of sound separation. The glazing should be non-reflective to avoid the disturbing effect of reflections.

Downstairs Shower Room

- This area (Figure 7.22) is fully wheelchair accessible and includes a separate compartment for the washing machine/dryer
- Because of the need for provisional bathroom aids, washdown surfaces and so on, the room could have a more clinical or even institutional feel about it, but careful choice of tiling materials softens this effect. The design still aspires to be a home that everyone would like to live in
- The w.c. and sanitary fittings are white, contrasting by 30% LRV with the wall and floor tiling, and a horizontal band of darker-toned tiles accentuates the contrast with the white grab rails. It was felt that this more subtle approach was more conducive to the project objectives than the brightly coloured toilet seat sometimes encountered in more institutional projects
- The shower curtains have magnetic closing, and the shower enclosure is equipped with a retractable seat to ease assisted bathing if that is required.

GROUND FLOOR SHOWER ROOM

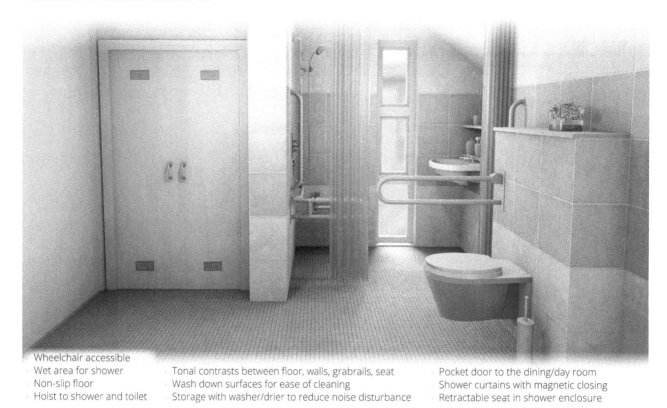

Wheelchair accessible
· Wet area for shower   · Tonal contrasts between floor, walls, grabrails, seat   · Pocket door to the dining/day room
· Non-slip floor   · Wash down surfaces for ease of cleaning   · Shower curtains with magnetic closing
· Hoist to shower and toilet   · Storage with washer/drier to reduce noise disturbance · Retractable seat in shower enclosure

Image HLP

Figure 7.22 Ground floor shower room, Chris and Sally's House

Lift and Stairs

- Both the lift and stairs rise from the kitchen/diner area to the first-floor landing. They are open plan, clearly visible and accessible. The lift shaft space is a future provision at this stage but could provide the best means of access to the upper floor for Chris in particular as his condition progresses. The stairs have a half landing as a rest point and to minimise risks of falls and are equipped with handrails on both sides.

Main Bedroom

- As Figure 7.23 shows, the intrusion of the roof line creates an interesting ceiling profile which imposes some constraints on the design and layout of the rooms, and the bed has been carefully positioned to facilitate access to allow for the future provision of a hoist
- The bedroom has an adjoining kitchenette area which could be used for preparing drinks and light meals as well as storage and administering medications
- The window is at a low height to achieve views from the bed position and also natural light, increasing awareness of daytime and reinforcing natural circadian rhythms. Windows are fitted with curtains including a highlight at the edge and should also have blackout blinds to assist natural sleep patterns
- Wardrobes and chests of drawers are accommodated to the sloping ceiling and should ideally have glass doors and glass drawer fronts or dropped draw fronts so that their contents are visible.

Bedroom 2

- The second bedroom (Figure 7.24) is viewed as a potential respite space or as a spare bedroom for a carer or visiting relative. The room is wheelchair adaptable with 900 mm space around the bed

MAIN BEDROOM

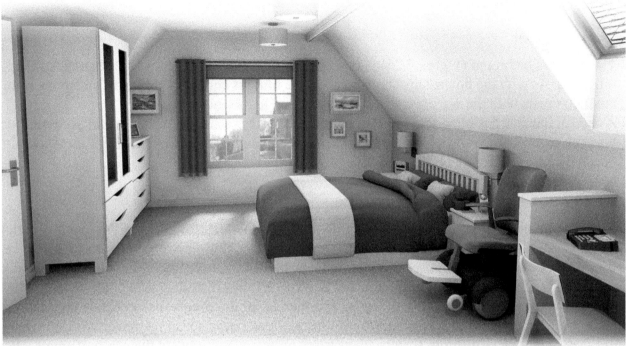

- Fully wheelchair accessible
- 'View to Green'
- Hoist to shower room

- Curtains and blackout blinds
- Wheelchair charging position
- Ambient and task lighting

- Adjoining kitchenette area – for preparation of light meals and drinks and storage of medication

Image HLP

Figure 7.23 Main bedroom, Chris and Sally's House

BEDROOM 2

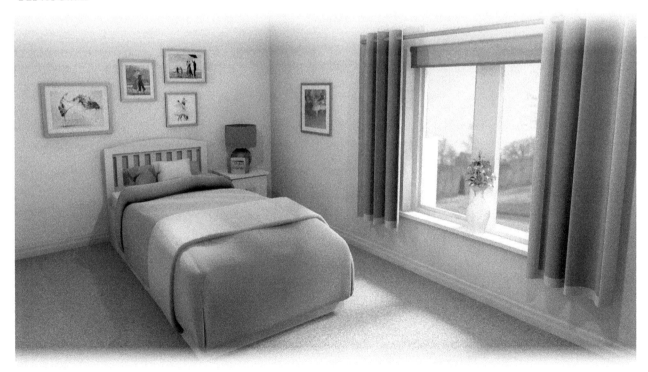

- Respite for carer
- 'View to Green'

- Blackout blinds
- Tonal contrasts for easy visibility

- Wheelchair adaptable

Image HLP

Figure 7.24 Bedroom 2, Chris and Sally's House

- As before, the curtains are shown with a contrasting edge, and the bed itself has a cover with the correct 30% LRV contrast with the floor and walls.

Upstairs Bathroom

- The upstairs bathroom (Figure 7.25) is equipped with a shower but could be adapted to a bath if needed. As with the downstairs shower room, the tiling is carefully chosen to create the right tonal contrasts with the w.c., washbasin and necessary grab rails
- A careful balance has been sought between the needs for washdown surfaces and accessibility features such as grab rails which tend to create a clinical impression and the brief for a homely house that anyone would be happy to live in.

Landscape Design of Chris and Sally's Garden

Sitting out and external activities such as gardening are beneficial for people living with dementia. Exposure to sunlight develops Vitamin D, and experiencing daylight helps to regulate the body's natural circadian rhythms. Nature stimulates all of the senses, including the visual stimulus of colour and the movement of foliage and flowers. A water feature provides additional visual sound and touch experience. Rustling leaves and the feel of the breeze also enhance the sensory experience. The garden should contain fruit for taste, for example, an apple tree or wild strawberries. Plants which have a strong scent such as roses or lavender stimulate the sense of smell.

The garden is laid out with a circular movement route to encourage exercise and interest in the garden all year round.

The garden is enclosed by hedges and shrub beds to provide protection from the wind and a sense of enclosure. A number of sitting opportunities are provided, including space for eating outside on a good day.

UPSTAIRS SHOWER ROOM

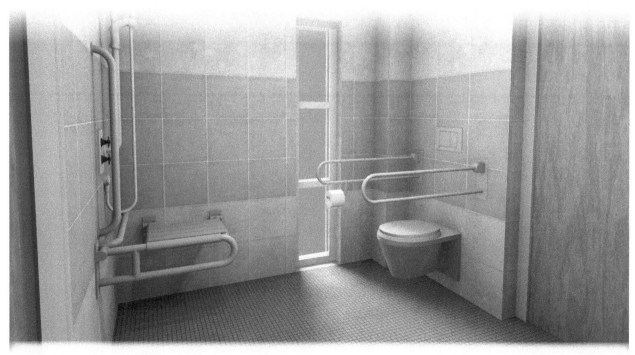

- Wheelchair accessible
- Wet area for shower
- Non-slip floor
- Hoist to shower and toilet
- Tonal contrasts between floor, walls, grabrails, seat
- Wash down surfaces for ease of cleaning
- Shower curtains with magnetic closing
- Retractable seat in shower enclosure

Image HLP

Figure 7.25 Upstairs shower room Chris and Sally's House

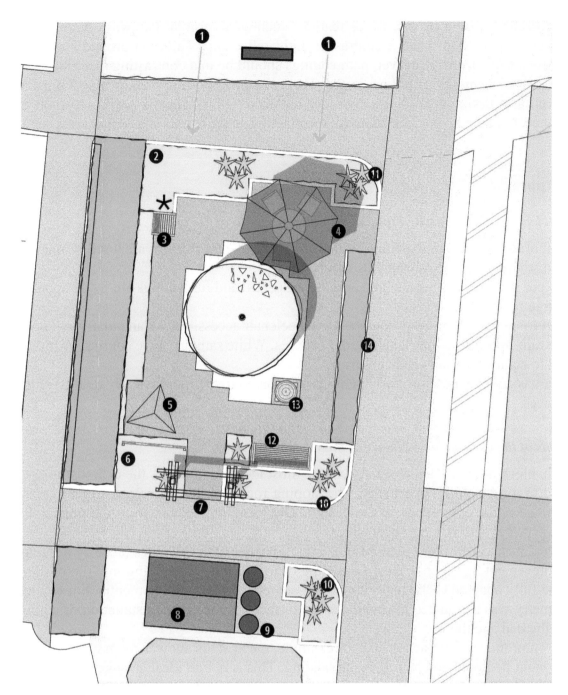

1   View from Chris and Sally's House

2   Raised planter with sensory planting

3   Seating edge with visual focus

4   Patio - 'alfresco' dining area

5   Rotary drier

6   Ornamental screen

7   Pergola acts as threshold and frames views of shed door

8   Potting and tool shed

9   Compost bin and water butt

10   Raised planters

11   Eye catching planting (foliage, colour and texture)

12   Timber bench with back and arm rest

13   Water feature

14   Hedge enclosure

Image HLP

Figure 7.26 Chris and Sally's garden

Thresholds are created by the use of features such as a pergola. Pathways have a consistent tonal materials palette to avoid a contrast in light reflectance value on ground surfaces which might cause a trip hazard. However, path edgings should be in a contrasting material.

The functional elements are not neglected. There is a small potting shed, compost bin and water butt as well as a drying area. Grass areas are replaced with permeable paving to reduce heavy maintenance. Shading is provided through tree planting, a patio umbrella, ornamental screens and a pergola.

Design Appraisal

A House That Anyone Would Be Pleased to Live in

Many visitors have expressed their appreciation of this. The adaptations are low key, non-intrusive and avoid stigmatising the dwelling as special needs.

The colour schemes are tasteful and enrich the spaces, and furnishings are fresh, appealing and comfortable.

The wet room spaces are fully equipped to wheelchair accessibility standards, including necessary grab rails and 1.5-m wheelchair turning circles. White sanitary ware contrasts with the beige wall tiles to achieve a good visual contrast.

These areas could appear somewhat clinical compared to the more homely quality of the main living spaces.

Constraints of the Conversion – Nature of the Project

The stable block at the BRE site was never the most ideal building for the demonstration project compared to a new build opportunity. The sloping rooves at the first floor, in particular, introduced an additional complexity to the design. The location, isolated from the potential garden area by a service road, was not ideal either.

However, these constraints are representative of the real-life challenges faced by designers, and a key achievement has been to incorporate the charm of the old building into the design vision of a home fully adapted to the requirements of someone living with dementia. For example, the roof geometry was negotiated to provide a flat surface for the future installation of a hoist track between the bed and the w.c.

Some compromises were necessary; for example, the upstairs shower room has two doors, one from the main bedroom and one from the landing. This is not an ideal arrangement for someone living with dementia, who could potentially be confused by being confronted with two doors from the bathroom. However, the potential use of the second bedroom as a respite bedroom for Sally or as a visitor bedroom necessitates bathroom access for the occupants without going through the main bedroom.

There is a design choice here. If this was perceived as a real problem, then the landing door could be permanently locked, blocked off or painted the same colour as the wall to provide a degree of camouflage which will deter its use by those living with dementia.

The Dayroom

One space which has caused comment is the dayroom space adjoining the living room. Some visitors thought this was unnecessary because the main bedroom upstairs and its en-suite wet room are more than adequate for end-of-life care.

However, the alternative uses of a quiet room, hobby room or dining space do provide useful flexibility in use for Chris and Sally. The sociability of the design allows Chris and Sally to be in close contact while being potentially engaged in different activities through the day.

The Kitchenette at the First Floor

Another space which caused comment was the kitchenette alcove adjoining the main bedroom. This might be perceived as unnecessary, given there is a well-equipped kitchen downstairs. However, in the imagined scenario, Chris or Sally could be confined to bed for certain periods. Carrying a tea tray upstairs, even in the lift, could present a potential risk of accidents. In some scenarios, the kitchenette could be very useful.

Visiting carers or medical staff might also find a space like this with a sink and worktop useful for preparing medication or treatments.

Adaptive Plan

The design achieves this through its open plan arrangement and through the provision of flexible spaces such as the dayroom/dining room/quiet room/hobby room adjoining the living room and kitchenette upstairs which could be used as an area for providing nursing care as well as light meals.

The second bedroom allows flexible use as visitor's or carer's accommodation or as respite for the Sally persona.

The space allowed for the future provision of a lift between the ground and first floors also provides a potential dining space at the ground floor and a potential sitting space upstairs.

Legibility and Walkability

The open plan arrangement allows visibility and navigability between the spaces on the ground floor. Access is via the kitchen dining area or the living room. The spaces are walkable as well as accessible, enabling Chris and Sally to move around the house using furniture or fixed objects to steady themselves.

'Long Life, Loose Fit'

The design achieves its 'long life, loose fit' objective by being flexible in use through its adaptive plan form but also demonstrates that it is possible to achieve a dwelling which is inherently designed for dementia while also being a home that anyone could wish to live in. Incorporating 'Design for Dementia' design principles into housing design could be a pre-adaptation which facilitates living well at home with or without dementia. Dementia compatibility in housing design should be a significant part of design briefs to provide greater flexibility in the housing stock to cater for all needs throughout our lifetimes.

Reference

Halsall, W., and MacDonald, R., 2015. Volume 2 – Design *for* Dementia – research projects, outlines the research projects and describes the participatory approach. ISBN 978-0-9929231-2-9.

8 Indoor Environmental Quality Studies

Ahmad Aladawi, Ben M. Roberts, Eef Hogervorst and Malcolm Cook

Introduction

Indoor environmental quality (IEQ) has a direct effect on the comfort, health and wellbeing of the people occupying the space due to their exposure to temperature, humidity, pollutants and airborne pathogens (Jin et al. 2020b). For people with dementia, however, the indoor environment is particularly important because vulnerable people may spend up to 100% of their time indoors (Torfs et al. 2008), compared to 90% for healthy adults, and so their health and wellbeing are greatly affected by IEQ parameters (Jin et al. 2020a). IEQ is characterised by thermal comfort, indoor air quality (IAQ), acoustic comfort and visual comfort (Valderrama-Ulloa et al. 2020). The focus of this chapter is illustrated in Figure 8.1 and concentrates primarily on thermal comfort parameters and CO_2 concentration, which is an airborne pollutant that can be taken as a proxy for ventilation effectiveness. The importance of ensuring an appropriate internal environment for people with dementia cannot be understated, and the significant impact of sub-optimal indoor environments is potentially significant. This chapter seeks to explain the linkage between wellbeing of people with dementia and the environmental physics underlying the creation and maintenance of an appropriate level of IEQ.

The chapter is structured as follows. The first section reviews the current body of literature to identify the impact of the indoor environmental quality parameters on people with dementia and their caregivers. The second section describes the optimal indoor environmental parameters for people with dementia and their caregivers. The third section summarises the current understanding and findings, and finally, the chapter concludes with a summary and reflections on future directions of research.

Impact of Indoor Environmental Quality Parameters on the Health and Wellbeing of People With Dementia

Four main IEQ parameters directly affect people with dementia's health and wellbeing (Dodd and Donatello 2021): (1) temperature, (2) relative humidity, (3) air velocity and (4) indoor air quality, which may be adversely affected by elevated CO_2 concentration in the air (Malki-Epshtein et al. 2023). Whilst there are other environmental and personal factors that might be considered in relation to human comfort in general, such as clothing insulation and metabolic activity, the aforementioned four have been directly linked to the comfort, health and wellbeing of people with dementia (Khan et al. 2021). Hence, the discussion within the following sections is restricted to these four main parameters.

Impact of Indoor Temperature on the Health and Wellbeing of People With Dementia

Older people are most vulnerable to low and high temperatures and heat waves (Nunes 2020), which increases the risks of hospital admission (Zhang et al. 2023). At present, there are an

DOI: 10.1201/9781003306054-8

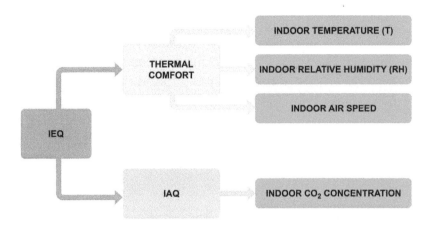

Figure 8.1 IEQ parameters

estimated 2000 deaths annually in the UK related to high temperatures, and this number is expected to rise to 7000 by 2050 due to global warming and an ageing population (Tham et al. 2020).

It has been found that for each 1°C increase in the indoor temperature, human body temperature increases by 0.21°C (Tham et al. 2020). It has also been recognised that body temperature regulation is less efficient with age, and this is even more pronounced in dementia (Venneri et al. 2021). This can lead to dysfunction of cellular metabolism via enzymatic dysregulation, leading to vulnerability to disease. The main health issues related to high indoor temperature are elevated blood pressure (Hansen et al. 2022), blood glucose and core temperature, as well as reduced respiratory function and, subsequently, reduced engagement in physical activities, further contributing to poor health and possibly dementia (Tham et al. 2020).

High indoor temperatures can also cause respiratory problems, such as shortness of breath and coughing, as a result of the fact that blood oxygen levels decrease when the indoor temperature increases (Palmer 2020). In contrast, it has also been found that indoor temperature has an inverse relationship with blood oxygen level but that higher blood pressure is associated with higher body temperature (Tham et al. 2020). Similarly, investigations of the impact of indoor temperature in nursing homes in some EU countries have suggested that low temperature causes bronchial hyperresponsiveness (Bentayeb et al. 2015). It has also been noted that both high (>26°C) and low (<20°C) indoor temperature have a significant impact on people with dementia, both physically and mentally, and are directly related to poor respiratory health, as well as issues with psychosis and diabetes management (Tham et al. 2020). Other symptoms related to high temperature include headache due to dehydration and/or blood pressure fluctuations, dizziness and fatigue exacerbated by sleeping problems (Quinn and Shaman 2017).

Both high and low indoor temperatures have negative impacts on people's health and wellbeing. At present, there are no international standards that identify the optimal range of indoor temperature specifically for people with dementia. This knowledge gap increases the concerns around health issues for older people in the future, and it is recognised that this needs to be addressed by different stakeholders and included in design strategies and building regulations or standards.

Impact of Indoor Humidity on the Health and Wellbeing of People With Dementia

Humidity has a direct effect on the health and wellbeing of people with dementia. Older people who live in a dry environment have a high risk of dry skin and dehydration (Chen et al.

2019). It has been observed that people with dementia have higher dehydration risks, leading to potential itching and discomfort, with low humidity when compared to healthy older people (Jin et al. 2020b). Furthermore, low humidity increases the frequency of wheezing and coughing (Bentayeb et al. 2015). Some studies have found that low humidity directly affects functional vision and causes dry eyes, which then causes discomfort and limits the ability of people with dementia to perform their daily tasks accurately (Wolkoff et al. 2021). Ensuring people with dementia are living at an optimal humidity level will not only assist in preventing these symptoms but will also aid in making them more productive and independent (Childs et al. 2020).

The Impact of Indoor Air Velocity on Health and Wellbeing of People With Dementia

Air velocity is another factor that affects the thermal comfort of people with dementia (Jiao et al. 2017). Many studies have found that a high air velocity can directly affect the health and wellbeing of people with dementia; for instance, it has been observed that high air velocity has a negative impact on the health of people with dementia and can cause thermal discomfort. The combination of high air velocity and low relative humidity decreases body temperature and increases the risk of having dry eyes (Hashiguchi and Tochihara 2009).

Some studies have found that high air velocity impacts on the health of people with dementia, causing dry skin and throat symptoms (Yang et al. 2020). Others have investigated the impact of air velocity on people with dementia and found that living with an optimal air velocity decreased sick building syndrome (SBS) symptoms such as headaches, blocked or runny nose, dry, itchy skin, dry, sore eyes or throat, cough or wheezing and improved the health and wellbeing of residents (Melikov et al. 2012).

Air velocity is an important factor in thermal comfort. Ensuring people with dementia and their caregivers can live with optimal air movement levels will assist in optimising their health and thermal comfort and protecting them from other diseases and sick-building syndrome.

Impact of the Indoor CO_2 Concentrations on the Health and Wellbeing of People With Dementia

CO_2 concentration in inhaled air significantly impacts the health and wellbeing of people with dementia (Ma et al. 2022) and is an indicator of ventilation rate and effectiveness (Adzic et al. 2022), as well as being associated with coughing and, often, breathlessness (Bentayeb et al. 2015). Many health symptoms are associated with high CO_2 concentration. For example, it can affect sleep quality and concentration levels during daily tasks (Serrano-Jim Enez et al. 2020). CO_2 concentrations between 1000 and 2000 parts per million (ppm) indicate poor ventilation relative to the number of occupants in the space Malki-Epshtein et al. (2023). Furthermore, concentrations between 2000 and 5000 ppm can cause headaches and decrease attention levels, while concentrations above 5000 ppm damage the brain and worsen the health and wellbeing of older people, including those with dementia (Serrano-Jim Enez et al. 2020).

Optimal Indoor Environmental Parameters for People With Dementia and Their Caregivers

Optimal Indoor Temperature for People With Dementia

The perception of thermal conditions on the part of people with dementia differs from non-demented adults (Serrano-Jim Enez et al. 2020), and various studies have been conducted to identify the optimal indoor temperature for people with dementia during different seasons. For instance, studies undertaken in China investigated winter thermal comfort of 200 elderly people in two cities in China, Qiqihar in the northeast and Shanghai in the southeast. These studies showed that the average indoor temperatures in Qiqihar were 14.5 ± 4.3°C, higher than that of Shanghai at 10.4 ± 1.5°C. They suggested that the optimal indoor temperature during the winter for elderly people at risk of dementia ranged between 16 and 24°C (Chen et al. 2019).

Studies in Australia investigated thermal comfort in nursing homes and compared thermal comfort of residents with that of non-residents in both the summer and winter seasons (Tartarini et al. 2017). The nursing homes' windows were single glazed, with metallic frames, and the external walls were solid brick with no insulation. The temperature was measured on an hourly basis, and sensors were installed in external walls of the rooms that the residents spent most of their time in. The average indoor temperature was 21.6°C in winter and 22°C in the summer. Results showed that the nursing homes were not appropriately equipped to provide thermal comfort for their residents in either the summer or winter seasons (Tartarini et al. 2017). The residents preferred warmer temperatures (+0.9°C) and wore more clothes compared with the non-residents. The minimum measured temperature in the winter was lower than 20°C, and the results suggested that the optimal indoor temperature for people with dementia is 23.2°C (Tartarini et al. 2017).

In the European Union (EU), studies investigated the optimal indoor temperature in nursing homes in seven EU countries: Poland, Sweden, Greece, France, Italy, Denmark and Belgium. The indoor temperature was measured for 1 week to investigate the impact of thermal quality on 600 older people's health. The optimal assessed temperature ranged between 22.4 and 25.1°C, and the results showed that people over 80 years of age were most vulnerable to indoor thermal changes (Bentayeb et al. 2015). This study suggested the optimal temperature to be 23°C in all countries except Greece, where 22°C was considered preferable. Several limitations were identified in this study, however; first, the measurements were taken at different times in each country and were limited to a short period of 1 week. Second, no responsiveness test was conducted. A responsiveness test is needed because it generates more accurate thermal sensation data and helps to clarify the impact of indoor thermal quality on older people. (Yu et al. 2020). Last, people with dementia who were incapable of answering the questionnaire were excluded from the study.

Between July and September 2019 in Spain, a study investigated the thermal comfort of 623 participants in six nursing homes, including residents and non-residents (Forcada et al. 2020). As recommended in the ASHRAE 55 standard (ASHRAE 2020), the temperature sensors were placed away from windows and local heat sources at a height of 1.5 m from the floor. Participants were interviewed to examine their thermal sensations using an ASHRAE 7-point thermal sensation scale (Forcada et al. 2020). The measured temperature ranged between 23.14 and 28.46°C, and results also showed that residents did not change their clothes to adapt to thermal changes. Moreover, thermal sensations were found to be different by gender, as female residents felt warmer than male residents while wearing light clothes at higher temperatures. Thermal sensations for all were found to be dependent on the climate and outdoor conditions. For instance, the highest recommended temperature for older people, including people with dementia, in this study, which took place in a Mediterranean climate, was 28.4°C, whereas it was 26.2°C in the temperate oceanic climate and 26.3°C in the humid subtropical climate (Forcada et al. 2020). Similarly, Jin et al. (2020) confirmed that gender difference is a primary factor affecting thermal sensation, as females feel colder than males in winter.

In the UK, a year-long study of residential care homes was conducted to investigate thermal sensation in older people with and without dementia. The Abbreviated Mental Test (AMT)

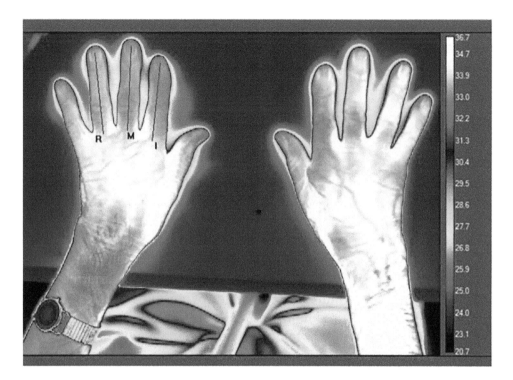

Figure 8.2 Thermal map image for both hands (Childs et al. 2020)

was used to classify whether the patient had dementia. Each patient completed a survey based on the 7-point thermal sensation scale, and people who could not answer simple questions were excluded from the study. The participants placed their hands on an imaging-long wave infrared (LWIR) detector, with indigo/blue colours representing the lowest temperatures and bright colours (white/yellow/orange) representing the highest temperatures (Figure 8.2) (Childs et al. 2020).

The measured temperature ranged between 21.4°C and 26.6°C. Results showed that most participants with dementia rated this 'cool/cold' for the thermal sensation scale, while the non-dementia residents rated this as 'neutral' or 'comfortable', which suggested that people with dementia have a lower thermal sensitivity level compared with non-demented residents. In addition, 37% of residents and 60% of non-residents exposed to operative temperatures higher than 26°C reported feeling warm or hot, respectively. The recommended temperature ranged between 23 and 27°C. This study proved that infrared thermography has potential as an assessment technology to identify thermal comfort for those with dementia who are not able to communicate or express their comfort verbally. Similarly, examination of optimal thermal perceived quality in a Scottish nursing home recommended 22.7°C as an optimal indoor temperature in the winter (Jin et al. 2020b).

Numerous studies have investigated thermal comfort in older people across the globe. The majority have suggested that older people have different thermal perceptions and that the range of comfortable temperatures varies from one country to another. This is affected by several factors such as outdoor climate, geographical location, participants' gender and experimental designs and conditions. Based on the previous discussion, the optimal temperature for people with dementia that is considered within this chapter ranges between 23.3 and 26.0°C.

Optimal Relative Humidity for People With Dementia

Relative humidity (RH) has a high impact on the health and wellbeing of people with dementia. Therefore, identifying the optimal range of relative humidity for people with dementia is vital (Serrano-Jim Enez et al. 2020). To achieve this, many studies have sought to identify this range. Some have adopted a range identified in internationally recognised publications, such as Chartered Institution of Building Services Engineers (CIBSE) Guide A (CIBSE 2021) and ASHRAE 55–2020 (ASHRAE 2020). For example, an investigation of the RH comfort range for people with dementia in a nursing home in Australia between 2015 and 2017 recommended the optimal range to be between 30 and 60% (Tartarini 2017). The same range was recommended after investigating the optimal relative humidity in 200 older people in China (Chen et al. 2019), whilst a study in seven EU countries recommended a range of 37 to 57% (Bentayeb et al. 2015)

Another study examined the optimal humidity comfort in female residents aged 83 to 94 years old in a Scottish care home during winter (Jin et al. 2020b). Measurements were taken at the skin surface alongside measurements of indoor relative humidity. Measurements were taken in four periods to cover different relative humidity levels. In the first period, no environmental intervention was applied. In the second period, the humidity was adjusted to 40% in all rooms. In the third period, there was no intervention. In the fourth period, the relative humidity was set to 50%. Interviews with participants and a questionnaire survey were conducted to examine their indoor environmental comfort. Results showed that the minimum range of RH recommended by ASHRAE (30%) was not high enough and could cause dry skin (Jin et al. 2020b). The study suggested a range from 43 to 70% as an optimal range of RH for older occupants. However, different studies have suggested a narrower range and recommended 50 to 60% as an optimal RH range when the indoor temperature ranges between 23 and 28°C (Forcada et al. 2020), with others suggesting an optimal RH value of 45% (Serrano-Jim Enez et al. 2020).

Whilst the studies reviewed do not focus exclusively on people with dementia, many of these were conducted in care homes. It has been estimated that people with dementia represent 70% of care home residents in the UK (Alzheimer's Society 2023). Thus, the studies in care homes are likely to capture the humidity preferences of people with dementia but also identify the opportunity for future studies to focus solely on people with dementia or to design a study that allows the preferences of people with dementia to be extracted from the wider sample.

Different studies have been proposed to investigate the optimal RH range for older people, including people with dementia, and some of these studies adopted internationally recognised standards as a guideline. However, other studies highlighted different humidity ranges for older people, as these standards did not consider the perceptual differences between younger and older adults. Based on what has been discussed, a range of 45 to 60% is recommended in this chapter for people with dementia.

Optimal Indoor Air Velocity for People With Dementia

A review of contemporary literature reveals a lack of studies focusing on the effect of air velocity on the comfort of people with dementia. Two studies are selected for review in this chapter which took place in nursing homes or special homes for older people but do not specify whether the subjects are people with dementia. It has been estimated, however, that people with dementia represent 70% of care home residents (Alzheimer's Society 2023). Thus, it could be assumed that the two studies reviewed capture the preferences of at least some people with dementia, although there is clearly an opportunity for further studies which focus solely on the indoor air velocity preferences of people with dementia.

A study of participants aged 70 and over measured indoor air velocity during different seasons in China. In winter, this varied from 0.00 to 0.31 m/s with a mean of 0.05 m/s, whilst in the summer, the air velocity varied from 0.01 to 1.06 m/s and between 0.00 to 0.34 m/s in mid-season. The study recommended an optimal air velocity of 0.1 m/s, as recommended by the European Standard EN15251 for older people (Jiao et al. 2020).

Another study measured the indoor thermal parameters in 25 common rooms of five nursing homes in winter in Spain. The average age of older participants was 87 years. The recorded air velocity ranged from 0.00 to 0.39 m/s, and results showed that older people have lower thermal perception, recommending an air velocity level of 0.1 m/s as advised by the Thermal Environmental Conditions for Human Occupancy ASHRAE Standard 55 (Forcada et al. 2021). The same level was also recommended in a separate study after investigating the thermal comfort of older people in China (Yu et al. 2020).

Based on this discussion, the optimal air velocity level that will be considered for people with dementia in this chapter ranges between 0.1 and 0.3 m/s

Optimal Indoor CO_2 Concentrations for People With Dementia

Elevated CO_2 concentrations have an impact on the health of people with dementia because they indicate insufficient ventilation relative to the occupancy levels. It is therefore essential to identify the optimal CO_2 concentrations during different activities of daily living (Bentayeb et al. 2015). People with dementia and their caregivers engage in indoor activities, with people with dementia having more sedentary time, which affects the CO_2 concentrations of the occupied environment (Camp et al. 2021). Some observers have identified four factors that affect the CO_2 concentrations in the room: room volume, occupancy level, type of activity that the people are doing and type of ventilation system. Activities vary from sleeping to resting, low-activity work, normal work and hard work (Adincu et al. 2020).

The sleep quality of an Alzheimer's patient was shown to qualitatively improve if CO_2 concentrations were kept below 800 ppm in the sleeping room, as indicated by fewer periods of restlessness, teeth-grinding and apnoea (Cremers et al. 2015). In addition, an investigation of the impact of CO_2 concentrations on sleep quality during the summer in China was conducted. In the study different CO_2 concentrations were applied: 800, 1800, and 3000 ppm in a chamber decorated as a bedroom (Figure 8.3).

Twelve participants were included in the study, and measurements were taken over 54 consecutive days. During the study period, participants answered questionnaires to rate their sleep quality after experiencing different CO_2 concentrations. The average sleeping time was 8 hours, the CO_2 concentrations were recorded every 30 seconds and the results showed that, first, sleep quality decreases when the CO_2 concentrations increase in the bedroom. Second, men had better sleep quality than women, and there was a significant gender difference at 800 ppm. However, the optimal range of CO_2 concentration recommended was below 800 ppm for better sleep quality for both genders (Xu et al. 2020).

Similarly, another study investigated the CO_2 concentrations in 200 older people in China and recommended the optimal range to be below 800 ppm (Chen et al. 2019). A different study investigated the air quality for people with dementia a nursing home in Australia for 1 year. During the study period, the highest CO_2 concentration measured was 1183 ppm, and 18% of the measured data exceeded 800 ppm. The authors concluded that CO_2 concentration should be maintained below 800 ppm as suggested by the Australian Standard AS 1668.2–2012 (Tartarini 2017).

Another factor that affects CO_2 concentration is the type of ventilation. McGill et al. (2015) measured the CO_2 concentration in eight newly constructed homes in the UK with two different ventilation strategies: mechanical ventilation with heat recovery (MVHR) systems and naturally ventilated dwellings. The measurements were taken in the summer and winter in bedrooms and living rooms (Table 8.1).

The results showed that naturally ventilated living rooms had a lower maximum CO_2 concentration than bedrooms with MVHR in summer, but this was higher in winter. Naturally ventilated bedrooms had a higher maximum CO_2 concentration than MVHR in both summer and winter (McGill et al. 2015). MVHR, therefore, may lead to lower CO_2 in bedrooms, without any change in window opening behaviour, and could be recommended to people with dementia.

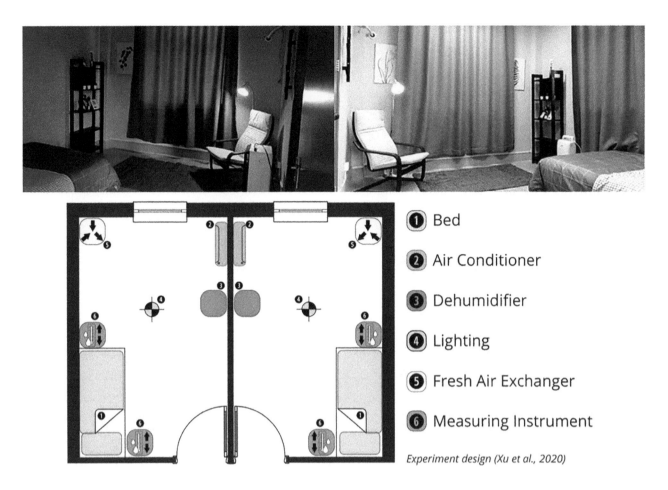

Figure 8.3: Experiment design (Xu et al. 2020)

Table 8.1 Summer and winter CO_2 measurements in naturally ventilated and MVHR dwellings (McGill et al. 2015)

Season	Ventilation system	Living room		Bedroom	
		Min (ppm)	Max (ppm)	Min (ppm)	Max (ppm)
Summer	Naturally ventilated	427	1696	405	4173
	MVHR	431	2558	412	1153
Winter	Naturally ventilated	503	3427	531	4456
	MVHR	481	1539	548	1578

In summary, the optimal CO_2 concentration for people with dementia ranges from 600 to 800 ppm, and MVHR may be best situated to achieve these levels in bedrooms rather than natural ventilation.

Summary of Optimal Indoor Environmental Quality Parameters for Caregivers of People With Dementia

CIBSE Guide A (CIBSE 2021) can reasonably be taken as a guideline for IEQ for caregivers because it is a trusted source of guidance in the UK, and it is illustrated in Table 8.2. As recommended by CIBSE Guide A, the optimal indoor temperature in winter ranges from 17 to 19°C in the kitchen and bedrooms, 22 to 23°C in living rooms and 23 to 25°C in summer, and the relative humidity is 40 to 60%, the CO_2 level below 1000 ppm, and indoor airspeed 0.1 to 0.3 m/s.

Table 8.2 Summary of IE parameters included in this review comparing measured (M) with recommended (R) values

Authors/year	Study location	Number of participants	Indoor temperature (°C)		Relative humidity (%)		CO₂ concentration (ppm)		Airspeed m/s	
			M	R	M	R	M	R	M	R
(Chen et al. 2019)	Qiqihar and Shanghai, China	200	Qiqihar: 11.4 to 14.5 ± 4.0. Shanghai: 10.0 to 11.1 ± 1.4	16 to 24	All rooms >60%, especially for toilets, with a higher range of around 80%, which might be caused by water usage	30 to 60	Qiqihar: ~1250; Shanghai: ~500	<800	NA	NA
(Tartarini et al. 2017)	Southeastern NSW, Australia	509 (322 residents and 187 non-residents)	Winter: 21.6; summer: 22	22.9 to 26; (median 23.2)	NA	NA	NA	NA	NA	NA
(Bentayeb et al. 2015)	Seven EU countries; Poland, Sweden, Greece, France, Italy, Denmark and Belgium	600	22.4 to 25.1	All countries (excl. Greece): 23.0; Greece: ~22.0	17.5 to 56.7	37 to 57	430 to 742	<1000	NA	NA
(Forcada et al. 2020)	Five nursing homes in Spain	623, including 476 residents (343 female and 133 male) and 147 non-residents (124 female and 23 male)	23.1 to 28.4	24.4	52.3 to 69.3	50.0 to 60.0	NA	NA	NA	NA
(Childs et al. 2020)		69	21.4 to 26.6	23.0 to 27.0	32 to 78	32.0 to 58.0	NA	NA	NA	NA
(Jin et al. 2020b)	UK	11 females from 83 to 94 years old	22.9	22.7	35.1	43.0 to 70.0	NA	NA	NA	NA
(Serrano-Jim Enez et al. 2020)	Spain	5	Spring: 13.4 to 22.2; winter: 13.0 to 16.2	22–26	Spring: 49.8 to 67.1; winter: 54.5 to 68.5	55	Spring: 600 to 1687; winter: 864 to 1384	<900	NA	NA

(Jiao et al. 2020)	Shanghai, China	1040 older people (479 male 561 female) aged from 70 to 95+	Winter mean: 12.8; summer mean: 29.2; mid-season mean: 20.2	Winter: 14.1 to 19.4; summer: 23.8 to 27.0: mid-season: 20.6 to 31.7	Winter mean: 49.8; summer mean: 65.3; mid-season mean: 57.7	NA	NA	Winter mean: 0.05; summer mean: 0.20; mid-season mean 0.02	NA
(Forcada et al. 2021)	Five nursing homes in Spain	881 [737 residents (559 women and 178 men), and 157 non-residents (127 women and 30 men)]	Mean 23.4	21.6 to 22.9	Mean 47.2	NA	NA	Mean: 0.22	0.1 m/s
(Xu et al. 2020)	Shanghai, China	12	24 to 27	NA	65 to 75	Three scenarios were investigated with the CO_2 measurement of 800, 1900 and 3000 ppm	<800	NA	NA

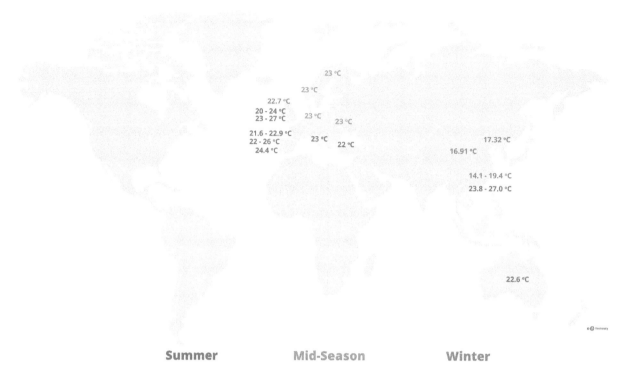

Figure 8.4 Optimal dry bulb temperature for older people based on seasons.

Source: Designed by the authors using data from Bentayeb et al. (2015); Tartarini (2017); Childs et al. (2020); Forcada et al. (2020, 2021); Jiao et al. (2020); Jin et al. (2020); Serrano-Jim Enez et al. (2020); Yang et al. (2020)

Table 8.3 Preferred IEQ parameters for people with dementia and their caregivers

IEQ parameter	People with dementia	Caregivers (CIBSE 2021)
Indoor dry bulb temperature	23.3 to 26°C	In winter, from 17 to 19°C in the kitchen and bedrooms, 22 to 23°C in living rooms. In summer, 23 to 25°C
Relative humidity	45 to 60%	40 to 60% in domestic environments and mechanical cooled, and 40 to 70% elsewhere
CO_2 concentrations	600 to 800 ppm	Below 1000 ppm
Air velocity	0.1 to 0.3 m/s	0.1 to 0.3 m/s

Several studies have been reviewed within this chapter to determine the optimal indoor environmental parameters for people with dementia and their caregivers. Table 8.2 summarises the main studies and illustrates the location and the indoor environmental quality parameters included in each one.

The recommended indoor temperatures for people with dementia in summer, mid-season (spring and autumn) and winter by location are shown in Figure 8.4 based on this review.

People from different climate zones live and adapt to their climate conditions, so they have different thermal comfort expectations, even within similar age and groups, including people with dementia. For example, the optimal temperature for people with dementia in China in winter ranges between 14.1 and 19.4°C compared with 22.7°C in the UK in the same season. People with dementia in Australia and Europe share similar optimal summer temperatures at around 22.6°C. Moreover, most of the studies focus mainly on the summer and winter seasons, and more studies are still needed in the mid-seasons. Table 8.3 summarises the optimal IEQ parameters for people with dementia and their caregivers in the UK as determined by the chapter.

The review presented in this chapter, whilst comprehensive, does have some limitations. First, across the various studies, the participants were exposed to different climate zones, so their thermal sensations were affected by their acclimatisation to different environments. Thus, the results cannot be generalised to different climate zones. Second, the clothing insulation and the metabolic rate were different between the participants in the studies involved. Finally, although the chapter illustrates the essential impact of four IEQ parameters, none of the studies considered all these parameters in combination. In the future, indoor IEQ studies should consider the combination of all IEQ parameters to include both laboratory and field studies to achieve reliable results that can be generalised for specific climate regions and adopted across the globe.

Considering the limitations of previous work, a new facility has been developed to test and evaluate the design and operation of future dementia-friendly homes, which is described within the case study chapter. Chris and Sally's House (Jais et al. 2019) offers a unique opportunity to design a dementia-friendly environment that delivers energy efficiency, thermal comfort and good indoor air quality. This is achieved by implementing a smart Internet of Things (IoT) system which includes temperature, RH and CO_2 sensors as well as door and window actuators programmed to optimise the indoor environment, quality of life and well-being of people with dementia and their caregivers. Not all windows are actuated, enabling some user control, which is known to be of benefit for thermal comfort. The IoT system monitors the position of all window actuators and so can vary the opening sizes depending on user behaviours. When taken together, this system offers a healthy, user-centred solution able to deliver an energy-efficient home for people with dementia and their caregivers. Such facilities are vital for use in future research to discover the optimum IEQ parameters desired by people with dementia and their caregivers and devise ways to deliver satisfactory IEQ with the minimum consumption of energy.

Summary

People with dementia have different perceptions of the indoor environment compared with adults without dementia (Childs et al. 2020), which might include their caregiver. However, no internationally recognised standard considers these perceptual and physiological differences between people with dementia and their caregivers in terms of IEQ and the effect on their function and wellbeing, nor their impact on building design and operation. This chapter identified the need for bespoke standards by illustrating the impact of IEQ parameters on people with dementia and their caregivers' health and wellbeing and established the optimal IEQ parameters for both people with dementia and their caregivers.

People with dementia are more vulnerable to temperature variations and prefer warmer temperatures (23 to 26°C) compared to younger healthy adults (18 to 22°C). They also prefer slightly higher relative humidity (45 to 60%) compared with their caregivers (40 to 60%). People with dementia and their caregivers share similar preferences for CO_2 concentrations and air velocity values of 600 to 800 ppm and 0.0 to 0.1 m/s, respectively.

Further work is needed to address the general lack of research which focuses on the comfort, health and wellbeing of people with dementia. Identifying the optimal IEQ parameters for people with dementia and their caregivers is the first step in designing and creating an optimal indoor environment for them. Achieving this environment will not only improve the comfort, health and wellbeing of people with dementia and their caregivers, but it will also encourage them to engage in society, make them more independent and productive and reduce the pressure on the healthcare sector.

References

Adincu, D.A., Popescu, A., and Atanasiu, M., 2020. Experimental measurements of CO2 concentrations in sleeping rooms. *IOP Conference Series: Materials Science and Engineering.* doi: 10.1088/1757-899X/997/1/012137.

Adzic, F., et al., 2022. A post-occupancy study of ventilation effectiveness from high-resolution CO2 monitoring at live theatre events to mitigate airborne transmission of SARS-CoV-2. *Building and Environment*, 223, 109392.

Alzheimer's Society, 2023. Facts for the media about dementia | Alzheimer's Society. www.alzheimers.org.uk/about-us/news-and-media/facts-media [Accessed 2 Mar 2023].

ASHRAE, 2020. ASHRAE standard 55 2020 – Thermal environmental conditions for human occupancy. www.ashrae.org/technical-resources/bookstore/standard-55-thermal-environmental-conditions-for-human-occupancy [Accessed 1 May 2021].

Bentayeb, M., et al., 2015. Indoor air quality, ventilation and respiratory health in elderly residents living in nursing homes in Europe. *European Respiratory Journal*, 45 (5), 1228–1238. doi: 10.1183/09031936.00082414.

Camp, N., et al., 2021. Technology used to recognize activities of daily living in community-dwelling older adults. *Public Health*, 18, 163. doi: 10.3390/ijerph18010163.

Chen, Y., et al., 2019. Winter indoor environment of elderly households: A case of rural regions in northeast and southeast China. *Building and Environment*, 165, 106388. doi: 10.1016/j.buildenv.2019.106388.

Childs, C., et al., 2020. Thermal sensation in older people with and without dementia living in residential care: New assessment approaches to thermal comfort using infrared thermography. *International Journal of Environmental Research and Public Health*, 17 (18), 1–23. doi: 10.3390/ijerph17186932.

CIBSE, 2021. Environmental design CIBSE guide a. www.cibse.org/knowledge/knowledge-items/detail?id=a0q20000008I79JAAS [Accessed 1 May 2021].

Cremers, M., et al., 2015. Aggregate jump and volatility risk in the cross-section of stock returns. *The Journal of Finance*, 70 (2), 577–614. doi: 10.1111/JOFI.12220.

Dodd, N., and Donatello, S., 2021. Level(s) indicator 4.1: Indoor air quality User manual: Introductory briefing, instructions and guidance (Publication version 1.1). *JRC.* https://ec.europa.eu/jrc [Accessed 28 Feb 2023].

Forcada, N., et al., 2020. Summer thermal comfort in nursing homes in the Mediterranean climate. *Energy and Buildings*, 229, 110442. doi: 10.1016/j.enbuild.2020.110442.

Forcada, N., et al., 2021. Field study on thermal comfort in nursing homes in heated environments. *Energy and Buildings*, 244, 111032. doi: 10.1016/j.enbuild.2021.111032.

Hansen, A., et al., 2022. The thermal environment of housing and its implications for the health of older people in South Australia: A mixed-methods study. doi: 10.3390/atmos13010096.

Hashiguchi, N., and Tochihara, Y., 2009. Effects of low humidity and high air velocity in a heated room on physiological responses and thermal comfort after bathing: An experimental study. *International Journal of Nursing Studies*, 46 (2), 172–180. doi: 10.1016/j.ijnurstu.2008.09.014.

Jais, C., et al., 2019. Chris and Sally's House: Adapting a home for people living with dementia (innovative practice). *Dementia and Geriatric Cognitive Disorders*, 20 (2), 770–778. doi: 10.1177/1471301219887040.

Jiao, Y., et al., 2017. Thermal comfort and adaptation of the elderly in free-running environments in Shanghai, China. *Building and Environment*, 118, 259–272. doi: 10.1016/j.buildenv.2017.03.038.

Jiao, Y., et al., 2020. Adaptive thermal comfort models for homes for older people in Shanghai, China. *Energy and Buildings*, 215, 109918. doi: 10.1016/j.enbuild.2020.109918.

Jin, H., Liu, S., and Kang, J., 2020a. Gender differences in thermal comfort on pedestrian streets in cold and transitional seasons in severe cold regions in China. *Building and Environment*, 168, 106488. doi: 10.1016/j.buildenv.2019.106488.

Jin, Y., Wang, F., Carpenter, M., Weller, R.B., et al., 2020b. The effect of indoor thermal and humidity condition on the oldest-old people's comfort and skin condition in winter. *Building and Environment*, 174, 360–1323. doi: 10.1016/j.buildenv.2020.106790.

Khan, M., et al., 2021. Thermal comfort and ventilation conditions in healthcare facilities – Part 2: Improving indoor environment quality (IEQ) through ventilation retrofitting. *Environmental Engineering and Management Journal*, 19 (11), 2059–2075.

Ma, C., et al., 2022. Monitoring the indoor environment for older people with dementia. *CLIMA 2022 Conference*. doi: 10.34641/CLIMA.2022.277.

Malki-Epshtein, L., et al., 2023. Measurement and rapid assessment of indoor air quality at mass gathering events to assess ventilation performance and reduce aerosol transmission of SARS-CoV-2. *Building Services Engineering Research and Technology*, 44 (2), 113–133. doi: 10.1177/01436244221137995.

McGill, G., Oyedele, L.O., and McAllister, K., 2015. Case study investigation of indoor air quality in mechanically ventilated and naturally ventilated UK social housing', *International Journal of Sustainable Built Environment*, 4 (1), 58–77. doi: 10.1016/j.ijsbe.2015.03.002.

Melikov, A.K., and Kaczmarczyk, J., 2012. Air movement and perceived air quality. *Building and Environment*, 47 (1), 400–409. doi: 10.1016/j.buildenv.2011.06.017.

Nunes, A.R., 2020. General and specified vulnerability to extreme temperatures among older adults. *International Journal of Environmental Health Research*, 30 (5), 515–532. doi: 10.1080/09603123.2019.1609655.

Palmer, S.J., 2020. Measuring oxygen saturation in homecare. *British Journal of Community Nursing*. MA Healthcare Ltd, 408–410. doi: 10.12968/bjcn.2020.25.8.408.

Quinn, A., and Shaman, J., 2017. Health symptoms in relation to temperature, humidity, and self-reported perceptions of climate in New York City residential environments. *International Journal of Biometeorology*. doi: 10.1007/s00484-016-1299-4.

Serrano-Jim Enez, A., et al., 2020. Indoor environmental quality in social housing with elderly occupants in Spain: Measurement results and retrofit opportunities. *Journal of Building Engineering*, 30, 101264. doi: 10.1016/j.jobe.2020.101264.

Tartarini, F., 2017. Impact of temperature and indoor environmental quality in nursing homes on thermal comfort of occupants and agitation of residents with dementia. https://ro.uow.edu.au/theses1 [Accessed 5 Mar 2021].

Tartarini, F., et al., 2017. Indoor air temperature and agitation of nursing home residents with dementia. *American Journal of Alzheimer's Disease and other Dementias*, 32 (5), 272–281. doi: 10.1177/1533317517704898.

Torfs, R., De Brouwere, K., Spruyt, M., Goelen, E., Nickmilder, M., and Bernard, A., 2008. *Exposure and Risk Assessment of Air Fresheners*. VITO, Document No2008/IMS/R/222.

Tham, S., et al., 2020. Indoor temperature and health: A global systematic review. *Public Health*, 179, 9–17. doi: 10.1016/j.puhe.2019.09.005.

Valderrama-Ulloa, C., et al., 2020. Indoor environmental quality in Latin American buildings: A systematic literature review. *Sustainability*, 12 (2), 643. doi: 10.3390/su12020643.

Venneri, A., Motta, C., Zhang, G.-W., Ferreri, F., Rossini, P., Guerra, A., . . . Corbetta, M., 2021. TMS-EEG biomarkers of amnestic mild cognitive impairment due to Alzheimer's disease: A proof-of-concept six years prospective study. *Frontiers in Aging Neuroscience*, 13. https://doi.org/10.3389/fnagi.2021.737281.

Wolkoff, P., Azuma, K., and Carrer, P., 2021. Health, work performance, and risk of infection in office-like environments: The role of indoor temperature, air humidity, and ventilation. *International Journal of Hygiene and Environmental Health*, 233. doi: 10.1016/j.ijheh.2021.113709.

World Health Organization, 2021. *Towards a Dementia Inclusive Society: WHO Toolkit for Dementia-Friendly Initiatives (DFIs)*. World Health Organization: Geneva, 67.

Xu, X., et al., 2020. Experimental study on sleep quality affected by carbon dioxide concentration. *Indoor Air*. doi: 10.1111/ina.12748.

Yang, J., et al., 2020. Effects of clothing size and air ventilation rate on cooling performance of air ventilation clothing in a warm condition. *International Journal of Occupational Safety and Ergonomics*, 2020. doi: 10.1080/10803548.2020.1762316.

Yu, J., et al., 2020. A pilot study monitoring the thermal comfort of the elderly living in nursing homes in Hefei, China, using wireless sensor networks, site measurements and a survey. *Indoor and Built Environment*, 29 (3), 449–464. doi: 10.1177/1420326X19891225.

Zhang, Y., et al., 2023. Short-term associations between warm-season ambient temperature and emergency department visits for Alzheimer's disease and related dementia in five US states. *Environmental Research*, 220, 115176. doi: 10.1016/J.ENVRES.2022.115176.

9 Post-Occupancy Evaluation

Mike Riley and Manisha Jain

Introduction

A critical factor in delivering successful building projects that support dementia sufferers in their physical environment is learning from previous successes and failures. Post-occupancy evaluation (POE) is a structured approach to the assessment of the performance of buildings and their role as enablers of creating an environment in which dementia sufferers can live well. A wide range of evaluation techniques based around quantitative and qualitative models of POE has been developed, although the degree to which they are considered effective is variable. This is particularly so when dealing with building users whose ability to provide lucid feedback on their experience is compromised by their condition. While POE has been established for many years within the UK and internationally, it has been subject to varying levels of support and acceptance. The role of POE as an effective tool for enhancing building performance and, more importantly in this context, for ensuring the best match with users' needs has been generally recognised. However, there has also been recognition that its effective implementation in the context of dementia-related facilities is inhibited by a series of barriers. There have also been differing viewpoints on the very purpose of POE. Some commentators view it as a method of gathering data to support design evolution, some see it as a method of evaluating project success and others perceive it to be a tool for evolving building functionality in use or ensuring best user experience. In the case of dementia-related facilities, all of these are relevant, but the latter point is crucial to achieving the best possible experience for building users who suffer from the condition.

Post-occupancy evaluation is a process used to assess the performance of a building or space after it has been occupied. In the context of dementia care facilities, it can be used to assess the effectiveness of the design in meeting the needs of people with dementia, as well as to identify areas for improvement.

The process of POE can be applied well for dementia care facilities and typically involves several steps, including:

- Collecting data on a variety of physical, functional and behavioural factors, such as energy usage, indoor air quality and the aspects of building/user interaction that impact the overall user experience
- Analysing the data to identify patterns and trends and to assess the effectiveness of the design in meeting the needs of people with dementia
- Sharing the results of the evaluation with stakeholders, such as the residents, family members and carers, as well as those responsible for designing and operating residential facilities in order to close the feedback loop
- Using the results of the POE to inform and improve the design of the facility, which might include making changes, such as modifying the layout, adding new features or changing the way services are delivered.

DOI: 10.1201/9781003306054-9

It is important to note that POE should be done in consultation with professionals in geriatric care, dementia care and architecture, as well as people living with dementia, their caregivers and other stakeholders. Additionally, POE should be conducted regularly.

This chapter seeks to identify some of the main approaches to POE that exist and to consider their application and efficacy in the evaluation of facilities that are specifically designed for dementia sufferers. Most of the POE models in existence attempt to evaluate building performance in the context of the physical aspects of the building, the functional requirements of its specific use and the satisfaction of end users. However, the degree to which they are perceived to succeed in this, and the extent to which they are valued by building designers and operators, are subject to considerable question (Turpin-Brooks and Viccars 2006). In particular, evaluating end-user satisfaction is challenging due to the nature of the condition and the ability to engage users in the qualitative evaluation process. As such, it requires the application of innovative techniques to gauge their satisfaction or otherwise. Some of the more functional or ergonomic aspects of design evaluation are, however, more easily assessed through direct observation of the interaction between users and their physical environment.

Context

Post-occupancy evaluation is the process of assessing a building's performance after it has been occupied and used. This type of evaluation is particularly important for buildings used for dementia care, as it allows for the identification of any issues or problems that may not have been apparent during the design and construction phases.

One of the main objectives of POE in dementia care facilities is to determine the extent to which the design and layout of the building support the well-being and safety of residents. This includes assessing ease of navigation, the effectiveness of wayfinding and the appropriateness of the physical environment for individuals with dementia.

Another important aspect of POE in dementia care facilities is to evaluate the effectiveness of any assistive technologies or safety features that have been incorporated into the building. For example, the effectiveness of electronic door locks in preventing wandering or the appropriateness of the temperature and sound controls in reducing agitation can be assessed.

POE can also be used to evaluate the effectiveness of staff training and the provision of specialised care and support for individuals with dementia. This includes assessing the effectiveness of staff in providing person-centred care and responding to the changing needs of residents.

One of the main benefits of POE in dementia care facilities is that it allows for the identification of any issues or problems that may not have been apparent during the design and construction phases. This information can then be used to make improvements to the building and the provision of care and support, which can lead to improved well-being and safety for residents, which is the ultimate goal of dementia care facilities.

It is also important to note that POE is an ongoing process and should be done regularly to identify new issues and evaluate the effectiveness of interventions over time. Additionally, involving residents, families and staff in the POE process can provide valuable insights and perspectives on the building's performance and help to ensure that any changes made are in line with the needs and preferences of the people who will be using the building. Post-occupancy evaluation is an essential tool for assessing the performance of buildings used for dementia care.

It may be taken as axiomatic that the ability of a person with dementia to experience good quality of life is supported by a well-designed environment, which provides a therapeutic and understandable environment and reduces condition distress (Landi and Smith 2019). The earlier chapters of this book have set out how this might be achieved and explored the process of engaging users to participate in a process of co-creation. This section focuses on the ways in which we might systematically evaluate the success or otherwise of such design interventions and how a process of fine-tuning might be enabled to ensure maximum user satisfaction. Designing and creating facilities for sufferers of the range of conditions that we broadly class as dementia presents specific challenges. These have been identified and discussed in previous chapters. The complexity of the condition and the various forms that residential and care facilities need to take, together with the differing needs of end users, result in the need to adopt well informed approaches to ensuring best fit between the facility and the occupier. This leans towards the adoption of a multi-skilled team approach that includes input from designers and experts in the dementia condition itself. It has been posited that POE offers a valuable role in this process; however, previous research suggests that the level of adoption is inconsistent and the perceived efficacy of the process within the care sector is subject to question. There is also a degree of scepticism regarding the extent to which existing models accurately reflect and assess the factors that influence user satisfaction within buildings within the very specific context of dementia. As a result, there are varying attitudes amongst designers and facilities operators regarding the extent to which POE can be considered an effective tool to support the enhancement of facility performance both in a general context and within the specific context of residential facilities for dementia sufferers.

It is generally acknowledged that four different living scenarios exist for older adults (Van der Voordt and Houben 1993), as follows:

- Independent housing: residents require a low level of care provision
- Intermediate facilities: residents require a medium level of care; these facilities provide catered private accommodation as well some common spaces
- Older adults' residential or care homes: residents require a high level of care. Private residents' rooms are supplemented by communal spaces as well supported care spaces
- Nursing home: residents require a very high level of care, including elderly, mentally infirm (EMI) residents.

The evaluation of such facilities in use has been attempted using various models of POE, and there are several examples of its use in the specific context of dementia. Key aspects of POE within this field include the facility's physical setting, which can be analysed by the specific case or wider context, and the timeframe of evaluation, which might be based on immediate data or a longitudinal compilation of data over time. In essence, the evaluation seeks to produce an insightful, investigative review comprising an in-depth assessment of the facility's performance, based partly on qualitative information and partly on quantitative data (Landi 2017).

What we understand as building performance lies at the overlap of physical building form or technology, user behaviour and functional need; these aspects can be difficult to assess in the case of dementia sufferers. However, a generic model of interaction is illustrated in Figure 9.1 White (1986).

Much of the focus of building performance assessment within facilities management (FM) has related to environmental psychology and evaluating building performance based on human perception. This has developed as a key subject area within FM (Becker 1990; Belcher 1997) and is considered one of the primary underpinnings of the POE process. However, the implications of such an approach in the context of dementia present very specific challenges, and a detailed understanding of the condition is important as well as an understanding of the nuances of building design. The rationale behind POE is to consider the extent to which a building meets the needs of its end users and also to recognise ways in which design, performance and fitness for purpose can be improved. If we adopt the approaches outlined in earlier sections of this book to engage with users and co-create at the design stage, it is logical to see the evaluation as a closing of this loop.

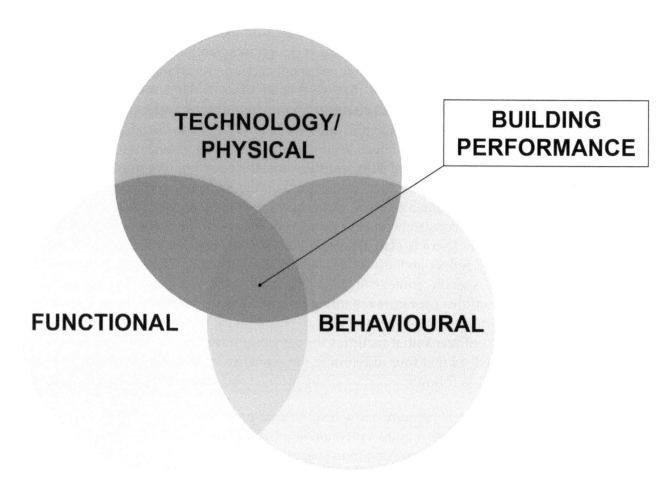

Figure 9.1 Building performance at the overlap of behaviour, function and technology (White 1986)

However, this early engagement and involvement in the design development is not always possible, and, in some cases, we are in the position of attempting to optimise pre-existing facilities or to transition between more traditional facilities and dementia-specific environments. If we see POE as a logical conclusion to the design process, with the feedback loop providing a valuable platform for lessons to be learnt from occupiers, this can be fed forward to inform future cases and allow a longitudinal knowledge base to be built (Zimmerman and Martin 2001). This approach is supported by numerous observers, including Steinke et al. (2010), who identified the importance of an effective feed-forward process to allow the benefits of lessons learnt to be maximised within a healthcare environment. This is where much of the application of POE has taken place, as illustrated in Figure 9.2.

To fully understand if a building is truly effective, feedback needs to be sought from those using it. In the case of dementia sufferers, the ability to provide such feedback is likely to be heavily compromised. However, this does not mean that it is not possible; simply that the techniques that we employ must be fit for purpose for that population set.

Historic Application and Evolution of POE

It is worthwhile to reflect on the origins and principles of POE and to translate the broad concept into a meaningful approach to ensuring the best outcomes in designing for dementia care. As we consider the origins, purpose and evolution of the process, the term 'building performance' is used to capture the various strands of the interaction between building and the degree to which the facility achieves its desired outcomes. This is at the interface between technical, functional and behavioural factors, as we noted in the earlier section of this chapter. The principles of evaluating

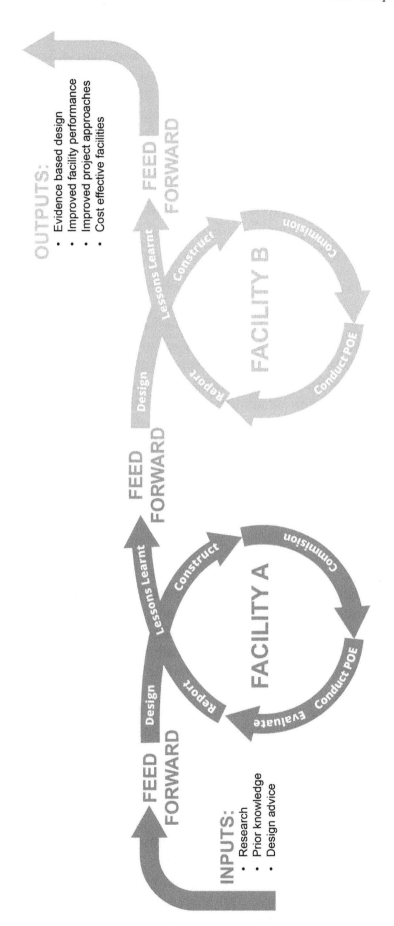

Figure 9.2 Traditional feed-forward model of POE

Source: Based on Steinke et al. 2010

the performance of buildings and the impact of this upon users and their satisfaction have been established for many years. Examples include the Burolandschaft office developments, undertaken by the Quickborner team in Germany, as early as the 1950s (de Dear et al. 1997). The term post-occupancy evaluation itself originates from the occupancy permit which was issued by building inspectors in the United States to confirm that a building was fit for occupancy once completed (Bechtel 1997). It has now gained more generic recognition as a process to systematically evaluate building performance in use. The concept originated as the application of one-off case study evaluations during its introduction in the 1960s, later evolving into a cross-sectional evaluation in the 1970s and 1980s. It came to prominence in the early 1960s, originating within architectural practice and being incorporated within RIBA's first handbook (1965). RIBA recognised that a lack of 'scientific exploration' existed into the successes and failures of construction projects. This led to the inclusion of the final stage of RIBA's 'Plan of work', Part M: feedback (RIBA 1965).

The notion of POE was formed as a direct response to problems associated with buildings within the care industry, such as mental-health hospitals and nursing homes as well as correctional facilities. Preiser (1995) states that that the performance of both existing and new buildings within the sector was considered to be having an adverse impact upon the rehabilitation of residents/inmates. Early adoption of POE was also prevalent within the residential environment as a direct result of rapid housing developments following the Second World War. Preiser and Vischer (2005) claim that a significant amount of construction of urban renewal projects in North America and much of the new town construction in Western Europe produced vast amounts of housing without really considering the needs and lifestyles of the occupants for whom they were developed. This approach caused both social and architectural issues, leading to the need for a systematic evaluation of the buildings and how they were being used (Vischer 2001). As such, the origins and intentions of POE make it logically grounded in the context of dementia facilities and their residents.

Over 150 POE techniques are available worldwide (Leaman 2003), with effectiveness dependent upon the following:

- Giving results which are easily comparable with previous studies
- The extent to which time and patience of respondents are encroached upon
- The perceived value of the process in terms of quality and content
- The degree of contextual relevance in a given situation
- The assurance of reliability, such that it gives similar results when used by different people within similar circumstances
- Importantly in the context of this work, the degree to which it addresses factors which are related to the needs, activities and goals of the building users (Preiser 2002; Leaman 2003).

The numerous existing POE methods that are available draw upon a number of techniques, which may be more or less appropriate in the circumstances associated with dementia facilities. The use of questionnaires to support quantitative approaches to analysis of data features heavily in the mainstream models. These established methods can be adopted and amended where necessary, and the potential exists to adopt entirely custom-made approaches in individual cases. Before discussing the specific approaches targeted at dementia care, it is worth briefly outlining some of the major and most prevalent models within current lexicon. Many of these focus on a particular building use class such as commercial, residential or education and may have limited scope for use in dementia care, but they are included for completeness of the discussion.

PROBE

Post-Occupancy Review of Buildings and their Engineering (PROBE) took the form of a research project which was funded by the UK government and the Builder Group. It ran from 1995 to 2002, with the results being made available to a wide audience through the Usable Buildings website. During this time, PROBE published the results of 20 POEs. The aim was to gather results from previous POEs and put them into the public domain to help designers and clients learn from them, as opposed to feeding the results back into the buildings' occupiers. The approach by PROBE was significant, as it was the first in the UK to publish its results, and as a result, it set a precedent for future publications (Cohen et al. 2001). It sought to gather both quantitative and qualitative feedback and used tools such as:

- TM22 energy survey method (for quantitative results)
- Building Use Studies occupant survey
- Interviews
- Walkthrough observations
- Review of technical issues.

The Building Use Studies Occupant Survey

Developed by Building Use Studies (BUS) Ltd alongside the Building Research Establishment (BRE), this method of benchmarking, based on a questionnaire survey, can be applied to a number of different building types. It has been in use for over 30 years and has a database available to compare results against other benchmarks. The questionnaire is applicable to buildings which are non-domestic, with permanent occupants, for example, offices, higher education buildings and schools. A small set of key performance indicators is used, which can be compared against other buildings. It tries to create a compromise between the needs of the user, data management, analysis, validity in terms of statistics and question answering (Cohen et al. 2001).

Topics that are typically included within this type of questionnaire cover such aspects as

- Physical conditions within the environment (lighting, noise, air movement, quality and temperature)
- Personal control over the physical conditions
- Management response to complaints
- Health and overall comfort
- Background and the overall quality of the building.

An issue which needs to be considered when contemplating using this method is that the questions are standardised and therefore not always relevant to a given building. This is so results can be compared to previous results gathered (Turpin-Brooks and Viccars 2006). This is a natural disadvantage to the method and effectively results in evaluating a building against somebody else's previously defined needs as opposed to those of current users or occupiers. This is particularly limiting in the case of evaluating purpose-designed facilities for dementia sufferers.

Construction Industry Council Design Quality Indicators

The Construction Industry Council Design Quality Indictors (CIC DQIs) is a questionnaire used for POE designed to suit a diverse range of people at almost any stage of the life cycle of a building. Developed by the University of Sussex alongside the Construction Industry Council, the nature of the questionnaire means that it can be used to gather feedback from anybody who is affected by the building, such as clients, occupiers, local residents and even passers-by.

The self-completion questionnaire consists of approximately 100 questions, with answers selected from a 6-point scale. The structure of the questionnaire is broken down into three main sections in terms of

- Functionality (in terms of use access and space)
- Build quality (in terms of performance, engineering systems and construction)
- Impact (in terms of form and materials, internal environment, urban and social integration, character and inspiration) (Usable Buildings website 2009).

This again is heavily compromised by the ability of dementia sufferers to engage in a meaningful and consistent way with such an extensive and heavily structured approach.

Overall Liking Score

The Overall Liking Score (OLS) is used to obtain feedback from occupants regarding what they like about a building and aspects which they find successful, as well as any concerns they may have. ABS Consulting, in collaboration with the University of Manchester Institute of Science and Technology (UMIST), developed the approach to address the three aspects of sustainable development: economic, environmental and social. This is often referred to as the triple bottom line. OLS has been used numerous times within the UK, of which many have been within the care sector as part of POE.

The flexibility and simplicity of this approach, together with its qualitative nature, make a potentially useful element of evaluation in the case of dementia-related facilities. Its greatest value comes when combined with other observational and quantitative components of a wider evaluation approach.

Soft Landings

Soft landings is a process which considers the lifecycle of a project, committing time and resources into briefing, pre-handover and the long term operation of the facility. The Soft Landings Framework is published jointly by BSRIA and the Usable Building Trust and is intended to provide a basis for managed transition of buildings from construction to use (BSRIA 2014). Projects undertaken using this framework feature a series of interlinked stages that are intended to bridge the potential schism between design, construction and occupation. These can be summarised as follows:

Stage 1: Inception and Briefing
Stage 2: Design Development
Stage 3: Pre-Handover
Stage 4: Initial Aftercare
Stage 5: Extended Aftercare.

(BSRIA 2014)

The soft landings concept seeks to ensure that designers and contractors are responsible for considering the whole-life performance of buildings rather than simply their creation. This model is intended to act as a 'golden thread' linking procurement, design, delivery and FM, with POE featuring as an integral part of the entire process (Rowland 2012).

However, the project delivery focus of this model means that, whilst potentially very valuable in dementia projects, the specificity of ensuring well-designed environments may be less prominent than overall project success in terms of delivery and handover factors.

Living Lab

One approach that is specific to dementia settings and which has liberated successful results is the living lab; this attempts to enhance the participatory element of the evaluation, focusing on user-led co-creation. This was discussed in the earlier chapter dealing with engagement with the dementia community. It derives from the work of the Innovate Dementia project (Woods et al. 2013) in which people living with dementia were actively and demonstrably involved in developing the evaluation approach, including validation of questionnaires and interview questions that were used to gather the qualitative information. This has been applied to design schemes in practice and grounded within an architectural context by applying the process of POE in three parts: 'thinking, making and living' (Landi 2017).

The three phases are as follows:

First, the 'Thinking' phase, which seeks to investigate the conceptual design process, including the care model applied in any specific case. This involves literature review relating to the chosen model of care, any linked design publications and any existing feedback relating to the selected facility. It also features qualitative semi-structured interviews and questionnaires to gather opinion and perceptions of the facility in use from managers and architects/designers. In addition, the physical elements of the environment are analysed.

This is followed by the 'Making' phase, which is intended to review and describe the actual physical setting based on site survey and fieldwork. In the case studies effected by Landi et al., video and photographic archives were generated to evidence the interactions between users and the physical environment. The purpose of this phase is to identify the relationship between the building and its physical environment, the care context and the experience of residents or occupiers. Crucially, this phase identifies and evaluates care-related activities and programmes and their spatial implications. As such, it is essential that input is provided from appropriately qualified care experts as well as building designers. Following the fieldwork and data gathering process the facility is analysed through available design tools such as plans, sections, schemes and configurations.

The final stage is the 'Living' phase, which aims to identify, describe and document the interactions within the facility that is being evaluated using several key activities. The first of these is behavioural mapping, which observes and interprets residents' daily activities over a specific observation period; typically, this is between 2 and 4 hours but can be tailored to suit individual cases. The second is the conducting of semi-structured, qualitative interviews and semi-structured questionnaires with a cross-section of residents, care givers and other relevant stakeholders. These are then triangulated with the physical assessments noted in the 'Making' phase.

A living lab is a term used to describe a real-world environment that is used to test and evaluate new products, services and technologies. In the context of architectural design evaluation, a living lab refers to a building or space that is used to test and evaluate new design concepts, materials and technologies. The goal is to create an environment that simulates real-world conditions as closely as possible in order to test and evaluate the effectiveness of the design concepts in a real-world setting.

One of the main benefits of using a living lab to support architectural design evaluation is that it allows designers and researchers to observe how people interact with the space and to collect data on the effectiveness of the design. This can include data on matters like energy efficiency, indoor air quality and the overall user experience.

Living labs can be used to evaluate design concepts for a wide range of building types, including residential, commercial and public buildings. The type of building will depend on the research question and the design concept being evaluated.

In the context of dementia care, living labs can be used to evaluate design concepts that are intended to support people with dementia. This can include evaluating design concepts for buildings and spaces that are intended to be safe, accessible and supportive for people with dementia. This can include evaluating the effectiveness of features such as lighting, colour and contrast, as well as the effectiveness of the floor plan and the overall user experience.

It is important to note that living labs should be designed and operated in a way that is inclusive and ethical. The process should involve individuals living with dementia, their caregivers and other stakeholders to ensure that the design concepts are tailored to their needs and preferences.

In summary, living labs are real-world environments that are used to test and evaluate new design concepts, materials and technologies. They provide a valuable opportunity to evaluate design concepts in a real-world setting and to collect data on the effectiveness of the design. In the context of dementia care, living labs can be used to evaluate design concepts that are intended to support people with dementia and to inform and improve the design of buildings and spaces.

Characteristics of POE Models and Their Application

Given the complexity of the interaction between dementia sufferers and their physical environments, it is vital that careful consideration be given when deciding an appropriate POE technique and model. While there are numerous tools and established approaches to POE available as outlined in the previous section, it is definitely the case that one size does not fit all. Given the potential challenges associated with gauging opinions and perceptions of residents, innovative approaches may need to be explored.

Use of Surveys and Questionnaires

The use of questionnaires can be beneficial in collecting data for the POE process, but it also encourages structured interaction with residents. POE questionnaires typically consider key physical and environmental dimensions of the facility and seek to quantify user perceptions of success. They often focus on the internal environmental factors that impact users and the ability to experience a satisfactory interaction with the building and its spaces. The impact of IEQ on the experience of dementia sufferers was discussed in an earlier chapter. The more established, generic models will tend to seek opinion on factors such as:

- Air quality
- Thermal control
- Spatial comfort
- Privacy
- Lighting comfort
- Noise control
- Building control.

Distribution of questionnaires in care settings such as dementia facilities is often supported by carers or some form of amanuensis but is clearly restricted to residents within certain levels of the condition. The adoption of supplementary questionnaires for carers and staff can be influential in assessing the experience of residents if appropriately crafted. The questionnaire is also seen, traditionally, as the least intrusive and disruptive method of gathering information. The principal advantage of this approach is that a large sample can be targeted, which supports the reliability of the results obtained, although this may be less the case in dementia care environments, where users may be low in number. It is recommended, as good practice, that when developing a questionnaire, it should be kept as simple as possible, and pilot questionnaires should be tested before wider application takes place. This forms a part of the potential co-creation approach to developing evaluations as described earlier.

There are several established questionnaire based models already in use for POE across the care sector and more widely in a number of industries. These include:

- The Building Use Studies Occupant Survey
- The Office Productivity Network (OPN) Survey
- Construction Industry Council Design Quality Indicators
- Healthcare Design Quality Assessment Method
- Overall Liking Score
- Building In Use (BIU)
- BRE – relating to sick building syndrome
- Living lab.

The principal mechanism by which these are analysed is through the use of quantitative analytical tools. However, there are also several qualitative approaches to POE data gathering, some of which are described in the following.

Use of Focus Groups and Workshops

Focus groups and workshops provide an arena for a sample to meet for in-depth discussion to extract feedback. This method can be advantageous in terms collecting information from a small number of building users in a short period of time. The same tools that are utilised in the engagement with the design process might usefully be deployed in evaluation. For example, the application of living lab approaches and photo cue cards to generate responses and discussion was described in an earlier chapter.

Interviews

Structured and semi-structured interviews are traditionally seen as effective ways of collecting invaluable feedback directly from users and staff. In order for interviews to be meaningful, a flexible approach is required in order to engage fully with dementia sufferers, but the adoption of a simple checklist of target issues may assist in extracting the most relevant issues.

The use of interviews allows the interviewer to probe areas and remove ambiguity in questions being asked. However, it is particularly important that, in the dementia setting, care is taken to ensure that bias is not incorporated into the interview. A way of overcoming this issue would be to bring in an impartial third party in the same way that might be considered for focus groups (Patton 1987).

Direct Observation

This method sees care facility operators and/or design team members evaluating through observation. As well as giving direct, observational feedback, the facility can also be triangulated and rated against the outcomes of questionnaires, focus groups or POE techniques.

This method can also gather both qualitative and quantitative results if approached properly. However, the methodology needs meticulous application – for instance, repeating observations at different periods of the day. Unless a structured methodology is developed and kept to, comparisons can also be difficult to obtain. Finch (1999) encourages observation as a technique for POE through empathetic design. This sees direct expert observation of users and feeding back through a report incorporating their innate understanding of building usage.

Whitemyer (2006) reinforced this view in his article 'Anthropology in Design', stating that observation offers a more accurate account of how people act within their given environments.

Such observation not only discovers activities that are carried out but also what additional interactions take place at the same time.

Therapeutic Environment Screening

One approach to systematic evaluation that is specific to residential care is the Therapeutic Environment Screening Survey for Nursing Homes (TESS-NH). This was commissioned by the National Institute on Aging (NIA) and embeds within it the Special Care Unit Environmental Quality Scale (SCUEQS). It features a set of tools and procedures to collect and evaluate data, one of which focuses specifically on the physical environment. Because it is aimed specifically at nursing home environments and facilities that house sufferers of dementia, it is a tailored and valuable evaluation tool.

Based on direct observation of dementia sufferers within their physical environment, it works on the basis of mapping specific indicators of sensory and spatial properties (Lawton et al. 1984; Weisman 1981). It also features the notion of 'consensus goals' of the physical environment and the facility overall. These are identified as:

- provision of safety, security and physical health
- orientation
- provision of privacy, control and autonomy
- stimulation (both positive and negative)
- enhancement of socialisation (social milieu)
- personalisation/familiarity.

In order to capture these consensus goals, 84 discrete attributes are assessed, together with a further global item. These attributes are set within 13 'domains', which are:

- exit control, which facilitates safer circulation and wandering
- maintenance, which reduces hazards and improves aesthetics
- cleanliness, which reduces infection risk and increases satisfaction
- safety in the environment, which reduces risk of injury, trips and falls
- orientation and cueing, which reduces confusion
- privacy, which improves satisfaction and reduces agitation
- unit autonomy, which reduces interruption and noise, enhancing mood
- outdoor access, which reduces agitation and improves vitamin D levels
- lighting, which can reduce depression and improves wayfinding
- noise, which improves sleep and ability to focus
- visual/tactile stimulation, which supports the development of a 'homelike' environment
- space/seating, which improves circulation, reduces confusion and agitation and enhances social interaction
- familiarity/homelikeness, which reduce agitation and improve functionality.

(Day et al. 2000; Netten 1989; Cruise et al. 1998; Cohen and Weisman 1991; Lawton et al. 1984)

Behaviour Mapping

One method that can be used to examine a person with dementia's engagement within a space is through observations made with behaviour mapping. This is also known as place-centred behaviour mapping. It was formulated from the behaviour setting theory which posited that the environment acts as a setting for different behaviours to be developed and organised and demonstrates the interaction between people and their environment. As such, behaviour mapping utilises this and observes patterns of behaviours within a space and time at set intervals (Schwarz et al. 2004). Observations can also be made using architectural drawings to create a visual representation of the location and behaviour which can be considered beneficial for POE (Smith et al. 2011). While behaviour mapping is typically done by hand and accompanied by direct observations, perhaps there is scope for extending this to confidential video recordings to examine behaviours and interactions at a deeper level.

Research has highlighted that this particular method of observations is well suited for evaluating engagement from those with dementia. One study in the United States used this tool to examine patterns of behaviours among residents with Alzheimer's disease and staff across five residential-style care centres that were specifically designed for those with dementia. The activity categories that were observed included sitting, activities of daily living, light housekeeping, leisure, walking, watching, behavioural and psychological symptoms and other miscellaneous activities. The author's key finding from behaviour mapping indicated that across all locations, leisure was the most frequently observed activity. They discussed the fact that another difference noted was between a 12-resident and a 20-resident house design, whereby the latter had more activities held within the house rather than the communal spaces. Comparatively, they found that the former held more activities in the communal spaces. This demonstrated how the residents' behaviour was shaped by the house design, and this can further influence future design of dementia settings and how residents and staff engage within the space and organise activities.

Another study in Australia used behaviour mapping pre- and post-POE to examine engagement in residents who moved from a residential care home to purpose-built dementia care cottages (Smith et al. 2011). The authors used behaviour mapping techniques with architectural drawings to highlight engagement from residents and positive and negative or neutral affect when engaged, plus staff engagement and activities, in conjunction with other environmental assessments. Overall, the behaviour maps showed increased engagement in all dementia cottages within the first 3–4 months after the move, and this further increased after staff-training workshops. It was highlighted that the features of the dementia cottage design, such as provisions for wandering, homestyle kitchen and hidden institutional stimuli, allowed for this increased engagement and lower distress amongst the residents. It was further found that this most benefited those with moderate-to-severe BPSD, who had the largest mean difference between baseline and post staff-training workshop. These findings demonstrate that behaviour mapping is indeed a useful tool for observing and subsequently evaluating behaviours of those with dementia in care settings, and more specifically in purpose-built dementia houses.

Behaviour mapping appears to be a beneficial tool that can be used to assess a person with dementia's experiences within a place and understand how home design can influence patterns of behaviour. Nevertheless, observations made with behaviour mapping may be influenced by the subjectivity of the observer. Therefore, it may be required that specific behaviours be operationalised correctly to ensure inter-rater reliability.

Behaviour mapping is a method used to observe and document the behaviour of individuals with dementia in a specific environment, such as a building or care facility. It involves creating a map or diagram of the physical space and then noting the behaviour of the individuals with dementia as they move through the space. This information can then be used to identify areas where the environment may be contributing to challenging behaviour, such as confusion, agitation or wandering. By making changes to the physical environment, such as adding clear signage or reducing clutter, the care facility can improve the well-being and safety of individuals with dementia. Additionally, behaviour mapping can also be used to identify and address staff-related issues that may be contributing to challenging behaviour.

The process of behaviour mapping for evaluating building design for dementia care typically involves the following steps:

- Defining the goals and objectives of the mapping study: This includes identifying the specific behaviours that will be observed and the areas of the building that will be evaluated
- Preparing the mapping materials: This includes creating a detailed map or diagram of the building, and any necessary forms or tools for recording the observations
- Conducting the observations: A team of trained observers, such as staff members or researchers, will systematically observe and document the behaviour of individuals with dementia as they move through the building
- Analysing the data: The observations are then analysed to identify patterns and trends in the behaviour of individuals with dementia
- Identifying areas for improvement: Based on the observations and analysis, specific areas of the building and environment that may be contributing to challenging behaviour are identified
- Developing an action plan: A plan is developed to address the identified issues, such as making changes to the physical environment or addressing staff-related issues
- Implementing the changes and re-evaluating: The changes are made and the building is re-evaluated to determine the effectiveness of the interventions in improving the well-being and safety of individuals with dementia.

It is important to note that behaviour mapping is an ongoing process and should be done regularly to identify new issues and evaluate the effectiveness of interventions over time.

The factors that are typically evaluated during behaviour mapping for dementia facility design are the physical environment, the social and emotional environment, behavioural patterns, cognitive abilities, communication and personal preferences. Consideration of the physical environment might include the layout and design of the space, including circulation patterns, lighting and the use of colour and contrast. This is evaluated to identify potential hazards, such as tripping hazards or poor lighting, and to assess how easy it is for people with dementia to navigate the space. Consideration of the social and emotional environment might include the interactions between people with dementia and their caregivers, as well as the overall atmosphere of the space. This is evaluated to identify areas where people with dementia may feel isolated, confused or agitated and to assess how well the space supports social interactions and engagement. Consideration of behavioural patterns might include the specific behaviours that people with dementia exhibit, such as wandering, agitation or repetitive behaviours. These are evaluated to identify patterns that may be triggered by specific features of the environment, such as noise levels, lighting or the presence of certain objects. Consideration of cognitive abilities includes consideration of the level of cognitive impairment of the people with dementia, as well as the specific cognitive abilities that are affected by the condition. These are evaluated to identify areas where people with dementia may have difficulty, such as with memory, language or spatial awareness, and to assess how well the environment supports their cognitive abilities. Consideration of communication includes the ways in which people with dementia communicate and understand language, as well as the ways in which caregivers communicate with them. These are evaluated to identify areas where people with dementia may have difficulty understanding or expressing themselves and to assess how well the environment supports communication. Finally, consideration of personal preferences includes the individual's personal preferences, such as their likes, dislikes and routines. These are evaluated to identify ways to personalise the environment and to make it more comfortable and familiar for the individual.

Behaviour mapping is a comprehensive approach that takes into account the diverse needs of people with dementia and helps to create an environment that is safe, comfortable and supportive for all. It is important to involve professionals in geriatric care, dementia care and architecture to conduct behaviour mapping and the design of the facility.

Considerations to be Made in Conducting POE

It is considered that greater accuracy is gained when combining a number of techniques within a chosen POE method. This allows feedback to be gained during one and explored further during another. With this in mind, Jaunzens et al. (2002) feel that when considering supporting techniques, it is essential that:

- It is holistic, looking at the relationship between the physical environment, provision of facilities and organisational attitudes
- Both cause and effect of issues are explored
- The results are verified subjectively, through either objective measurements or balanced subjective opinions from a broad range of stakeholders
- All parties are included, assessing perceptions against reality
- The methodology is transparent so that results can be interpreted with assurance, limitations can be understood and can be repeated if benchmarking and tracking is to be carried out over a period of time.

Each organisation will approach POE differently, dependent upon their objectives and the availability of both time and resources. Considering these factors, Langston and Ding (2001) offer a breakdown in terms of the level of effort an organisation allocates to the process, categorised as *indicative*, *investigative* and *diagnostic*.

Steinke et al. (2010) developed upon the work of Amaratunga and Baldry (2000) to propose the use of a balanced scorecard, directed specifically at building performance evaluation (BPE) in healthcare facilities. This is referred to as the BPE scorecard and encompasses four performance dimensions as follows:

- Service: How can facilities enhance client experience in healthcare?
- Functional: How can facilities enhance the quality of the work environment?
- Physical: How can facilities achieve and exceed current building standards?
- Financial: How can facilities add value financially and improve operational efficiency?

The methodology that was proposed by Steinke et al. (2010) was aimed specifically at public-sector healthcare facilities and involves a ten-stage approach that evolves through the design, delivery and use of a building or facility as follows:

In the mental health sector, the conditions for the occupiers need to be assessed from various perspectives in order to ensure that patients, staff and visitors are able to make the most of the services the building offers. Orstein et al. (2009) evaluated the performance of a psychiatric hospital in Brazil as it was being refurbished to ensure that a more pleasant environment would emerge, which would in turn promote well-being and health among its users. This research used various tools in order to gain a better perspective of the various groups of users by conducting walkthroughs, interviews with stakeholders, focus groups and behavioural maps. In their concluding remarks, the researchers stated that not only was POE essential in the improvement of psychiatric hospitals but that the implementation of pre-design evaluation was also important so that adequate time is spent in the planning process.

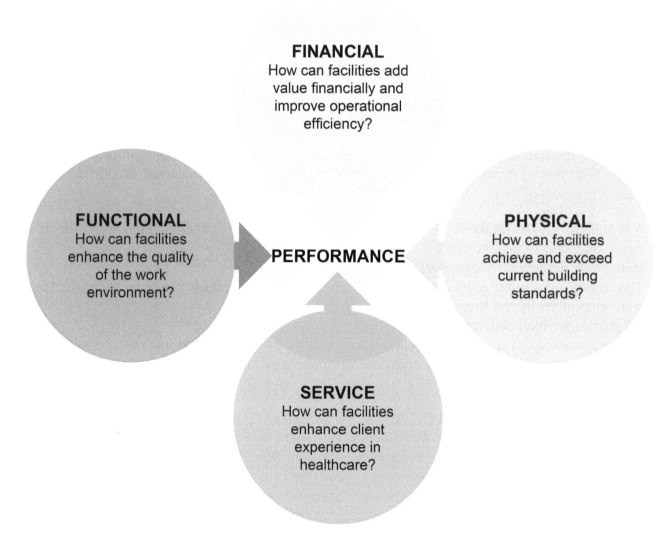

Figure 9.3 Building performance balanced scorecard (Steinke et al. 2010)

Table 9.1 Stages of building performance evaluation model (Steinke et al. 2010)

Project phase	Stage of model	Activity
Direction setting	**Stage 1**	Identify project/facility with associated project 'champions' at provincial government and organisational board level.
	Stage 2	'Champions' liaises with organisational executive to identify challenges and goals for the project.
	Stage 3	'Champions' nominate core team to effect evaluation project This team to comprise key stakeholder representatives including designers, project managers, contractors, facilities managers, client representatives and end users.
Scorecard creation	**Stage 4**	Scorecard created to encompass:
		Current challenges to be addressed
		Key objectives to respond to challenges and opportunities Review of existing research and published literature Collection of objectives into four performance dimensions Development of propositions for each objective Determination of performance indicators for each objective
		Establishment of targets and interim milestones for each objective Establishment of data collection methods
		Establishment of data analysis methods
		Approval of plan at executive level
	Stage 5	Ethical approval achieved for study

Project phase	Stage of model	Activity
Design and construction	**Stage 6**	Continual reference to scorecard during design and construction of facility
Evaluation and lessons learned	**Stage 7**	Evaluation team conduct evaluation of facility
	Stage 8	Analysis and interpretation of data from evaluation
	Stage 9	Peer review of initial findings
Report and documentation	**Stage 10**	Final report to executive/board with knowledge sharing through publication and presentation of findings

It is widely recognised that there are many other factors beyond the quality of the space which play a role in shaping user experience, although these are not necessarily reflected within existing POE models.

There are two distinct approaches available to evaluate building performance: quantitative and qualitative. Each of these form the bases of various established POE models, each with their own advantages and disadvantages.

Qualitative Methods

While there are several different quantitative methods available, there are only a handful of building performance methods which take into account less quantifiable criteria. Preiser and Schramm (2002) identified that there are certain circumstances, often stemming from cultural differences, in which qualitative methods are more appropriate. This is because the evaluator is able to engage in interactive communication to help gather the data needed. In the setting of dementia care, understanding these qualitative factors is vital to ensuring the creation and maintenance of an environment that is conducive to living well.

Depending on the breadth of information sought, qualitative methods can serve as a general evaluation tool to aid the evaluator to familiarise themselves with the building in question. In these situations, the evaluator speaks to the building users and observes what they do and how they behave within the built environment (Preiser and Schramm 2002). Preiser and Vischer (2005) developed the Building Performance Evaluation, which focuses on the qualitative assessment of performance. BPE looks at the building's life cycle and delivery through a list of nine performance criteria in order of priority which include health, safety, security, function, efficiency, work flow, psychological and social and cultural performance (Preiser and Schramm 2002). The methods of acquiring this data include direct observation, still photography and survey questionnaires of building users as well as interviews (Preiser and Wang 2008). Therefore, performance can be assessed through expert observation and consumer feedback.

User Perceptions of Building Performance and User Satisfaction

A building should be able to perform functions in a way that ensures occupant satisfaction – that is, the provision of the facilities needs to support the operations carried out by the users of that facility (Khalil and Nawawi 2009). The way in which an individual perceives his or her environment is dependent on emotive as well as perceptive-cognitive aspects. The emotive response to the building will determine how the user treats it – that is, do they find it pleasant or unpleasant (Gonzalez et al. 1997, 69)? On the other hand, there is the perceptive-cognitive aspect which accounts for an individual's awareness of the building's physical properties such as noise, air, illumination and temperature (Gonzalez et al. 1997). The perspective of building users is important to help researchers understand how intelligently designed buildings are hoped to function better for users (Vischer 2009).

User perceptions are important, as well as the extent to which the user can interact with actual performance of the building. Bordass et al. (2001) found themes from PROBE studies which had been identified as being success factors in building – one of them being that users like buildings that can respond to their activities. Good outcomes arise when the building, its systems and its management are matched accordingly to the requirements of the users, the brief and the site (Bordass et al. 2001). Good designs therefore allow the user to take action in an attempt to rectify a problem, or the building needs to have a management team which responds quickly to performance issues.

Summary

A wide range of POE techniques is available to assess building and facility performance. Many of these have been applied, with varying levels of success, in the context of dementia care. The very specific characteristics of dementia care environments and the needs of their residents make it essential that appropriate evaluation be effected when developing and evolving design. The qualitative factors that impact the experience of users must be fully appraised as well as the more metric-based quantitative measures. For this reason, the versions of POE that incorporate both quantitative and qualitative consideration are most effective in delivering meaningful evaluations of dementia-related environments. In order to derive the best possible benefit and outcomes from the evaluation, it is important to ensure that there is input from designers, clinicians and care professionals in designing and effecting the POE process. Similarly it is crucial to ensure that appropriate feedback loops are embedded so that the process is fully applied and outcomes reviewed.

References

Amatunga, D., and Baldry, D., 2000. Assessment of facilities management performance in higher education properties. *Facilities*, 18 (7/8), 293–301.

Bechtel, R., 1997. *Environment and Behavior: An Introduction*. Sage: Thousand Oaks, CA.

Becker, F., 1990. *The Total Workplace*. Van Nostrand Reinhold: New York.

Belcher, R., 1997. Corporate objectives, facilities measurement and use: A university model. RICS Cobra Conference, Portsmouth, RICS Books.

Bordass, B., Leaman, A., and Ruyssevelt, P., 2001. Assessing building performance in use 5: Conclusions and implications. *Building Research & Information*, 29 (2), 144–157.

BRIA, 2014. The soft landings framework for better briefing, design, handover and building performance in use (Mar). BSRIA BG 54/2014. ISBN 978 0860.

Cohen, R., Standeven, M., Bordass, B., and Leaman, A., 2001. Assessing building performance in use 1: The PROBE process. *Building Research & Information*, 29 (2), 85–102.

Cohen, U., and Weisman, G., 1991. *Holding on to Home*. Johns Hopkins University Press: Baltimore.

Cruise, P.A., Schnelle, J.F., Alessi, C.A., Simmons, S.F., and Ouslander, J.G., 1998. The nighttime environment and incontinence care practices in nursing home residents. *Journal of the American Geriatrics Society*, 46, 181–186.

Day, K., Carreon, D., and Stump, C., 2000. The therapeutic design of environments for people with dementia: A review of empirical research. *The Gerontologist* 40: 397–416.

de Dear, R., Brager, G., Cooper, D., 1997. *Developing an Adaptive Model of Thermal Comfort and Preference*. ASHRAE FINAL REPORT RP- 884, Macquarie Research Ltd., Macquarie University: Sydney, NSW.

Finch, E., 1999. Empathetic design and post-occupancy evaluation. *Facilities*, 17 (11), 431–435.

Gonzalez, M., Fernandez, C., and Cameselle, J., 1997. Empirical validation of a model of user satisfaction with buildings and their environments as workplaces. *Journal of Environmental Psychology*, 17 (1), 69–74.

Jaunzens, D., Cohen, R., Watson, M., and Picton, E., 2002. Post occupancy evaluation; A simple method for the early stages of occupancy. www.usablebuildings.co.uk/fp/OutputFiles/PdfFiles/FR4p1POEFYCIBSEpaperOct02.pdf [Accessed 11 Jan 2022].

Khalil, N., and Nawawi, A., 2009. Performance analysis of government and public buildings via post occupancy evaluation. *Asian Social Science,* 4 (9), 103–111.

Landi, D., 2017. Towards new architectural and urban typologies: Thinking, making and living as a post occupancy evaluation method. *Conscious Cities Journal*, 3. www.ccities.org/towards-new-architectural-urban-typologies-thinking-making-living-post-occupancy-evaluation-method/ [Accessed 7 Jan 2023].

Landi, D., and Smith, G., 2019. The implications of a new paradigm of care on the built environment. The Humanitas© Deventer model: Innovative practice. *Dementia: The International Journal of Social Research and Practice*, 1–8. https://doi.org/10.1177/1471301219845480.

Langston, C., and Ding, G., 2001. *Sustainable Practices in the Built Environment*. Butterworth Heinemann: Oxford.

Lawton, M.P., Fulcomer, M., and Kleban, M., 1984. Architecture for the mentally impaired elderly. *Environment and Behavior*, 16, 730–757.

Leaman, A., 2003. Post occupancy evaluation. Paper presented at Gaia Research Sustainable Construction Continuing Professional Development Seminars.

Netten, A., 1989. The effect of design of residential homes in creating dependency among confused elderly residents: A study of elderly demented residents and their ability to find their way around homes for the elderly. *International Journal of Geriatric Psychiatry*, 4, 143–153.

Ornstein, S., Moreira, N., Ono, R., França, A., and Nogueira, A., 2009. Improving the quality of school facilities through building performance assessment: Educational reform and school building quality in São Paulo, Brazil. *Journal of Educational Administration*, 47 (3), 350–367.

Patton, M.Q., 1987. *How to Use Qualitative Methods in Evaluation*. Sage: Newbury Park, CA.

Preiser, W., 1995. Post-occupancy evaluation: How to make buildings work better. *Facilities*, 13 (11), 19–28.

Preiser, W., 2002. *Learning from Our Buildings: A State of the Practice Summary of Post Occupancy Evaluation*. National Academy Press: Washington, DC.

Preiser, W., and Schramm, U., 2002. Intelligent office building performance evaluation. *Facilities*, 20 (7/8), 279–287.

Preiser, W., and Vischer, J., 2005. *Assessing Building Performance*. Elsevier, Butterworth Heinemann: Oxford.

RIBA, 1965. *Handbook of Architectural Practice and Management*. RIBA Publications: London.

Preiser, W., and Wang, X., 2008. Quantitative (GIS) and qualitative (BPE) assessments of library performance. *International Journal of Architectural Research*, 2 (1), 212–231.

Riley, M., Wordsworth, P., et al., 1995. *Post-Occupancy Evaluation: A Pragmatic Framework for Building Surveyors. Focus for Building Surveying Research*. RICS Books: Salford.

Rowland, D., 2012. *Government Soft Landings and the Benefits of BIM to FM*. ThinkBIM, Leeds Metropolitan University: Leeds, UK.

Schwarz, B., Chaudhury, H., and Tofle, R.B., 2004. Effect of design interventions on a dementia care setting. *American Journal of Alzheimer's Disease and Other Dementias*, 19 (3), 172–176.

Smith, J.C., Nielson, K.A., Woodard, J.L., Seidenberg, M., Verber, M.D., Durgerian, S., . . . Rao, S.M., 2011. Does physical activity influence semantic memory activation in amnestic mild cognitive impairment? *Psychiatry Research*, 193 (1): 60–62. https://doi.org/10.1016/j.pscychresns.2011.04.001. Epub 2011 May 23. PMID: 21601432; PMCID: PMC3105157.

Steinke, C., Webster, L., and Fontaine, M., 2010. Evaluating building performance in healthcare: An organizational perspective. *Health Environments Research & Design Journal*, 3 (2), 63–83.

Turpin-Brooks, S., and Viccars, G., 2006. The development of robust methods of post occupancy evaluation. *Facilities*, 24 (5/6), 177–196.

Usable Building, 2009. *For Feedback and Review*. Usable Building. www.usablebuildings.co.uk/.

Van der Voordt, D.J.M., and Houben, P.P.J., 1993. New combinations of housing and care for the elderly in the Netherlands. *Netherlands Journal of Housing and Environmental Research*, 8 (4), 301–325.

Vischer, J.C., 2001. Post occupancy evaluation: A multi-facetted tool for building improvement. *Learning from Our Buildings: A State of the Practice Summary of Post-Occupancy Evaluation (Federal Facilities Council)*. National Academies Press: Washington, DC.

Vischer, J.C., 2009. Applying knowledge on building performance: From evidence to intelligence. *Intelligent Buildings International*, 1, 239–248.

Weisman, G.D., 1981. Modelling environment-behavior systems: A brief note. *Journal of Man-Environment Relations*, 1, 82–87.

White, E., 1986. Post-occupancy evaluation. *CEFP Journal*, 24 (6), 19–22.

Whitemyer, D., 2006. Anthropology in design. www.designmatters.net/pdfs/0406/0406anthropology.pdf [Accessed 3 July 2008].

Woods, L., Pendleton, J., Smith, G., and Parker, D., 2013. *Innovative Dementia Baseline Report: Shaping the Future for People with Dementia*. Liverpool John Moores University Press: Liverpool, England.

Zimmerman, A., and Martin, M., 2001. Post-occupancy evaluation: Benefits and barriers. *Building Research and Information*, 29 (2), 16.

10 Design Guidance

Bill Halsall

Introduction

Building on the research base of the previous chapters and on the experience of the demonstration project – Chris and Sally's House – as well as the broader knowledge and experience of the team, design guidance has been formulated which aims to assist people with dementia to live well at home.

The design guidance offered reflects current thinking and is evidence based as far as possible through the various research initiatives described.

Living Well With Dementia

This design guidance is specifically addressed to the needs of people living with dementia. It's estimated that 70–80% of people diagnosed with dementia live at home. While a considerable amount of research and development has been directed at extra care, residential care homes and other specialist care facilities which provide care tailored to the needs of people with dementia, in fact most people living with dementia continue living in their own homes and using the same spaces in their neighbourhoods and cities as everyone else.

Therefore, awareness of the issues associated with dementia should inform the design of all new dwellings and new neighbourhoods and the design of the public realm in general. Shops and other businesses serving the wider community should consider the specific needs of people living with dementia. Existing homes and neighbourhoods may be adapted to respond to this new awareness. In the longer term, this approach (aging in place) will reduce pressure on health and social services and help prevent accidents, improving safety and security for all.

The principles of Design *for* Dementia should be built in to design briefs and management strategies for the public realm as well as the private domain to enable people living with dementia to age in place, to live in supportive neighbourhoods and to use local and town centre facilities. The research and design theories underlining the approach have been described in Chapters 5 and 6. This chapter tackles the design guidance we have drawn from the research base.

Whom Is the Design Guidance Aimed At?

The guidance is aimed at everyone involved in the design and management of the built environment: to stimulate awareness, raise the profile, explore the issues and promote integrated thinking about the design of housing, public buildings and the environment of streets and public spaces. It is formatted to be accessible to service users and carers and to help to advance the debate about accessibility for all.

DOI: 10.1201/9781003306054-10

Accessibility for All

This is an integrated concept. We cannot look at the needs and aspirations of one group in isolation.

There is already in existence a complex legislative framework and advisory standards covering a wide range of topics. Some of these standards are summarised and explained later in this chapter.

The Design Guidance

- The purpose of the design guidance is to raise awareness and to stimulate design responses to the issues associated with Design *for* Dementia
- The design approach should be participatory rather than bureaucratic
- The key design principles are applicable to the public realm in general and to public buildings and facilities in particular as well as the private domain of extra care and residential schemes
- New developments should incorporate imaginative design responses, reflecting the needs and aspirations of those living well with dementia (e.g., the Design *for* Dementia Bungalow)
- Existing dwellings can be modified and extended in accordance with these principles to enable people to live well with dementia (e.g., the adaptation of traditional Victorian terraced houses).

Impairments of Dementia – Potential Design Responses

Sight

- Impaired vision due to yellowing of the lens
- Colour perception at the blue end of the spectrum deteriorates first; red/orange colours are retained longer
- Blurring of vision and increased sensitivity to glare – surfaces may appear differently; avoid black or shiny finishes
- Use high contrast – highlight key features, edges and hazards
- Need for higher lighting levels
- Reflections can be disturbing.

Hearing

- Noise disturbance causes distress
- Reduce ambient noise level
- Good sound insulation within the structure and between rooms
- Soft finishes and furnishing for acoustic absorbency.

Circadian Rhythm (Body Clock)

- Confusion of night and day
- Maximise natural light to increase awareness of daytime
- Easy access to outdoor open space – outdoor experience
- Green view from key rooms, especially from seating positions.

Impaired Memory (Especially for Recent Events)

- Open shelves and glazed cupboard/drawer fronts can ease the anxiety of losing things
- Avoid confusion of doors that all look the same but have different functions
- Memorable objects and images to assist navigation and sense of identity
- Visual linkage and permeability to assist orientation.

Impaired Learning

- Simple, straightforward designs and layouts
- Use landmarks and wayfinders
- Avoid changes that could cause disorientation.

Musculo-Skeletal Problems

- Reduce risks of falls by using level access with tonal continuity at thresholds
- Reduce the number of doors where possible
- Provide handrails and aids, made visible with high contrast.

Impaired Reasoning

- Keep things simple; reduce choices which could cause stress
- Logical, easy-to-understand routes.

Visuo-Perceptual Problems

- Difficulty judging distances
- Avoid steps where possible. If unavoidable, clearly distinguish treads and risers to reduce risks of falls
- Carefully considered use of glass – reflections can cause disturbance
- Are glazed doors and glazed screens clearly distinguishable?
- Considered use of tonal contrast; for example, avoid all-white bathrooms.

Responding to the Challenge

Designers working in the built environment can respond to this challenge through their work. Some responses may be very simple to achieve, such as avoiding the use of black rubber mats at thresholds. If this type of response can be achieved with a bit of consideration but no additional cost, then this is a first but potentially very liberating step for people with dementia, who may perceive the black mat as a hole or a change of material as a step.

In the built environment, the impact of design decisions on people living with dementia needs serious consideration. However, these environments are used by everyone; people of all abilities and all disabilities must be considered, as must the needs of all age groups. The built environment must respond to the needs of all groups in the community, potentially making for a quite complex design brief.

There are many guides already in existence which deal with, for example:

- The needs of wheelchair users
- The needs of sight or hearing-impaired users
- Servicing and access constraints
- Safe play for children
- Reducing traffic speeds
- Open space and play requirements.

In general, the design guidelines involved concur with each other, but there can also be conflicting requirements which need to be reconciled and resolved through a rigorous design process. The interrelationship of the many applicable standards, design guides and design audit methods are discussed in detail later in this chapter.

However, the authors believe that the objective is not to tick all the boxes or to produce more tick boxes or point scoring systems. Our objective is to address the needs of all groups in the community and to base designs on a set of considerations which build awareness and foster an empathy for the perceptual difficulties encountered by those living with dementia, difficulties which are not as self evident as physical disabilities but which are no less real. We must design for cognitive impairment as well as physical disability.

Living Well With Dementia in the Community

This concept implies consideration of accessibility, safety and security but also importantly providing the stimulus and conviviality of a mutually supportive community environment. For example:

- Dementia-friendly accommodation in a mixed community environment rather than in a segregated area
- Avoiding an institutional approach or feel
- Design principles applied holistically to the design of all residential typologies – future proofing designs as far as possible
- Exploring the potential of the adaptation of existing housing to enable living well with dementia
- Consideration of the design and management of shops and other publicly accessible buildings to cater for people with dementia
- Streets, pathways and lighting rethought to encourage and facilitate use by everyone including those living with dementia
- Integrated design of parks and open spaces to foster uses by all age groups and abilities.

Design Principles

Six key integrated design principles guide our thinking about Design *for* Dementia, whether in the context of specialist care, housing design or planning the wider environment. These are illustrated in Figure 10.1.

1. Familiarity

People living with dementia relate to their environment through familiar places, objects or landmarks. Familiar faces of family friends and neighbours become very important. Memory of past times and events may be more easily recalled than recent events.

Designers can respond by considering:

- Use of local landmarks within the living environment and as a setting for new designs in the macro scale
- History and heritage are a stimulus to memory
- Memories stimulated by all the senses – sight, touch, smell, hearing, taste
- Essence of their era – familiar environment
- Recognisable room appearances – domestic feel rather than institutional
- Landscape setting including a stimulus all year round
- Biodiversity attracting wildlife, birds, bees, butterflies.

2. Distinctive Environments

To assist people with dementia to move freely and independently around their homes and their neighbourhood, environments must generate a sense of place through distinctiveness of design.

KEY DESIGN PRINCIPLES

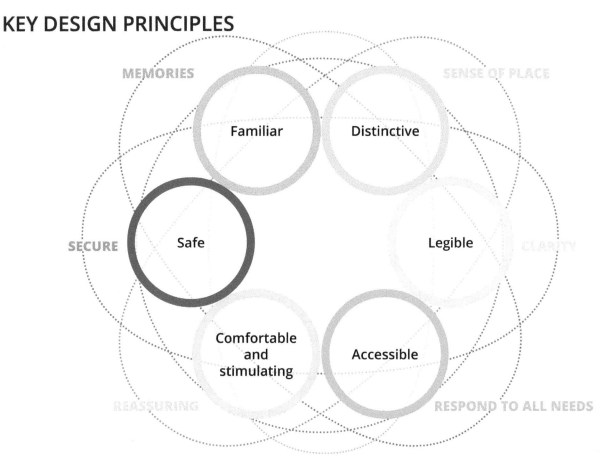

Six key design principles are the starting point for designing for dementia.
They assist designers to understand the needs, requirements and aspirations of
people living with dementia and to begin to develop imaginative design concepts
which are responsive to the experience of dementia.

Image HLP

Figure 10.1 Key design principles

Designers can respond by considering:

- Sense of place generated through character areas expressed through design. Think about their era of design, creating internal environments that relate to their memories
- Feels like home – personalisation
- Character – calm and reassuring environment
- Sense of identity – appropriate to the user
- Variety in size and design of spaces to inspire a range of indoor or outdoor activities
- Thresholds which define and soften the transition between character areas
- Clear gateways to generate a sense of place and identity both externally and internally.

3. Legibility

To navigate their surroundings, people with dementia need help in finding their way to where they want to go.

Designers can respond by considering:

- Clarity and legibility in design and layout. Easy visibility of destinations and entrances in obvious positions

- Visual integrated design using layout, colour, materials and lighting
- Wayfinders to aid orientation and act as landmarks between spaces
- Simple, clear movement patterns to make it easy to find the way around the dwelling or neighbourhood
- Entrances highlighted and identifiable
- Lighting to provide clear, well-lit routes
- Simple hierarchy of spaces internally and externally will help people to find their way around
- Orientation views out to the garden or the street views to green.

4. Accessibility

The design of all environments must respond to the needs of a full range of users, including those living with dementia.

Designers can respond by considering:

- Circulation wide enough for wheelchairs, mobility scooters and pedestrians to pass each other with ease and safety. Storage of mobility scooters and charging facilities are an important consideration in the design of dwellings and care homes
- Materials carefully selected to avoid reflective or dark surfaces which could confuse perception. Patterns in flooring or paving should be used with care to avoid perceptual difficulties. Avoid arbitrary patterns which could confuse and disturb
- Continuous level routes, with surface materials chosen to aid orientation and sense of direction
- Avoid steps; people living with dementia may have difficulty judging distance. Steps or escalators, if necessary, should have clearly visible alternatives – lifts or ramps at an acceptable gradient
- Reduce clutter and obstructions, particularly in footways, which should be dedicated for use by pedestrians, mobility scooters and wheelchairs
- The needs of other users should also be considered as part of a comprehensive and integrated design methodology. For example, the needs of the visually impaired and white stick users who require tapping edges and clearly identifiable demarcation of safe areas, including road crossing positions identified by tactile paving areas.

5. Comfortable and Stimulating Environments

Environments should reduce stress and disorientation and encourage participation, conversation and activity.

Designers can respond by considering:

- Comfortable domestic scale and reassuring, recognisable environments. Avoid an institutional feel and foster a sense of independence and control
- Green spaces, encouraging contact with nature. A view to green space is beneficial, as are walking and socialising in a green space
- Sensory stimuli, smell, touch, taste, sight and sound – considered use of colour
- Noise can be disturbing; position living spaces away from disruptive noise. Consider reverberation between walls and hard surfaces. Provide sound-absorbent materials both inside and outside
- Design circuits rather than dead ends to avoid frustration and provide views out to aid orientation.

6. Safety

The safety of people with dementia in both the home environment and the external spaces they use is obviously a critical design requirement.

Designers can respond by considering:

- Maximise active frontage and permeability to generate a flow of people and animate space
- Defensible space, clear delineation between private and public areas, but maintain good visibility of public space
- Tackle loneliness and isolation by providing informal rooms or spaces which will attract a mix of people and stimulate engagement and participation. Small intimate breakout spaces should also be well overlooked
- External spaces should be well overlooked. Natural surveillance of spaces creates 'eyes on the street' and contributes to a safe, secure neighbourhood, conducive to communal life
- Smart technology can assist safety and security, for example, sensory-operated lighting and secure systems providing discreet monitoring of vulnerable residents.

Summary of Guidance

These key principles provide a starting point for the development of the design process, which is described in more detail in subsequent chapters.

Design Approach

The design principles outlined in Figure 10.1 provide a simple structure to frame thinking about a design approach based on an understanding of the issues facing people living with dementia. We outline the opportunities presented to designers to enrich their designs through a considered and thoughtful approach based on empathy and awareness, particularly of the perceptual difficulties encountered by people living with dementia.

In our shared built environment of houses, neighbourhoods, towns and cities, we can not only design in response to an ever-growing catalogue of rules and regulations but pro-actively generate better designs.

Better design promotes better liveability and enriches our experience, providing stimulus to the senses and joy in our experience of life.

This experiential approach to design has a special relevance in Designing *for* Dementia, considering all the senses to produce responsive living environments which are safe and secure and conducive to community life.

Enhancing Enjoyment

A better approach to design enhances enjoyment of the environment for

- All age groups, including young people and families
- Children's play
- Those with reduced mobility
- Those with impaired vision or hearing
- Those with mental health issues
- People living well with dementia.

Framework of Constraints and Standards

Design takes place within a complex framework of constraints and standards applicable to different kinds of projects. Relevant statutory and advisory standards are summarised later in this chapter.

How Can This Approach Be Achieved?

The approach is participatory. This is fundamental and involves good communication, collaboration and involvement of all groups within the community, including people living with dementia.

- Working with end users – understanding the context and taking on board the experiences of end users to develop innovative and imaginative responses
- Involvement of communities from the outset – a strategy for community and stakeholder engagement should be agreed upon at the beginning of all projects
- Empowerment of local groups and initiatives along with stakeholders and agencies should be at the core of projects
- Involvement with the academic community and health professionals – sharing knowledge and experience towards a better understanding of the challenge
- An interdisciplinary design approach – planners, urban designers, highway engineers, architects, landscape architects and interior designers working together. Sharing expertise through design collaboration towards a consensus-based vision and an agreed-upon set of objectives is the best route to success.

Spectrum of Care

Figure 10.2 shows a spectrum of care provision based on the HAPPI report. The spectrum shows a graduation in care provision from less to more intensive levels of care. The focus of Design *for* Dementia is the question: How can the general environment, as well as housing provision, better respond to the needs of people with dementia?

The proposition is that this approach will, in the medium to long term, reduce pressure on the more intensive, specialised end of the spectrum and reduce the disruption and disorientation of moving people to the appropriate care facility. This approach generates greater independence and self-reliance, particularly in the early stages of dementia, potentially delaying or avoiding the need to move to a more intensive care facility.

Within this guidance, we have illustrated some general principles which should be followed in the design of care homes as well as general family housing, where the design approach is based on the design principles already outlined. We have not attempted to tackle the design details of more intensive facilities such as hospitals or hospices. There are references under further reading which can assist in these more specialised areas of design.

Ongoing Management

Design and implementation are only one part of the process; ongoing management is essential. The responsible bodies include local authority highway engineers, city centre managers, housing associations and private-sector landlords as well as retail chains and those responsible for public buildings.

Communities can be involved in managing their neighbourhoods and projects. That this process can be sustainable is demonstrated by the success of housing co-operatives, neighbourhood-based housing associations, development trusts, community land trusts and other neighbourhood management models.

Support networks, including dementia-friendly cafés, shops and businesses, represent a more broadly based and inclusive approach. Some businesses are already responding. People with dementia can have difficulty dealing with money, and supermarkets may have marked dementia-friendly aisles to assist people with dementia without embarrassment and to avoid queues and avoidable frustrations.

Public Realm and Private Gardens

This section develops a more detailed application of these principles to the design and layout of the external environment. A contextual design approach is demonstrated using well-established methodologies to illustrate a more analytical approach.

SPECTRUM OF CARE

Based on the HAPPI report. Housing Our Aging Population; Panel for Innovation

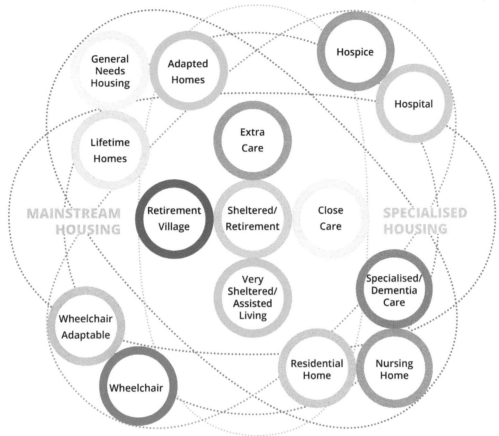

A spectrum of care is required – starting with the immediate home environment within mainstream housing but extending to specialised dementia care facilities and ultimately hospitals and hospices.

Image HLP

Figure 10.2 Spectrum of care

Tackling the design of the public realm involves reconciling the requirements of all groups in the community. Design *for* Dementia is only one facet of a more holistic design approach. The needs and aspirations of all must be considered as well as the constraints and safety requirements of highway design. Some of the applicable legislation and advisory standards are summarised later in this chapter.

Landscape design provides a unique opportunity to focus on the specific implications and opportunities of Design *for* Dementia. Enjoyment of the external environment has key benefits for people living with dementia, reducing stress and disturbance and creating stimulus and joy. Landscape design can manipulate all the five senses – touch, taste, smell, hearing and sight. This is an important consideration in Design *for* Dementia, and richly evocative and pleasurable landscape design can help people living with dementia to live well.

How Should We Address the Key Objectives of Public Realm Design to Be More Dementia Resilient

The well-being of people with dementia can be improved through the physical, cognitive, social and psychological benefits of being outdoors (Pollock and Marshall 2012). In our experience the planning and design considerations that support people to live well with dementia in the public realm can be categorised following the six inter-related design principles summarised in the following.

Familiarity

Improve the ability for independent movement within a familiar environment and enable people to recognise and understand their surroundings. This helps to reduce anxiety, increase a sense of security and prompt memory recall (Mitchell and Burton 2012)

Design considerations:

- Person-centred design ethos recognising that there is no 'one size fits all' approach
- Own clearly visible front door to engender dignity of the individual
- Design spaces of varied size and nature to inspire a range of outdoor social activities, including a choice of destination such as small break-out spaces for reflection or conversation
- Consider that spaces for small groups of less than ten people are better than larger spaces
- Include spaces and routes to promote physical exercise
- Design to inspire and evoke memories, that is, sensory planting.

Distinctiveness

Neighbourhoods with character and identity help to maintain levels of attention and concentration. Reinforce spatial experience, spatial distinctiveness and special sense of place – visuospatial distinctiveness.

Design considerations:

- Design a sense of place within an environment – contextual analysis
- Place-making design approach
- Person-centred sense of scale
- Use distinctive wayfinders/landmarks to enable intuitive movement, including clear easy-read signage and public art
- Include an inter-connected, rich variety of spatial types and character areas
- Promote sensory distinctiveness using plants with colour and fragrance.

Legibility

Help an individual to understand a place's layout and what goes on in it by providing clear legibility for orientation and navigation. This is important at two levels: physical form and activity patterns (Bentley and McGlynn 1985). This can reduce feelings of disorientation, confusion and anxiety.

Design considerations:

- Wide paths with even surface materials and defined edges, free of obstacles and confusing decision points
- Routes should guide people past points of interest which can provide opportunities to engage in activities and social interaction, as well as places to stop and rest, and opportunities for play in which children both visiting and from the neighbourhood can have fun
- Encourage spatial awareness/mind maps. People with dementia may have reduced spatial awareness and less capacity for sense of direction. Therefore, design the strongest visual cues to indicate direction
- Include clearly displayed signage at a lower level, approximately 1.2 m above ground level, including dementia-friendly signs and symbols which should be well lit
- In communal gardens, include pathways that meander and return to terraces and building entrances to ensure people with dementia remain well-oriented and rested
- Avoid dead ends; paths should form continuous routes.

Accessibility

Enable people with dementia to access fresh air, sunlight and views of the natural environment. This also helps to improve and maintain general health through exercise and reduced levels of anxiousness and agitation (Mitchell and Burton 2012).

Design considerations:

- Research has proven that having a green view and access to external garden areas gives a 50% reduction in symptoms of dementia including stress, agitation and aggression, and the consequent need for medication, as seen in Figure 10.3

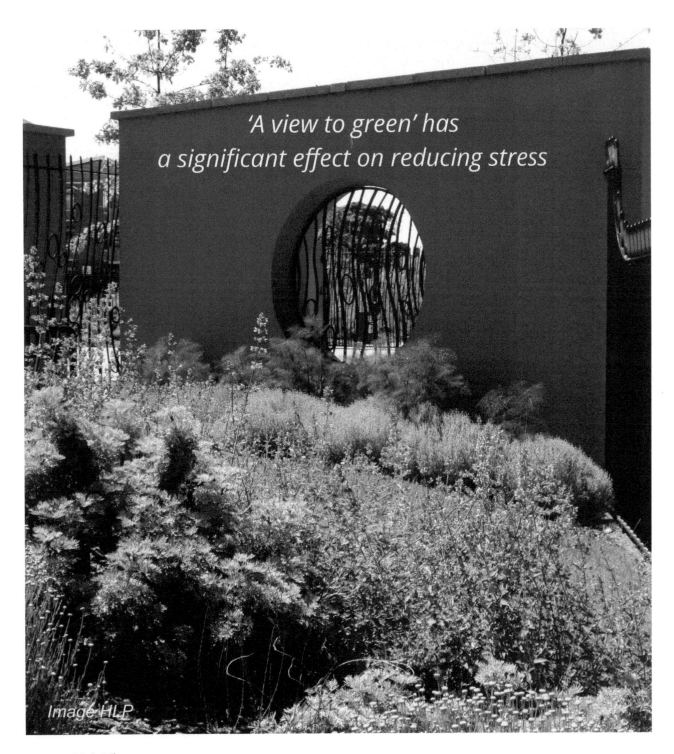

Figure 10.3 View to green

- Design for seamless interaction between internal and external spaces, bringing the outside in, both visually and physically
- Ensure visual accessibility to outside areas involving activity and movement
- Use care in the choice of materials; use tone, not colour, to guide movement
- Create level surfaces at building thresholds, free from visual or textural contrast
- Include appropriate visual and tactile contrasts used for paths, furniture and planting
- Ensure short walking distance between facilities – people over 75 take 10–20 mins to walk 400 m, younger people take 5–10 mins
- Lighting to enable the gardens to be enjoyed at night
- Raised beds to make planting more accessible
- Easily operable garden gates
- Handrails in compliance with building regulations
- Gentle gradients, avoiding steps
- Paths wide enough for pedestrians and mobility scooters to pass comfortably.

Comfort and Stimulus

Encourage people with dementia to enjoy their outdoor environment with physical and psychological comfort, dignity and independence of the individual through creation of person-centred spaces.

Design considerations:

- A view to, and awareness of, what's going on outside is important in terms of the passing of the seasons, time of day (circadian rhythm) and weather changes, as well as views of activities taking place
- Noise can startle and disturb. A tranquil environment is required that reduces noise, particularly sound next to windows, so utilise planting design and keep movement routes away from windows. Use the Meter-Pro App on a smart phone, which measures decibel levels
- Ensure design does not appear clinical or institutional
- Ensure the correct sunlight orientation of spaces
- Have regard to other micro-climatic considerations, that is, shaded and sheltered sitting points to maintain a comfortable body temperature
- Clear, easy access to a toilet should be provided
- Plenty of timber seating with back and arm rests; traditional designs can be recognised and identified as a seat better than contemporary styles
- Maximise stimulus – joy of the outdoor environment encourages relaxation and calm
- Use water in the landscape for both stimulus and calming effects (subject to safety considerations)
- Promote sensory stimulus – smell, touch, taste, sight, hearing
- Texture and forms of materials provide tactile experience and continuity of surface
- Encourage wildlife – design in wildlife corridors and plants which encourage bird life
- Provide sheltered bus stops with handrails and seating
- Incorporate handrails at crossings, safety islands and corridors.

Safety and Security in the Public Realm

Enable people with dementia to access and use the public realm without anxiousness and agitation.

Design considerations:

- Spaces should be fully secure and enclosed where necessary with appropriate railings. For instance, a transparent railing allowing views beyond, with planting to help camouflage the railing height and deter climbing
- Specify non-slip, non-reflective materials with defined edging to paths
- Take care using shared surfaces – a 'safe-zone' with defined edges is needed
- The impact of other users such as cyclists, motorists and emergency vehicles should be considered in detail. Any potential conflicts should be tackled at an early stage of design
- Include walking zones safe from traffic, including frequent marked crossing positions and visually distinctive kerbs
- In a street or public realm area – reduce obstructions
- Design wider pavements to accommodate a range of uses, including mobility scooters
- Specify visible kerbs to indicate changes of level
- Good lighting is essential
- Consider observation and natural surveillance of spaces from the buildings.

Activities

Plan and design for activities that might take place in outside spaces. Activities are recognised as a critical component of good-quality dementia care (Hazen and McManus 2012). Benefits include:

- The opportunity to reminisce and engage in familiar activities, such as gardening, laundry/hanging out the washing, crafts and hobbies
- Inspiring and evoking memories, such as work areas that reflect past interests and jobs
- Providing the satisfaction of entering and leaving different spaces
- Enabling interaction, enjoyment of other's company and spending quality time with families.

Design considerations:

Design for a range of outdoor activities:

- That encourage social interaction
- That assist physical health, activity, exercise and exposure to sunlight for essential vitamin D
- That engage the brain
- That allow relaxation – sitting, watching and reflecting
- That provide multi-sensory stimulation
- That restore and reinforce long-held skills, abilities and knowledge
- That enable people to achieve their creative potential and self expression
- That can be undertaken in the evening when the light is fading – probably need lighting and heating
- That can be intergenerational and/or entertain the children who are visiting.

Planting Choice

Plant choice is essential to the individual's perception, experience and enjoyment of the external environment, as well as influencing memory recall and association with natural timelines and chronology.

Design considerations:

- Develop a plant species palette which reflects seasonal change
- Sensory planting, including:
  - Touch/sight: texture such as bark, leaf
  - Colour: plants including lamb's ears and squirrel-tail grass
  - Smell: fragrant plants such as:
    - Groundcover, such as chamomile, sweet woodruff
    - Climbers, such as star jasmine, honeysuckle, rose
    - Shrubs, such as rosemary, lavender, mint

  - Use strongly scented plants beside paths so fragrance is released when people brush past, like lavender and sage
  - Sound: rustling plants such as bamboo, verbena and oats

- Locate groups of strongly scented or colourful plants as navigational markers
- Take care in choosing the height of species, that is, low-medium height next to windows to allow clear views from inside into the garden
- To enable a sense of involvement in the design process and to prompt memories, include individual species choice by the residents and their families, such as hydrangeas or roses
- Provide opportunity to experience the sights and sounds of wildlife by incorporating species attractive to wildlife like butterflies, birds, bees
- Incorporate nesting boxes and bird baths
- Plants with bright berries or inedible fruits should be located out of reach
- To avoid aggravating skin conditions, all plants should be non-toxic, thornless and without serrated leaves.

Sample Application

The private garden for the Design *for* Dementia Bungalow (Chapter 5) includes:

- Landmarks
- Colour contrast and lighting to help orientation
- Ergonomic raised bed planting to enable easy gardening
- Seating and working spaces protected from direct sunlight and wind
- Good visibility and visual access from inside the bungalow
- Opportunities for a variety of activities in a safe, attractive and familiar outdoor space
- Easy access to toilet facilities
- Wildlife opportunities – no diversity
- Design to stimulate all the senses.

Conclusion

Well-designed public and private outdoor spaces can respond to the six key design principles to produce responsive and stimulating living environments. The considerations can be applied to both micro and macro scales, that is, individual dwellings and the broader environment of the city. They can also be applied to both adaptation or modification of our existing built environments and the design of new neighbourhoods.

BRINGING THE OUTSIDE IN

Visual and physical access to natural outdoor spaces can reduce stress, improve an overall sense of well-being and can provide relief from pain. Elements of outdoor spaces can stimulate each of the five senses; touch, taste, smell, hearing and sight. Its positive benefits are proven for people with dementia, their visitors and members of staff.

A view to natural spaces and awareness of what's going on outside is also important in terms of the passing of the seasons, time of day, weather changes, as well as views of activities taking place.

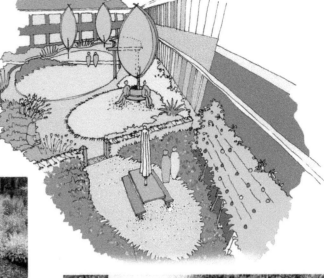

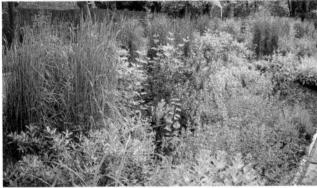

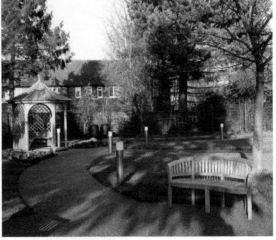

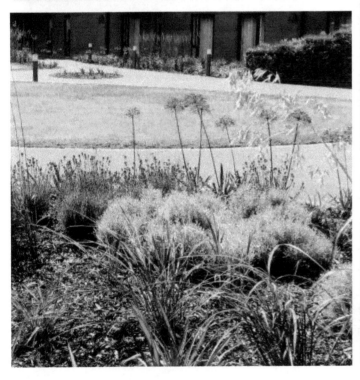

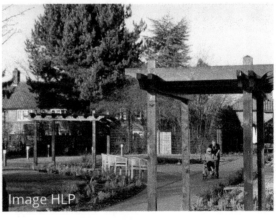

Figure 10.4 Bringing the outside in

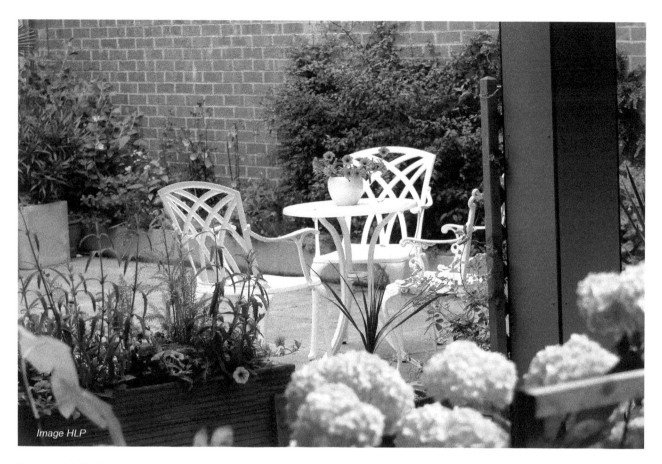

Figure 10.5 Communal patio surrounded by sensory planting

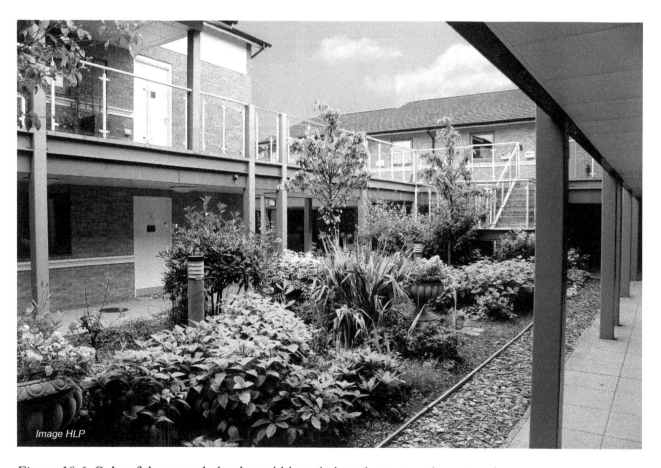

Figure 10.6 Colourful seasonal planting within a sheltered communal courtyard

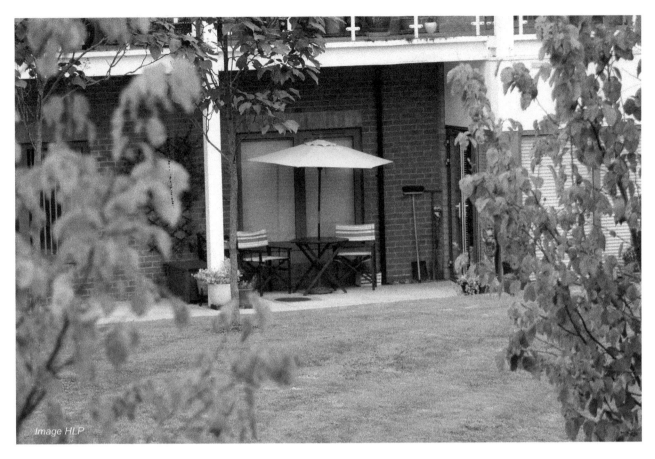

Figure 10.7 Private space overlooking gardens for quiet contemplation

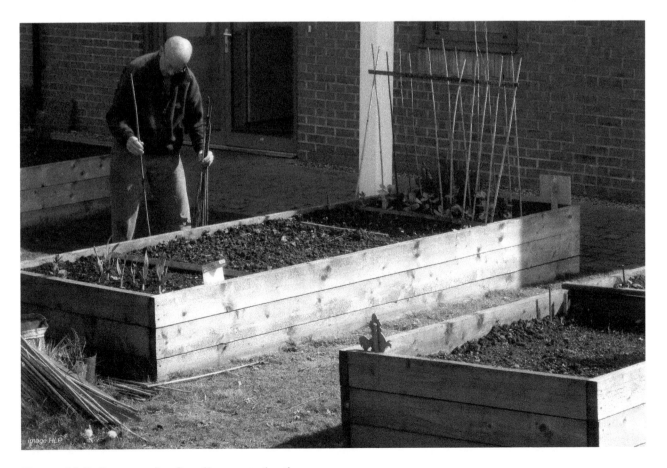

Figure 10.8 Opportunity for allotment planting

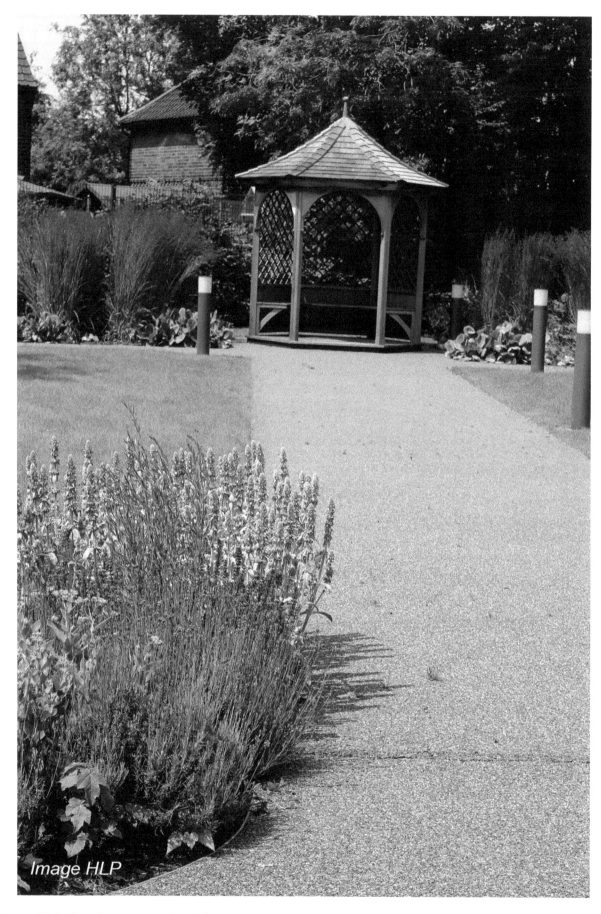

Figure 10.9 Gazebo acts as visual focus in the sensory garden, clear movement routes, wide paths with even surfaces

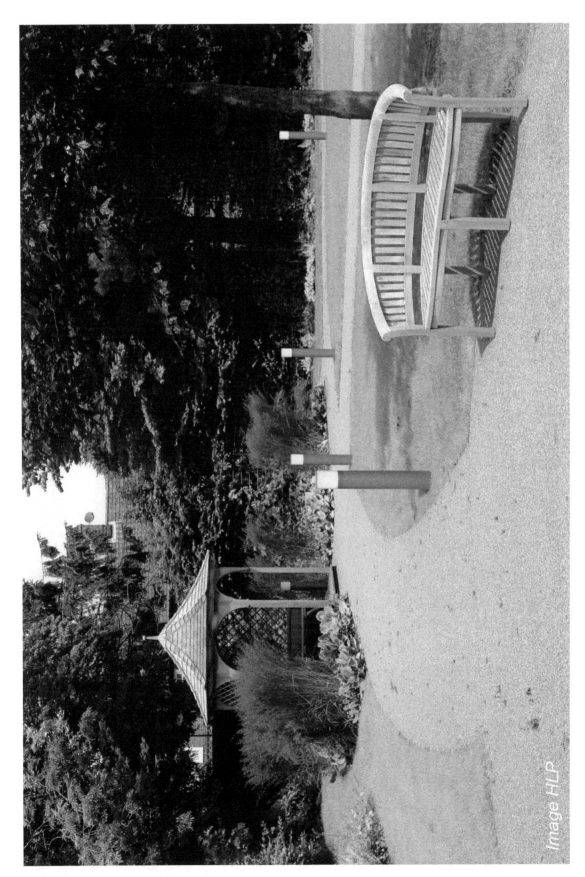

Figure 10.10 A gazebo acts as visual focus, located on wide paths with even surfaces that loop around sensory garden – conveniently located seats (that look like seats)

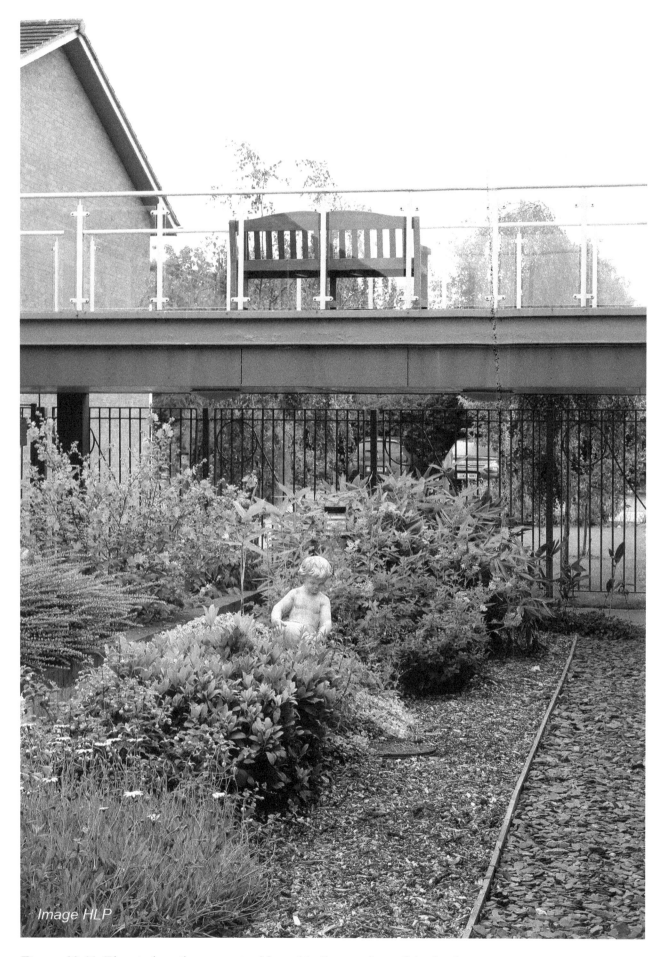

Image HLP

Figure 10.11 Elevated seating opportunities with distant view of the landscape

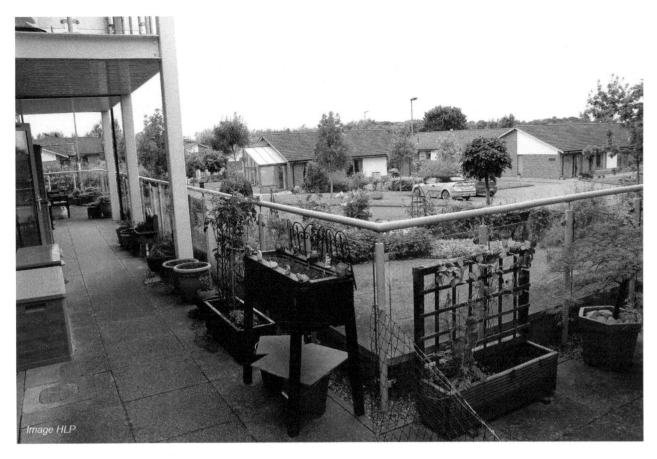

Figure 10.12 Balconies for individual planting overlooking colourful communal gardens

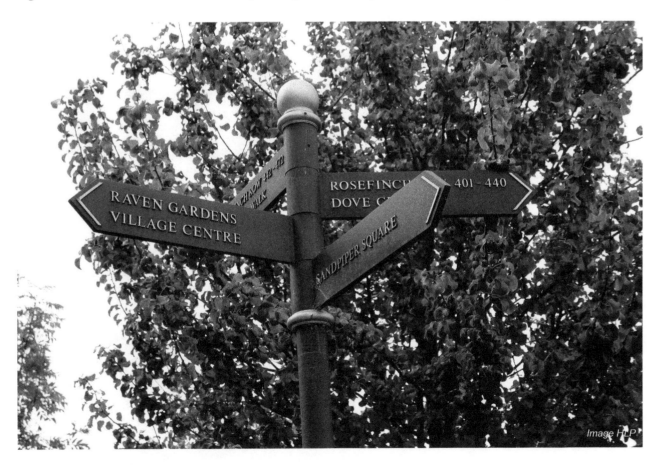

Figure 10.13 Clear fingerpost signs for wayfinding

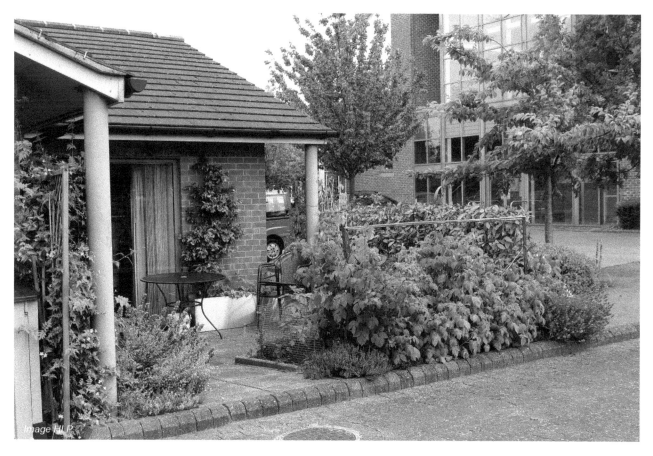

Figure 10.14 Homes are provided with patio spaces with opportunity for individual planting surrounded by colourful communal landscape

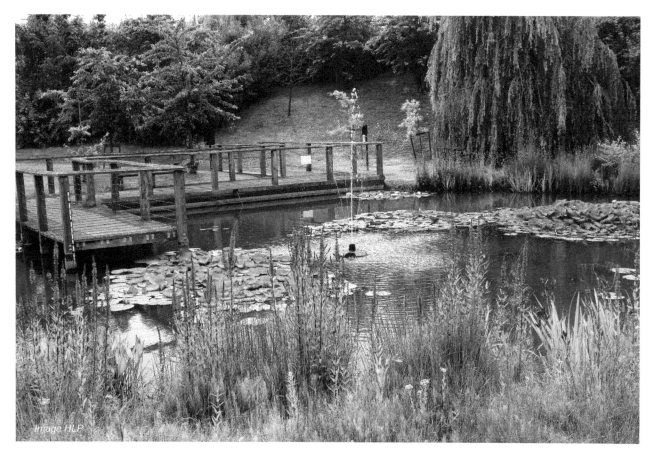

Figure 10.15 Safe access to water

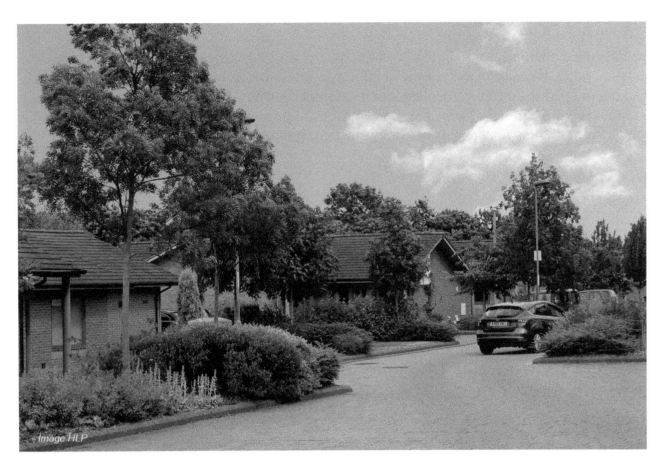

Figure 10.16 Dwellings sit within sensory communal planting

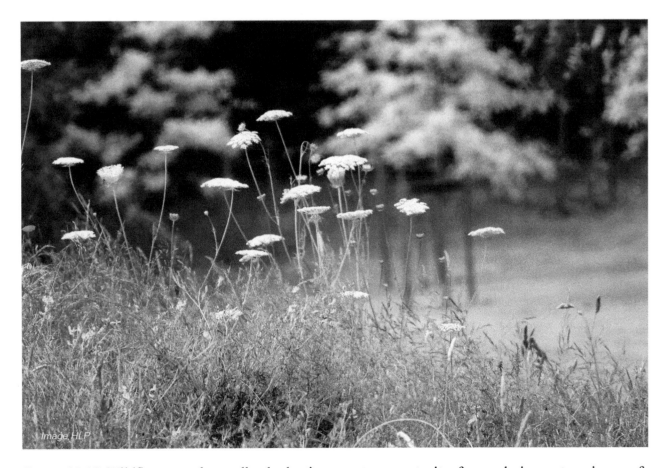

Figure 10.17 Wildflower and woodland planting create opportunity for exploring nature in a safe environment

Built Form

An integrated approach to design implies that the form of development should be considered a holistic design. Because of the beneficial effects for those living with dementia of a green view, walking in open space and gardening activity, the inter-relationship of inside and outside space is at the core of Design *for* Dementia. Built form frames space, and buildings sit in context. The complexities of these relationships are at the heart of good, responsive design.

Key Considerations

Site Layout

A person with impaired memory and reasoning will rely very heavily on what they can see. Creating a clear layout with lots of visual cues is important. Complex layouts and long corridors should be avoided.

Aspect and Prospect

Aspect considerations relate to the importance of sun direction in relation to room layout. Prospect considerations relate to the importance of views out to the natural landscape or street scene.

Internal Layout Factors

Orientation of rooms and spaces

- East-facing rooms can be rooms used in the mornings such as kitchens or bedrooms
- East- but preferably south- and west-facing rooms can be communal rooms, living rooms and gardens
- North-, northwest- or northeast-facing aspects may be better for access, parking and services
- However, consideration should also be given to the potential problems of overheating of south-facing rooms in summer, particularly in view of predicted climate change. Overhangs, brise soleil or special glass may be needed to mitigate these risks.

Internal Visibility

Open plan layouts, carefully planned so that residents can see the toilet from key positions in the house or apartment, work well. Also people living with dementia can mislay things easily, so good visibility of kitchen shelves, for example, will help. Glazed panels to drawers and cupboards with clear labelling indicating their contents will also help. But glass can produce reflections which may be disturbing to those living with dementia, so consider the use of non-reflective glass.

Waymarking and Navigation

Use landmarks within buildings or external spaces. These may be features of the building and will help people to find their way around. Signage should be very clear and pictorial. Personalisation in extra care or residential care schemes can help people to identify their flats. Familiar objects or pictures will help to create an individuality in their environment.

Within the scheme, designers should endeavour to create sense of place with distinct, easily identifiable spaces to assist navigation, particularly at changes of direction or destinations. Natural light introduced at key locations can assist orientation, as can views to external landmarks.

Privacy and Sociability

Design should be based on a clear hierarchy of spaces between public and private areas. A good separation is required between living areas and service areas which can be a source of noise, such as catering kitchens.

Clear definition should be achieved at dwelling thresholds, with opportunities for personalisation designed in. Connections with the outside, views to green space and access to patio, terraces or balcony should be considered from the point of view of people who may be confined to bed or seated, so windowsill levels should be low.

Courtyards

Courtyards, as illustrated in Figure 10.18, are a popular form; they are perceived to be safe and enclosed. However, they may be unsuccessful if there is insufficient sunlight. The height/width ratio is critical both for usage and planting design. Microclimatic effects of wind direction and behaviour are also a factor. In general in the UK, 2:3 is the minimum height/width ratio, but courtyards can also be too big with a risk of wind turbulence.

Scale

Avoiding an institutional feel is difficult, but domestic scale is important in achieving this, as illustrated in Figure 10.19. Single storey dwellings are preferred (see the Design *for* Dementia Bungalow Project). This might not always be possible. In flatted schemes there should be obvious staircases and lifts in prominently visible positions. There should always be an alternative; many people living with dementia have difficulty judging distance and are, therefore, uncomfortable with steps.

Spaces should be domestically scaled so communal areas should be broken down into smaller living room–sized spaces rather than larger communal rooms. Smaller spaces are better suited to the activities of daily living. Corridors should be kept short or avoided. If corridors cannot be avoided, there should be a clearly visible destination at the end.

Visibility/Permeability

Within the constraints of privacy, designs should be open plan but avoid directly facing bedroom doors or apartment entrances. Glazed screens can be useful in some situations to assist orientation, but the screens must be easily identifiable so as not to be confused with doorways and openings. Glazing can cause reflections which can be disorienting (use non-reflective glass). Ability to move freely without obstructions is important. Lighting levels must be enhanced, and signs should be at an appropriate level for wheelchair users.

Layout

Straight circulation systems enable residents to find their way better than layouts with lots of changes of direction. However, circuit layouts avoid the frustration of dead ends. Any turns in corridors should be marked by wayfinding events to assist orientation.

Corridors

Corridors, if unavoidable, should be short and wide enough to function as social spaces, possibly with informal meeting areas, seating and views to the garden. Natural light should be maximised. Wayfinding events and rest points with handrails should be designed in from the outset.

Wayfinders

Wayfinders are a useful way of establishing location and assisting orientation. Wayfinding events could include small seating areas, murals or pictorial signage, windows, views out or daylight.

Bathrooms

To assist easy usage, the layout should be highly visible, with contrast between floor and walls and fittings and surfaces. Light reflective materials should be limited, and lighting levels should be a minimum of 300 lux. Fixtures and fittings should be traditional and familiar, avoiding concealed on/off tap fittings, for example. Red and blue colours are used to denote hot or cold water. Cross-head taps are more familiar and easier to use by older fingers/hands.

Where possible, bathrooms should be designed to wheelchair accessibility standards including wheelchair turning circles, grab handles and level access showers – refer to Chapter 6. A shower is preferable for residents with disability issues, although some people living with dementia find the hiss of the shower disturbing and prefer a bath.

Designers need to achieve these features while still avoiding an institutional feel.

Lifts and Stairs

Although single-storey developments are preferred, multi-storey schemes may be necessary. In this instance, lifts and stairs should be clearly visible and alternative choices well lit and signed to aid navigation. Mirrors in lifts should be avoided. Reflections may cause distress.

Design for *Dementia audit tools*

Relevant publications which provide a checklist approach are:

- Dementia Design Audit Tool – Stirling University
- Dementia Design Checklist – NHS National Services Scotland
- HAPPI Audit
- Building for Life Standards
- Secured by Design
- Lifetime Homes.

Reflection on Design Principles

- These design principles can be applied to a range of types of schemes, including extra care and specialist residential care schemes
- They can also be applied to the refurbishment and adaptation of existing dwellings such as the Victorian terraced house, as shown in Figure 10.25
- The Design *for* Dementia bungalow research project demonstrates the principles applied to an ideal model archetype, as discussed in Chapter 5.

SUN PATH FOR COURTYARDS

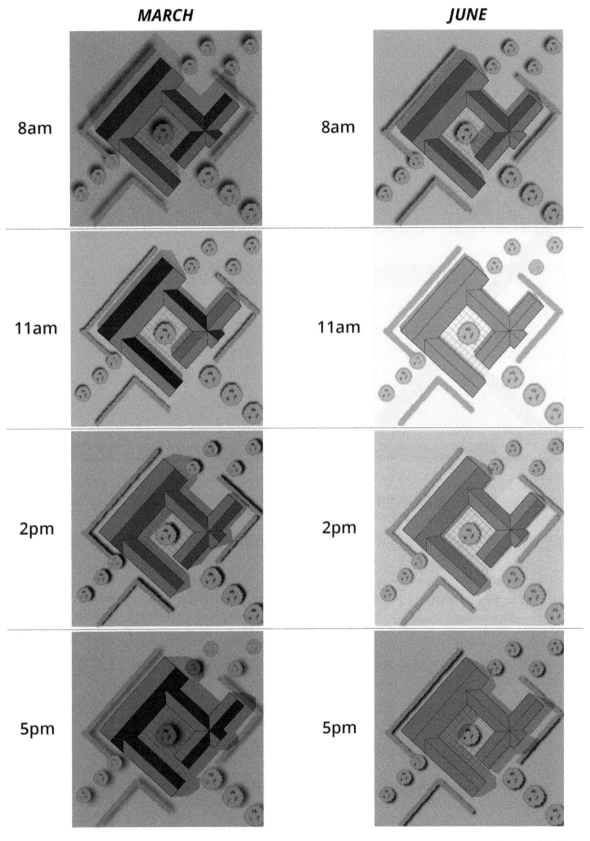

Image HLP

Figure 10.18 Key considerations

ASPECT RATIOS - HEIGHT/WIDTH

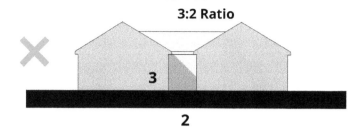

3:2 Ratio

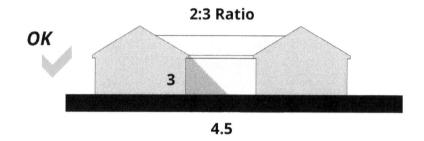

2:3 Ratio

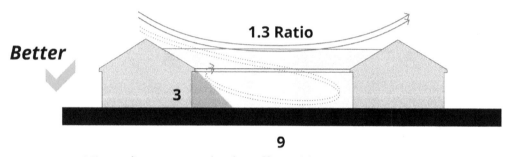

1.3 Ratio

Micro-climate can also be affected by wind and turbulence

Image HLP

Figure 10.19 Key considerations

CLUSTER CONNECTIVITY

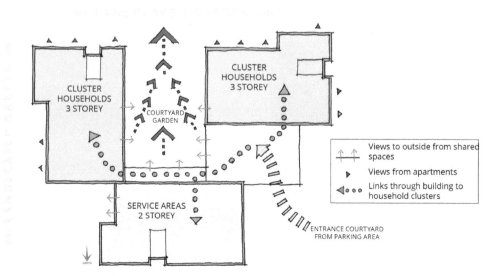

Image HLP

Figure 10.20 Design concepts for specialist residential care

TYPICAL LAYOUT OF A SPECIALIST
RESIDENTIAL CARE 'CLUSTER' OR HOUSEHOLD

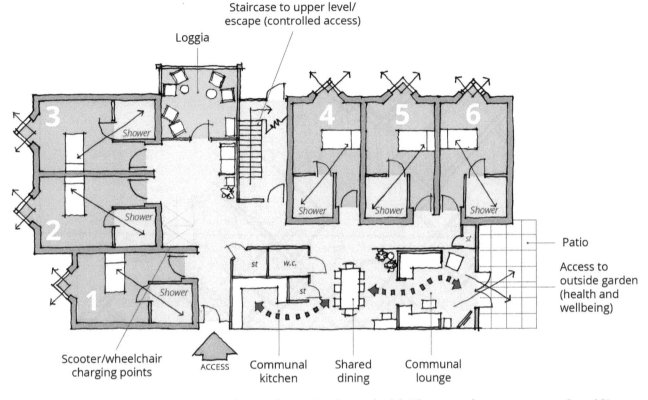

- Six residential apartments forming a 'cluster' or household *(There can be more - up to 9 or 10)*

- Open plan arrangement - no corridors

- Communal space for eating, food preparation and socialising

- Easy access to outdoor space

- Maximise 'views to green'

- Good internal sight-lines

- Good natural and artificial light

- Balance of 'privacy' with communal space

- Consider 'anti-ligature' design.

Image HLP

Figure 10.21 Design concepts for specialist residential care

CLUSTERS BLOCK OF 6 APARTMENTS

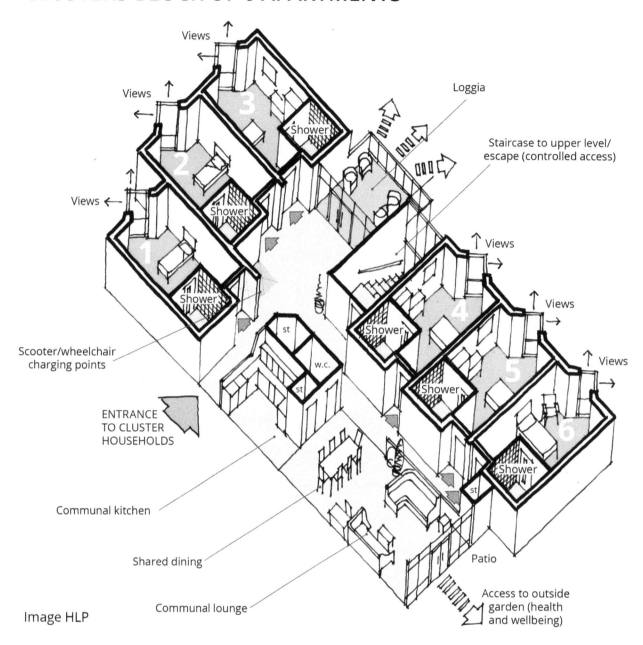

Image HLP

Figure 10.22 Design concepts for specialist residential care

TYPICAL APARTMENT LAYOUT

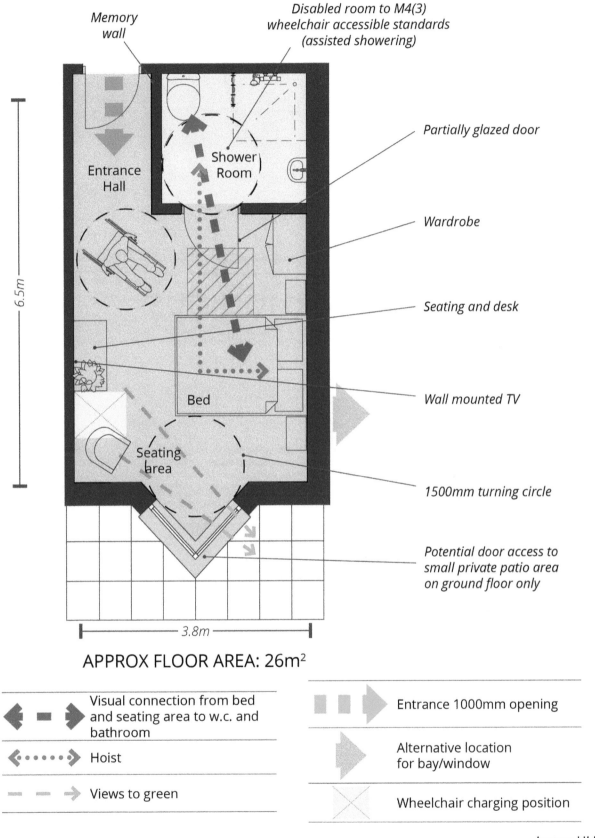

APPROX FLOOR AREA: 26m²

Visual connection from bed and seating area to w.c. and bathroom	Entrance 1000mm opening
Hoist	Alternative location for bay/window
Views to green	Wheelchair charging position

Image HLP

Figure 10.23 Design concepts for specialist residential care

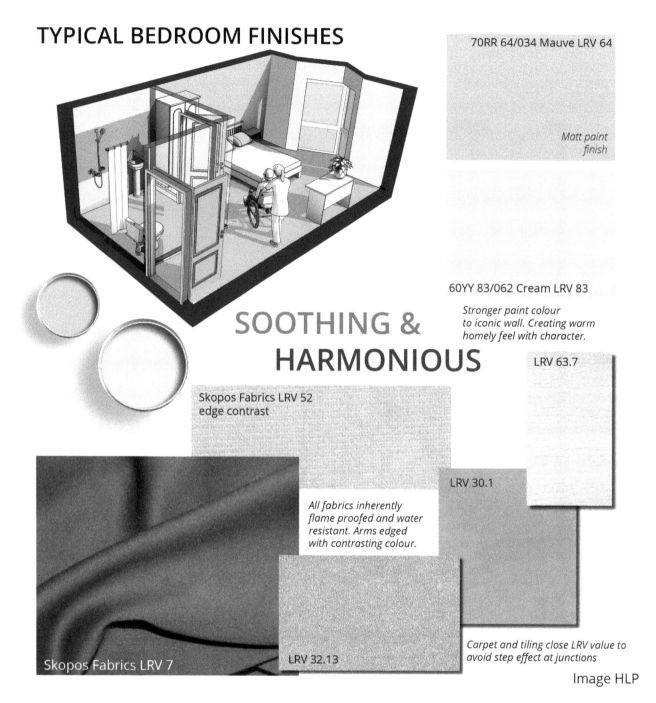

TYPICAL BEDROOM FINISHES

70RR 64/034 Mauve LRV 64

*Matt paint
finish*

60YY 83/062 Cream LRV 83

*Stronger paint colour
to iconic wall. Creating warm
homely feel with character.*

SOOTHING &
HARMONIOUS

LRV 63.7

Skopos Fabrics LRV 52
edge contrast

LRV 30.1

*All fabrics inherently
flame proofed and water
resistant. Arms edged
with contrasting colour.*

*Carpet and tiling close LRV value to
avoid step effect at junctions*

Skopos Fabrics LRV 7

LRV 32.13

Image HLP

Figure 10.24 Design concepts for specialist residential care

EXAMPLE OF A DESIGN *for* DEMENTIA ADAPTATION OF A TRADITIONAL VICTORIAN TERRACED HOUSE

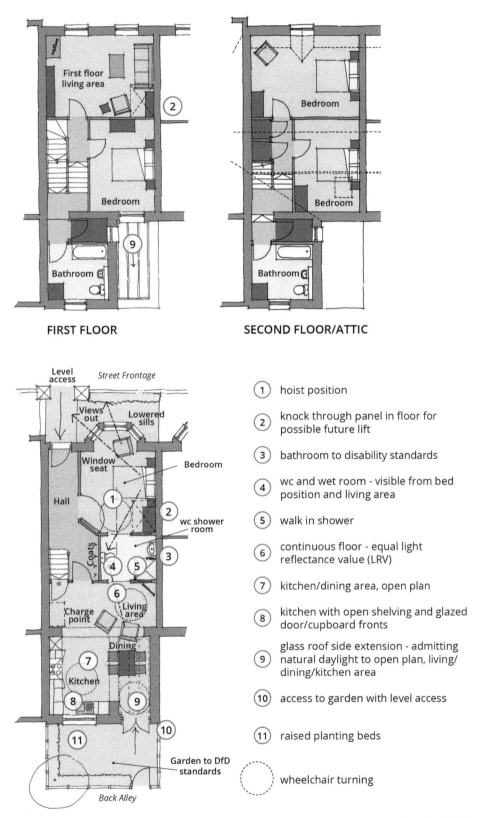

FIRST FLOOR

SECOND FLOOR/ATTIC

1. hoist position
2. knock through panel in floor for possible future lift
3. bathroom to disability standards
4. wc and wet room - visible from bed position and living area
5. walk in shower
6. continuous floor - equal light reflectance value (LRV)
7. kitchen/dining area, open plan
8. kitchen with open shelving and glazed door/cupboard fronts
9. glass roof side extension - admitting natural daylight to open plan, living/dining/kitchen area
10. access to garden with level access
11. raised planting beds

wheelchair turning

GROUND FLOOR

Image HLP

Figure 10.25 Example of a Design *for* Dementia adaptation of a traditional Victorian terrace house

TYPICAL BUNGALOW LAYOUT
2BED 3PERSON BUNGALOW M4.3 - 76m² - *wheelchair dwelling*

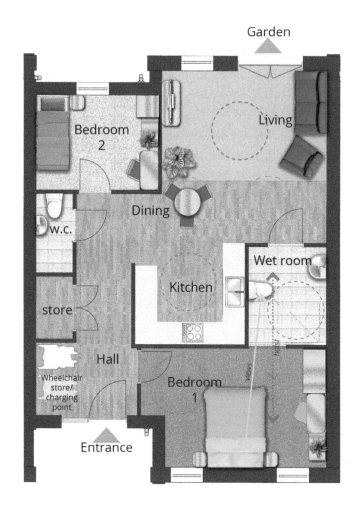

- Double bedroom with knock through panel to the wet room

- Single bedroom

- Living-dining kitchen area - open plan

- Bathroom with wet room/shower and visible w.c. from bedroom

- Second visitors w.c.

- Storage

- Wheelchair storage and charging

- Design for Dementia 'compatible'.

Image HLP

Figure 10.26 Typical bungalow layout

TYPICAL BUNGALOW LAYOUT

TYPE 2 - 2BED 3PERSON BUNGALOW M4.3 - 82m² - *wheelchair dwelling and Design for Dementia principle with accommodation for full time carer*

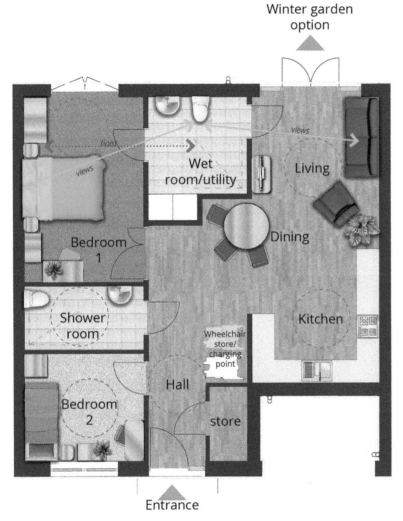

- Full Design for Dementia

- Single bedroom (for carer)

- Living-dining kitchen area - open plan

- Bathroom with wet room/ shower, visible w.c. from bedroom

- Second w.c./wet room

- Storage

- Wheelchair storage and charging

- Design for Dementia

Image HLP

Figure 10.27 Typical bungalow layout

VISUAL DEGENERATION - COLOUR

Due to the yellowing of the eye lens, the blue end of the spectrum is lost first. Therefore, it is easier to see warmer colours. More vivid colours should be used to compensate for the decline of the ageing eye.

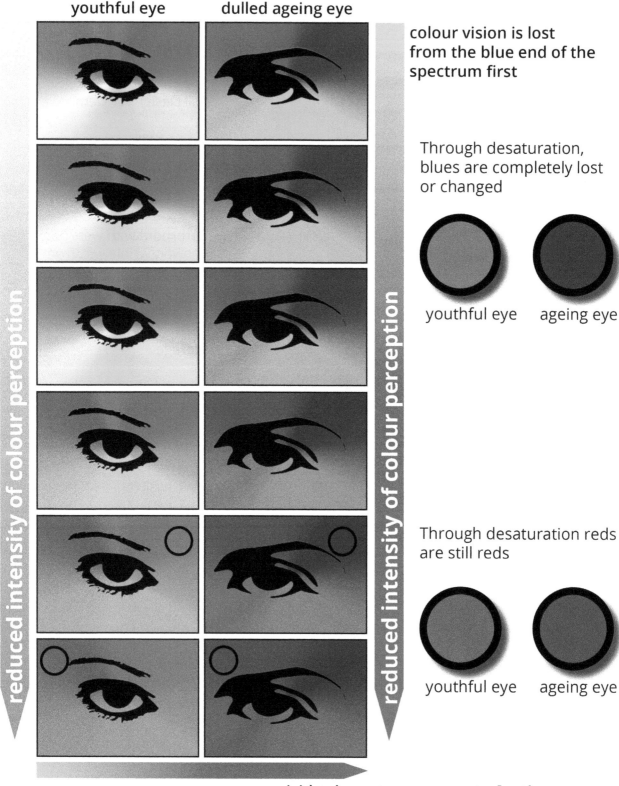

Figure 10.28 Visual degeneration – colour

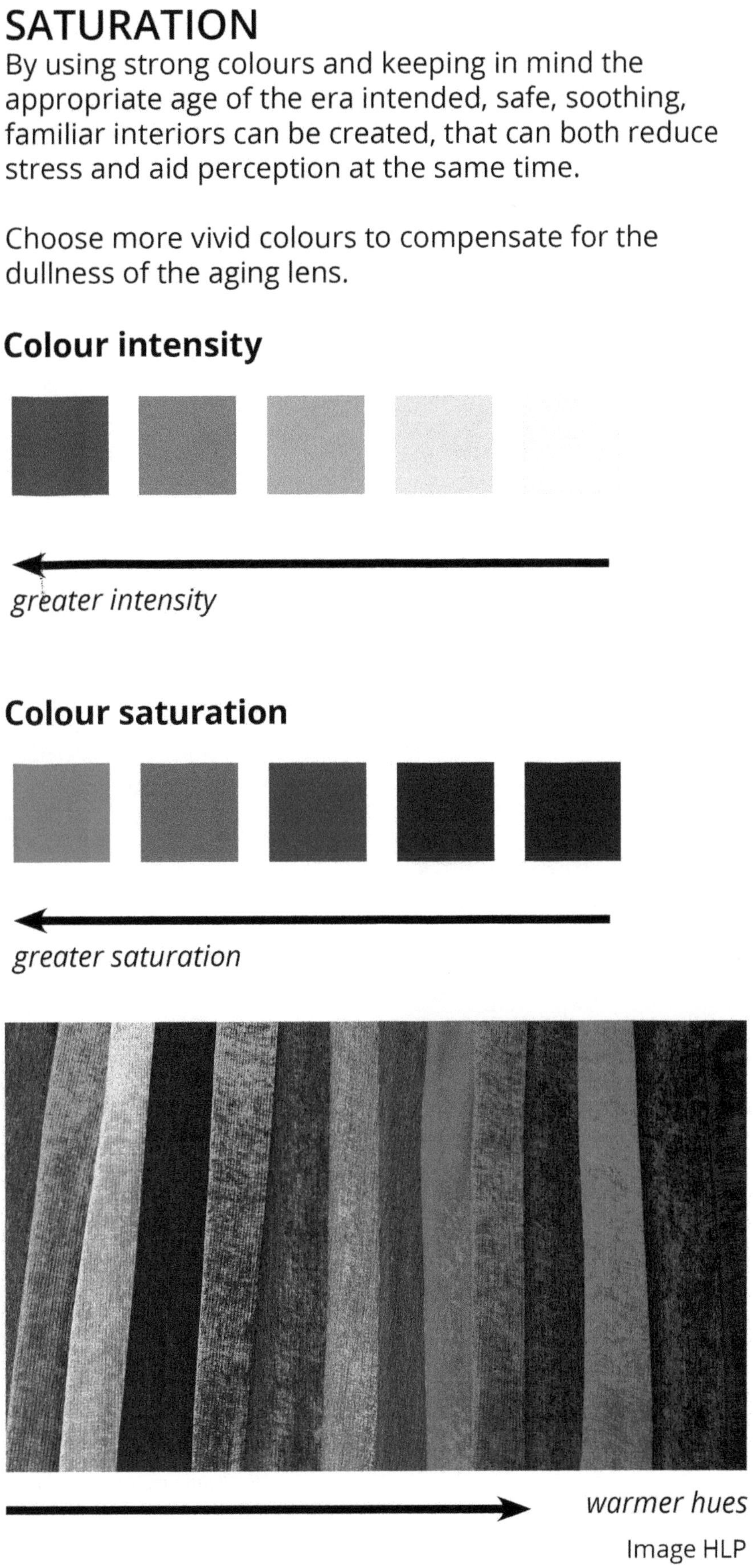

SATURATION

By using strong colours and keeping in mind the appropriate age of the era intended, safe, soothing, familiar interiors can be created, that can both reduce stress and aid perception at the same time.

Choose more vivid colours to compensate for the dullness of the aging lens.

Colour intensity

greater intensity

Colour saturation

greater saturation

warmer hues

Image HLP

Figure 10.29 Visual degeneration – saturation

VISUAL DEGENERATION - TONE AND CONTRAST

Understanding the importance of tone and contrast and how it can be used, is a vital tool as well as an aid to design.

The use of subtle traditional patterns will help keep the interior familiar to the end-users' era. Avoid using striped or swirling strobing patterns which could cause distress and agitation.

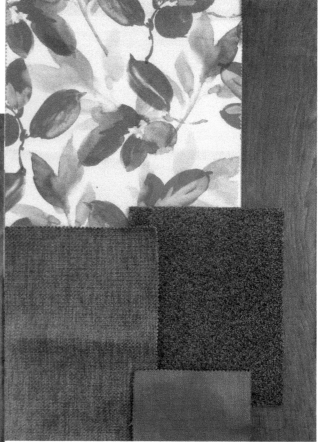

Materials in full colour

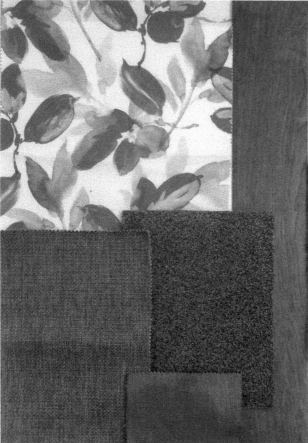

Monochrome image demonstrating comparative light reflectance value (LRV) of materials

The light reflectance value (LRV) of finishes is a useful method for designing and selecting materials to assist people living with dementia to perceive their environment more clearly. If the LRVs of adjacent materials are close in value then their appearance to the ageing eye will be consistent and unthreatening. This is particularly relevant to floor finishes because a change in LRV at floor level could be misinterpreted as a step.

Alternatively, contrast can be used to give definition to different surfaces, such as between walls and floors. A minimum of 30 LRV is required to create this contrast.

Contrast between walls and floors, skirting boards, architraves and doors will help people living with dementia to perceive their environment more clearly and help them to negotiate it. Doors which are accessible can also be distinguished from doors which are non-accessibl,e such as service rooms, by the applied use of colour.

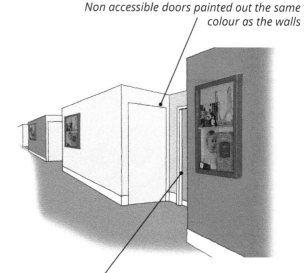

Non accessible doors painted out the same colour as the walls

Highlighting accessible doors with contrasting architrave and door colour

Image HLP

Figure 10.30 Visual degeneration – tone and contrast

VISUAL DEGENERATION - TONE AND CONTRAST

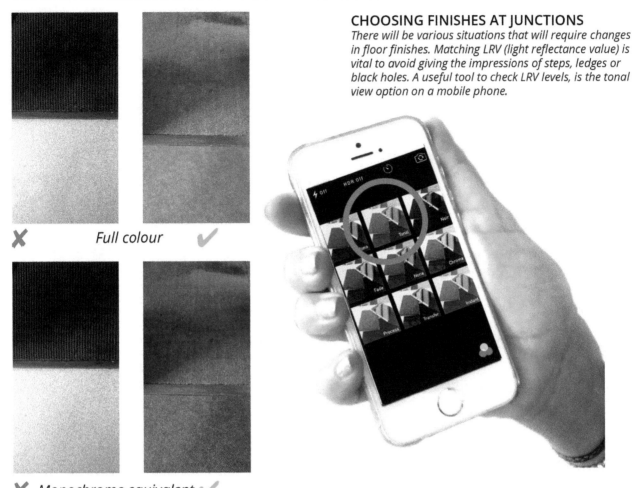

CHOOSING FINISHES AT JUNCTIONS
There will be various situations that will require changes in floor finishes. Matching LRV (light reflectance value) is vital to avoid giving the impressions of steps, ledges or black holes. A useful tool to check LRV levels, is the tonal view option on a mobile phone.

✗   *Full colour*   ✓

✗ *Monochrome equivalent* ✓

How can people be helped to live well in their own homes?

- Familiarity - neighbours - support community

- Possible adaptations as required

- Ramped access - comply with Lifetime Homes Standards; preferably with front and back level access

- Downstairs wc positioned where it is easily accessible from bedroom and living space

- Lighting levels - as much natural daylight as possible; 2x normal artificial lighting levels

- Continuous floor finishes, no trip hazards. Matching LRV (light reflectance value) at changes in floor finish so as not to create the visual impression of a step

- Contrast in colours used as a tool to aid definition e.g. architraves to the doors, or skirting in a contrasting tone

- Fully openable windows to encourage fresh air, increasing air quality

- Easy access to gardens - visual connection

- Kitchen - replace cupboard doors with glazed fronts to allow contents to be seen, graphic and lettered signage on drawers.

Image HLP

Figure 10.31 Visual degeneration – tone and contrast

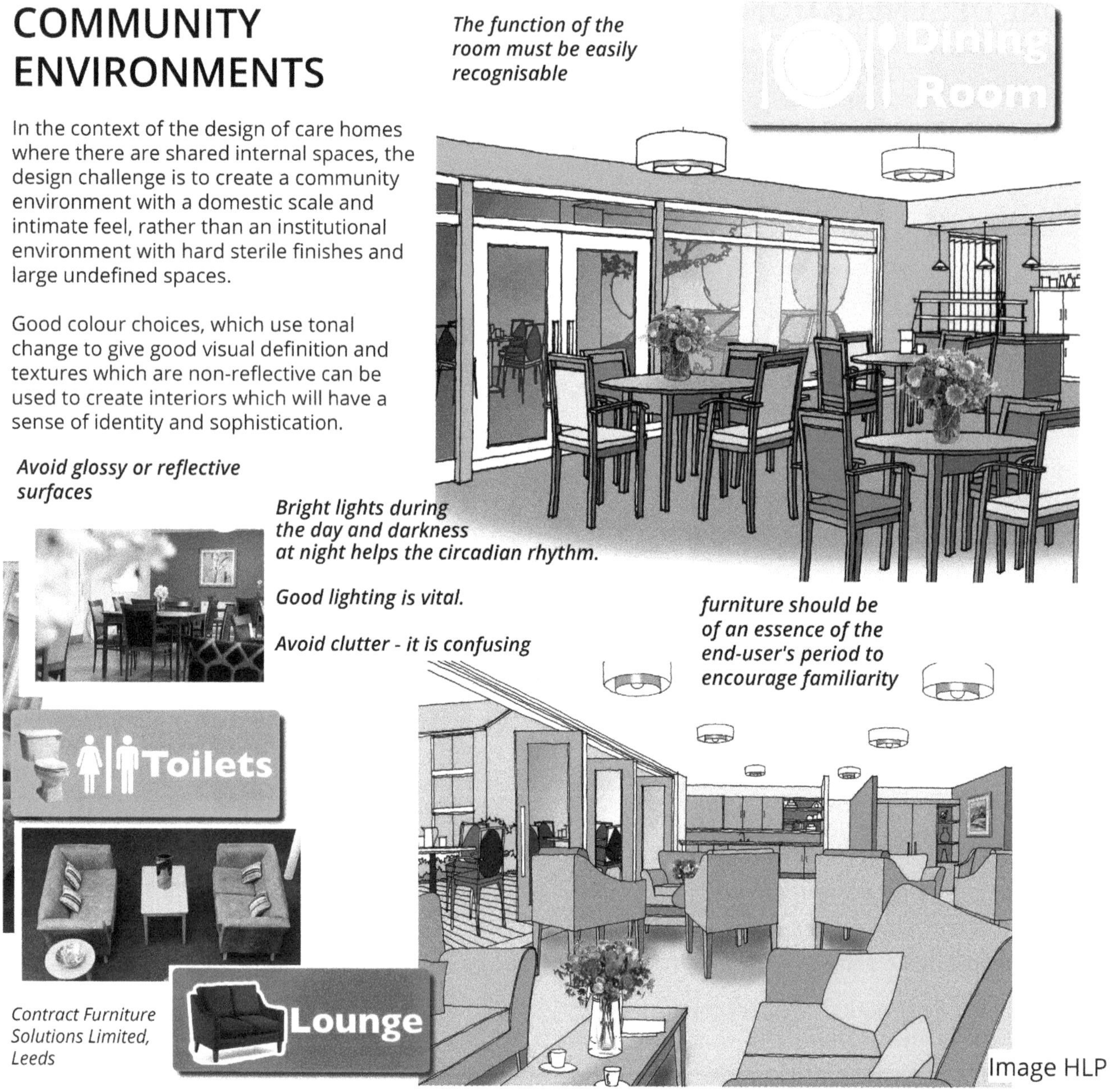

COMMUNITY ENVIRONMENTS

In the context of the design of care homes where there are shared internal spaces, the design challenge is to create a community environment with a domestic scale and intimate feel, rather than an institutional environment with hard sterile finishes and large undefined spaces.

Good colour choices, which use tonal change to give good visual definition and textures which are non-reflective can be used to create interiors which will have a sense of identity and sophistication.

The function of the room must be easily recognisable

Avoid glossy or reflective surfaces

Bright lights during the day and darkness at night helps the circadian rhythm.

Good lighting is vital.

Avoid clutter - it is confusing

furniture should be of an essence of the end-user's period to encourage familiarity

Contract Furniture Solutions Limited, Leeds

Image HLP

Figure 10.32 Community environments

COMMUNITY ENVIRONMENTS

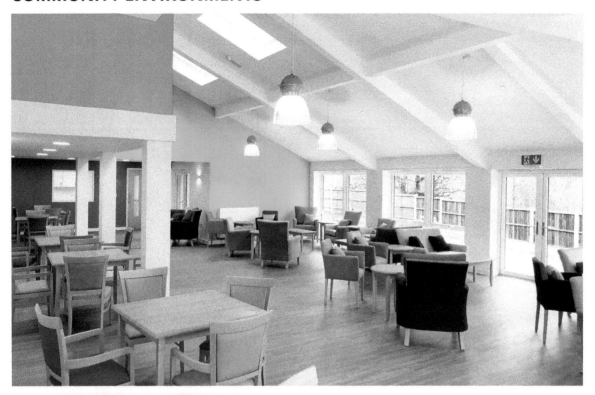

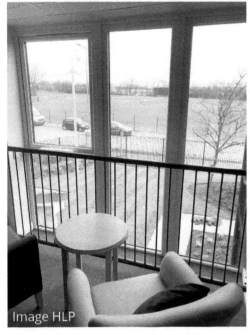

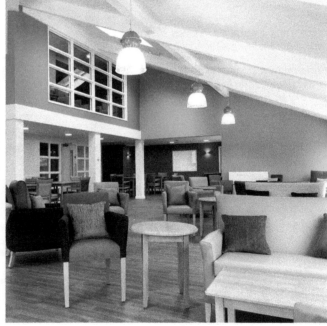

- Colour used to provide stimulus, interest and sense of place. Strong colours help to 'lift' the environment and avoid an institutional feel, keep colour around for those living with dementia

- Shades of beige and pastel colours are not the only choice

- Strong floral or geometric patterns are avoided

- Incidental sitting spaces with outward views.

Figure 10.33 Community environments

NAVIGATION

Good clear, clutter free navigation is important. Making the signage and wayfinders both graphic and in text form, helping those living with dementia find their way stress free.

position memory boxes adjacent to apartment entrances. A familiar object can mean a lot

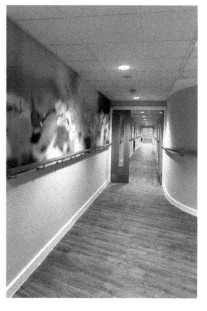

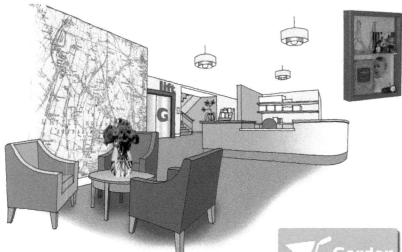

artwork should be meaningful

- *visual links between spaces helps promote independence and reduce anxiety*

- *tonal contrast (measured in LRVs) is critical for ensuring visual accessibility*

- *critical and trim elements should contrast significantly in tone where practically possible*

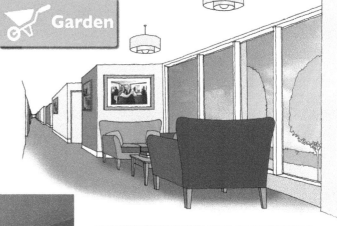

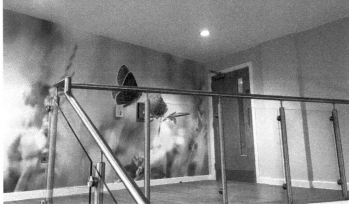

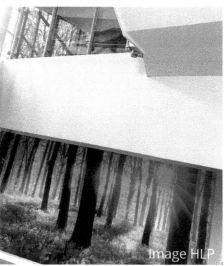

- *use building features, landmarks, objects, signage and colour together to give as many cues as possible*

- *signage should be consistent, clear, simple in text and format, with picture graphics to help those who cannot read*

Figure 10.34 Navigation

The Private Domain

The design of interiors requires intensive and detailed consideration of a range of factors in response to the difficulties people with dementia experience in negotiating their living environment. These difficulties include the visuo-perceptual aspects associated with dementia such as change in colour perception and difficulty in judging distance. Textures and patterns can cause disturbance as can reflectively surfaces and changes in floor colour.

Key Qualities for Successful Interiors

The creation of successful interiors in settings that support living well for people with dementia relies upon a set of key qualities:

- Simple – layouts should be clutter free and easy to understand
- Logical – designs should have a clear logic to ease navigation
- Functional – spaces should be appropriate to their use
- Quiet – noise can disturb; sound should be softened
- Living well – design should foster independence and control as far as possible and provide stimulus through all the senses.

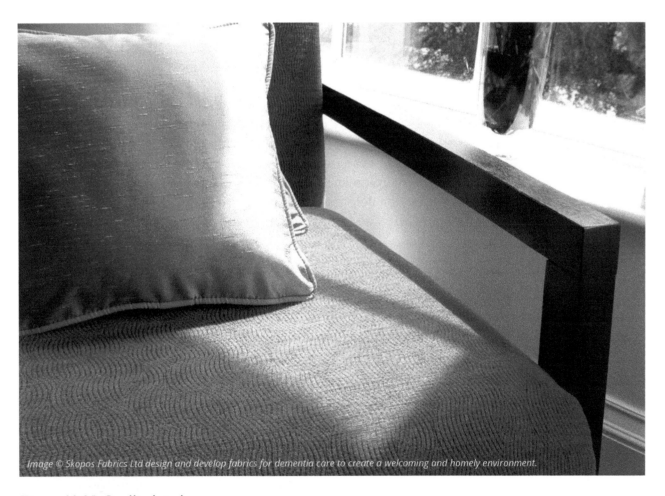

Figure 10.35 Quality interiors

Image Reproduced with Permission of Skopos Fabrics Ltd.

Factors That Need to Be Taken Into Consideration

The eyesight of the elderly and people living with dementia undergoes various changes, and their perception of their surroundings is altered. Understanding this is a good starting point when considering the design of the internal environment.

- Tone – how much light the colour reflects
- Hue – position on the colour wheel
- Saturation – depth or vividness of the colour.

Colour and Tonal Values

People with dementia have diminished ability to see contrast; therefore, good tonal contrast is needed between walls and floors. Ability to perceive colour may be reduced, so choice of colour finishes or signage is critical.

Visual Degeneration – Colour

Due to the yellowing of the eye lens, the blue end of the spectrum is lost first. Therefore, it is easier to see warmer colours, as illustrated in Figure 10.28. More vivid colours should be used to compensate for the decline of the ageing eye.

Saturation

By using strong colours and keeping in mind the appropriate age of the era intended, safe, soothing, familiar interiors can be created that can both reduce stress and aid perception at the same time. Figure 10.29 illustrates this.

Choose more vivid colours to compensate for the dullness of the aging lens.

The aged eye, whether the person is affected by dementia or not, starts to degenerate. This may produce interrelated issues. If additional lighting levels are provided to compensate for reduced acuity, then there may be a risk of glare. Other results of degeneration may be reduced perception of contrast and tone, reduced depth perception and perception of colour. On the colour wheel, the blue end of the spectrum is one of the first colours to be lost due to the yellowing of the eye lens. Therefore, using warmer tones and vivid colours will compensate for the dullness of the ageing eye.

Using stronger, more vivid colours is more interesting and attractive if the environment is still familiar to the end user. Beautiful interiors can still be created which can be appreciated by older people and people living with dementia as well as visitors or family members.

Private spaces should be personalised, taking care not to create a hotel or institutional feel. Small personal details create familiarity and help to reinforce identity.

Memory and Familiarity

- Memory can be aided through considerations of familiarity. Remembered styles and scenes may assist in reducing disorientation for end users
- Domestic scale of seating and dining areas is important. Pedestal tables should be avoided because they can be unstable when leant on. Wingback chairs restrict visibility and socialisation. Cushions should have a plain side so that they can be reversed if the pattern is causing disturbance
- Make mirrors reversible, as to some, their own reflections can be disturbing and confusing. Simply turning the mirror around to show a picture on the reverse can help reduce agitation

- Sanitaryware should be recognisable and visible, contrasting against floor and wall finishes
- Tableware may be 'of an era' to be more easily recognised and useable
- Interior design may be directed to a specific era for greater familiarity for the resident.

Spatial Use

Meaningful activities should be encouraged in spaces designed for specific purposes, such as:

- Reading – conveniently positioned open shelves, stable low tables, comfy chairs, quiet environment with good task lighting
- Games areas – social spaces, highchairs and tables, accessible visible shelves or cupboards, good lighting
- Cafe/bar areas – open sociable, inviting food smells, high tables and chairs
- Cinema/TV lounge – open, sociable, domestic scale, comfy chairs, high tables (TV with 4k screen)
- Gardens/allotments – raised planting beds, accessible, useable garden tools. Sitting-out areas should be visible, close and accessible
- Workshops – benches, high seats, good lighting levels. Tool racks should be on display
- Exercise routes – internal routes should be designed to encourage walking with resting areas, views out and fresh air. Natural light is important
- Dead ends should be avoided in favour of circuits. If dead ends are unavoidable, there should be views out and natural light. The end should have a significance, a meeting place, a place of interest. Routes and long corridors should include natural spaces for people to rest or to gather, creating small social spaces
- Art space – encouraging creativity provides stress relief; with accessible materials and implements on display
- Visitors' areas – space for visitors, including children, should be provided to encourage family engagement in safety.

Visual Degeneration – Tone and Contrast

Understanding the importance of tone and contrast and how it can be used is a vital tool as well as an aid to design. Figures 10.30 and 10.31 illustrate this.

The use of subtle traditional patterns may help keep the interior familiar to the end users' era. Avoid using striped or swirling strobing patterns, which could cause distress and agitation.

The light reflectance value of finishes is a useful method for designing and selecting materials to assist people living with dementia to perceive their environment more clearly. If the LRVs of adjacent materials are close in value, then their appearance to the ageing eye will be consistent and unthreatening. This is particularly relevant to floor finishes because a change in LRV at floor level could be misinterpreted as a step.

Alternatively, contrast can be used to give definition to different surfaces, such as between walls and floors.

A minimum of 30% LRV is required to create this contrast.

Contrast between walls and floors, skirting boards, architraves and doors will help people living with dementia to perceive their environment more clearly and help them to negotiate it. Doors which are accessible can also be distinguished from doors which are non-accessible such as service rooms by the applied use of colour.

Because of the difficulties in being too precise about LRV readings, a 10% tolerance either side should be allowed in achieving the recommended 30% contrast.

Spatial Awareness and Legibility

In response to the visuo-perceptual complications experienced with dementia, special consideration should be given to how people perceive their environment and negotiate it. Legibility can be assisted by:

- Providing clear sight lines with signage at lower levels
- Even lighting conditions, especially daylight
- Installing matt, even-coloured flooring. Light reflectance values can be measured using a mobile phone on mono to check whether tonal contrasts are excessive or disturbing
- Reducing noise and reverberation through using sound absorbent materials. Curtains and soft furnishings will help. Carpets are available which are moisture and dirt repellent and easy to clean.

Visual Degeneration

People with dementia are prone to visual impairment and may have a progressive diminishing ability to see contrast. Colour vision may also be impaired, tending to grey. Vision may be blurred.

Change in eyesight occurs with age, which affects vision and colour perception. Thickening and yellowing of the lens alter the way colour is perceived. People with dementia may experience:

- Reduction in contrast perception, resulting in difficulty differentiating between subtle changes in the environment such as carpets and steps
- Reduction in the perceived saturation or vividness of colours. For example, reds can start to fade to pink
- A progressive reduction in ability to perceive the blue end of the spectrum and dullness of the aging lens, so the use of warmer, brighter colours will help make things more visible
- Tonal contrast will aid perception, for example, floors to walls and walls to doors. Contrasting skirting boards and architraves.

Orientation in Time and Space

Orientation can be assisted through:

- Reflecting the seasons in decor or artwork
- Large calendars with time of day (i.e. morning or afternoon) and actual day and time
- Large clocks with large numbers (Arabic, not Roman, numerals)
- Natural daylight – assists in creating awareness of day/night cycle (circadian rhythm)
- Outside spaces – accessible and green
- Localisation – creating sense of place
- Wayfinders – landmarks within the building
- Legible, clear, simple design, clutter free
- Views to outside green spaces and to local landmarks.

Summary

- Reduce agitation and stress
- Facilitate independence – living well
- Community environment and social interaction
- Safety and security – reducing falls
- Enable routine activity through the day.

Community Environments

In the context of the design of care homes where there are shared internal spaces, the design challenge is to create a community environment with a domestic scale and intimate feel rather than an institutional environment with hard sterile finishes and large undefined spaces.

Good colour choices, which use tonal change to give good visual definition and textures which are non-reflective, can be used to create interiors which will have a sense of identity and sophistication.

Bringing the Outside in

Visual and physical access to natural outdoor spaces can reduce stress, improve an overall sense of well-being and provide relief from pain. Elements of outdoor spaces can stimulate each of the five senses: touch, taste, smell, hearing and sight. Its positive benefits are proven for people with dementia, their visitors and members of staff. This is illustrated in Figure 10.37.

A view to natural spaces and awareness of what's going on outside are also important in terms of the passing of the seasons, time of day and weather changes, as well as views of activities taking place.

Choosing Finishes at Junctions

There will be various situations that will require changes in floor finishes. Matching LRV is vital to avoid giving the impressions of steps, ledges or black holes. A useful tool to check LRV levels is the tonal view option on a mobile phone.

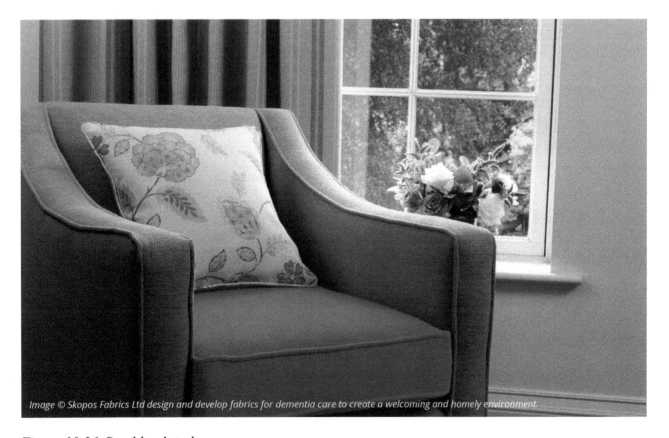

Image © Skopos Fabrics Ltd design and develop fabrics for dementia care to create a welcoming and homely environment.

Figure 10.36 Soothing interiors
Image used with kind permission of Skopos Fabrics Ltd.

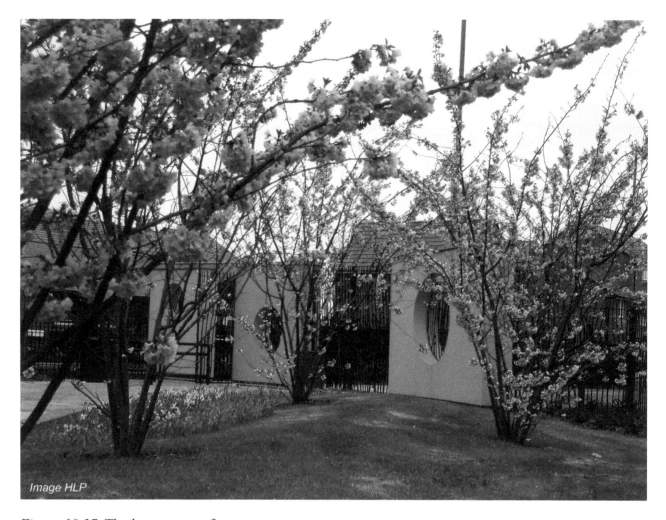

Figure 10.37 The importance of nature

How Can People Be Helped to Live Well in Their Own Homes?

- Familiarity – neighbours – support community
- Possible adaptations as required
- Ramped access – comply with Lifetime Homes Standards, preferably with front and back level access
- Downstairs w.c. positioned where it is easily accessible from bedroom and living space
- Lighting levels – as much natural daylight as possible, 2x normal artificial lighting levels
- Continuous floor finishes, no trip hazards. Matching LRV at changes in floor finish so as not to create the visual impression of a step
- Contrast in colours used as a tool to aid definition, such as architraves to the doors or skirting in a contrasting tone
- Fully openable windows to encourage fresh air, increasing air quality
- Easy access to gardens – visual connection
- Kitchen – replace cupboard doors with glazed fronts to allow contents to be seen, graphic and lettered signage on drawers.

Open plan layouts are preferred where possible (please refer to Chapters 5 and 6).

Navigation

Good, clear, clutter-free navigation is important. Making the signage and wayfinders both graphic and in text form helps those living with dementia find their way stress free.

Artwork should be meaningful.

- Visual links between spaces help promote independence and reduce anxiety
- Tonal contrast (measured in LRVs) is critical for ensuring visual accessibility
- Critical and trim elements should contrast significantly in tone where practically possible
- Position memory boxes adjacent to apartment entrances. A familiar object can mean a lot
- Signage should be consistent, clear and simple in text and format, with picture graphics to help those who cannot read
- Use building features, landmarks, objects, signage and colour together to give as many cues as possible.

Finishes

When choosing finishes, various things need to be considered:

- Are they fit for purpose, in that they do what they need to do in the area specified?
- The era, in that the end user will feel familiar and comfortable in the surroundings created
- With careful consideration and intuitive thinking based on the findings of research into dementia, risk-free interiors may be designed
- Creating an atmosphere free of clutter, easing decision making
- Clear and simple design, reducing agitation and confusion
- Is it free from risks, with subtle or heightened tonal changes to highlight hazards and to provide spatial definition?

Carpets – Considerations

- Noise reduction
- Soft underfoot, deadening sound
- Domestic feel of an era the end user will be familiar with
- Cleanability and durability
- Avoid strong busy patterns
- Continuity of tonal values throughout to help eliminate trip hazards. Strong tonal changes can appear as steps, creating confusion and distress
- Contrasting threshold strips can create trip hazards. Keep tonality the same across thresholds
- Different strong tonal values can be used as a tool to highlight hazards.

Vinyl/Sheet Flooring – Considerations

- Easy to clean
- Specify matt finish
- Avoid shiny/wet-look
- Slip resistance
- Match LRV at junctions
- Avoid chequerboard patterns
- Avoid dimples, which can be irritable underfoot.

Ceramic Tiles – Considerations

- Use in limited areas (hard, cold and noisy)
- If tiles are to be used, match the grout to the tile – joint lines can cause agitation.

Walls – Considerations

- Matt finish, avoiding shiny wet-look finishes
- Wallpaper will give a traditional feel better than painted walls, even if it's just one wall
- Limit aggressive patterns, look to feature tonal difference within patterns
- Make sure accessible doors are clearly highlighted with clear colours and accent architraves to help people see the doors
- Play down doors that don't need to be accessible by painting out in the same colour as walls, including architrave. This will reduce the number of doors the end user has to consider, reducing confusion and frustration
- Contrast walls with floor, LRV 30% difference (min).

Furnishings – Considerations

- Domestic feel considering the end user's era, a style which will be familiar to them
- Subtle patterns or plain fabrics – strong bold patterns can irritate and cause agitation
- Textures attractive to the touch, which can be soothing and reassuring
- Soft furnishings which absorb the noise will help to soothe agitation
- Many manufacturers are now supplying dementia-friendly products.
- Edges of curtains should be a different colour/fabric/texture, creating a contrasting edge that is easily seen
- Arms and seat cushions should be of a contrasting colour/texture to aid those living with dementia in finding secure seating, guiding them and therefore preventing falls due to misperception
- Chairs with arms to assist people standing up or sitting down.

Glazing and Doorways – Considerations

- Glazing should be used very carefully. Visibility between spaces can assist orientation, but confusion between a glazed door and side screen could cause confusion and potential accidents. Glazing should be distinguished using clear 'manifestations' (clearly visible patterns on glass). Fixed screens may have a transom to distinguish them from doors or openings
- Reflections from glass screens, doors or balustrades can also cause confusion and distress and can exacerbate visuo-perceptual difficulties
- Thresholds should provide an even transition, with continuity of LRV. Black rubber mats present difficulties and can appear as a hole. Steps should be avoided, if possible, but, if necessary, should be identified by contrast between treads and risers. For further reading, please refer to BS 8300:2009.

Conclusion

- People living with dementia, whether living in their own homes or care homes, can be enabled to have greater control and confidence within their environment through careful use of colour, materials and finishes as well as good lighting and acoustics
- Stress, confusion and disturbance can be reduced by making the right choices in the design of the interior domain
- Safety can be improved and accidents reduced
- Further information about the design of the interior domain can be obtained from a range of publications produced by Stirling University:

  - *Designing Interiors for People with Dementia* – Liz Fuggle, associate architect, DSDC

- *Light and Lighting Design for People with Dementia* – David McNair, director of lighting, DSDC; Colm Cunnigham, director, the Dementia Centre, Hammond Care; Richard Pollock, director of architecture, DSDC; Brian McGuire, managing director, Vision Call Scotland
- *Hearing, Sound, and the Acoustic Environment for People with Dementia* – Maria McManus, associate director, DSDC, and Clifford McClenaghan, associate architect, DSDC.

Summary of Design Standards

The inclusive approach to Design *for* Dementia implies that designers should not design for dementia in isolation. There are a wide range of standards which will apply; in the UK some are statutory, and some are advisory. Some of these are summarised over the following pages. The following is not exclusive. There are other advisory standards issued by different specialist groups; however, it provides a roadmap to the extent of the prevailing legislative and advisory framework which can come into play and which we must be aware of when we approach design for all.

Statutory Legislative Standards (UK)

Equality Act 2010

Key Areas

The Equality Act replaces the Equal Pay Act 1970, the Sex Discrimination Act 1975, the Race Relations Act 1976, the Disability Discrimination Act 1995, much of the Equality Act 2006, the Employment Equality (Religion or Belief) Regulations 2003, the Employment Equality (Sexual Orientation) Regulations 2003, the Employment Equality (Age) Regulations 2006 and the Equality Act (Sexual Orientation) Regulations 2007 (where applicable, as subsequently amended).

Comments

Gives guidance to all sectors of the community, employers and employees as to rights regarding discrimination and equality. Cross references to other legislative documents and guidance documents.

The act provides for 'detriment arising from disability', which clarifies and widens protection against disability discrimination. The act abandons the previous list of capacities, relying instead on the general requirement that impairment has a substantial and long-term effect on a person's ability to carry out normal day-to-day activities.

Consequently, we must assume that the impairment of dementia is covered by the Equality Act 2010.

The Building Act 1984

Key Areas

The Building Act 1984 is the primary legislation under which the building regulations and other secondary legislation are made.

Comments

The act allows for building regulations to be amended as and when required to ensure best practice and evolving technologies and systems can be incorporated.

Building Regulations 2010

Key Areas

Particularly Part M: Access to and Use of Building 2010 (2015 Edition incorporating 2016 amendments for use in England) Vols 1 and 2.

Comments

This section covers the technical guidance that supports Part M of schedule 1 of the Building Regulations, with the requirements with respect to access to and use of buildings.

Construction Product Regulations and CE Marking

Key Areas

Manufacturers, distributors and importers of construction products need to be aware of provisions that may govern the use of such products in the UK.

Comments

Under the CPR, from 1 July 2013, a construction product will need to be CE marked and accompanied by a declaration of performance if it is to be placed on the market in the European economic area. CE markings are applicable to construction products, and this includes any product designated for use by disabled people.

Post Brexit, all European Standards may be subject to change.

Highways Act 1980

Key Areas

This act provides for the creation, improvement and maintenance of roads and for acquisition of land. The act also deals with the management and operation of the road network in England and Wales.

Comments

The act, under Section 38, allows local authorities to adopt roads constructed by developers and for all future maintenance of the adopted road to be undertaken by the local authority. The act refers to *The Manual for Streets* for approved layouts and standards. These standards include requirements for roads to be designed and constructed to allow ease of use and safe use by vehicles and pedestrians, including the formation of safe pedestrian crossing points, traffic calming, lowered kerbs and so on to allow unrestricted access by all sectors of the population. Under Section 278 of the act, an agreement allows private developers to either fund or complete works to public highways outside or beyond the development site itself, such as traffic calming and capacity improvements.

Town and Country Planning (General Permitted Development) Order 2015

Key Areas

Forming part of the Town and Country Planning Act: 1990, Development Control is a key part of planning control and is exercised in the UK to prevent any significant development of property without permission by the local authority. In Part III of the Town and Country Planning Act 1990, under Section 59, the secretary of state delegates to public bodies the right to grant planning permission.

Comments

Under the General Permitted Development Order, householders are given rights to develop their property within strict guidelines without the need to obtain planning permission. This will include extensions, loft conversions and so on but must be within certain set size limitations.

However, these rights to permitted development may have been removed at the initial planning permission stage or if the property is within designated areas. The order will allow for adaptations to houses to accommodate a disabled occupier's needs without the need for prolonged periods of time taken to obtain formal permission. Consult the local planning authority regarding the scope of permitted development rights.

Advisory Legislative Standards

Building for Life 12

Key Areas

Building for Life is the industry standard endorsed by the government for well-designed homes and neighbourhoods that local communities, authorities and developers are invited to use to stimulate conversations about creating good places to live.

BFL 12 is a series of 12 questions which require a response to assess how successful a scheme will be:

- Connections
- Facilities and services
- Public transport
- Meeting local housing requirements
- Character
- Working with the site and its context
- Creating well-designed streets and spaces
- Easy to find your way around
- Streets for all
- Car parking
- Public and private space
- External storage and amenity space.

Comments

The 12 sections are split to more specific questions within the particular section. All answers are subjective, and each section should achieve a 'green' under a traffic light assessment system.

Building for a Healthy Life

Key Areas

Building for a Healthy Life is a new edition and new name for Building for a Life. It updates BFL, reflecting the Healthy New Towns programme and aspires to 'Putting Health in Place'. The new iteration focuses more on active travel, air quality and bio-diversity.

Comments

BFHL 12 offers a design code used by many local authority planning departments to appraise planning applications.

Manual for Streets

Key Areas

The *Manual for Streets* focuses on lightly trafficked residential streets, but many of its key principles may be applicable to other types of streets, for example, high streets and lightly trafficked lanes in rural areas. Advice is given to help ensure sustainable and accessible environments are included within the public realm.

Comments

The MfS gives advice to local highway authorities and developers on the layout of streets and roads to ensure public safety for all road users, pedestrian and vehicular. Advice is given on crossing points, pavement and road widths and safe access routes.

BS8300: 2009 Code of Practice for Access to Buildings for Disabled People

Key Areas

BS8300:2009 provides specific data and information concerning how people of all abilities and disabilities should expect a building to work in order to accommodate them.

Comments

Useful reference document giving clear advice via diagrams and text to help designers deliver buildings which are useable for all members of the community.

Dementia Design Audit Tools – Sterling University

Key Areas

A design audit tool for designers, comprising three parts:

Part 1 – Guidance and Notes
Part 2 – Work Book
Part 3 – Literature Review.

Part 1, Guidance and Notes, subdivides the building into basic areas. The environment within each area is then assessed and given a classification of essential or recommended; all essential items must be met. Each area is then scored (the weighting is on essential items), and the overall score totalled. Gold, Silver or Bronze can be awarded to the scheme depending on its overall success.

Comments

The design audit tool is an extremely useful document for designers and clients. It is an essential tool for use at the initial design phase of a project and then as a reference as the project progresses through to completion.

Secured by Design

Key Areas

Secured by Design is the UK police initiative supporting the principles of designing out crime. SBD goes through an extensive list of requirements and standards which must be met in order to achieve Secured by Design accreditation.

Comments

Most local authority planning departments expect that housing developments will follow the recommendations of SBD. Reference is made to SBD by the HCA Design and Quality Standards.

Housing Our Aging Population: Panel for Innovation (HAPPI Report)

Key Areas

Panel set up by the government to consider four key questions for the future development of dwellings:

- Improving the quality of life of our ageing population by influencing the availability and choice of high-quality, sustainable homes and neighbourhoods
- Challenging the perceptions of mainstream and specialised housing for older people for existing and future generations
- Raising the aspirations of older people to demand higher-quality, more sustainable homes
- Spreading awareness of the possibilities offered through innovative design of housing and neighbourhoods.

There are ten key components which should be considered for the design and use of housing for older people:

- Space standards
- Use of natural light
- Avoiding internal corridors and single-aspect flats
- Homes to be care ready
- Encourage interaction and social use of circulation spaces
- Multi-use space for casual meetings and interaction
- Public realm; encourage interaction with external environment
- Energy efficiency
- Adequate storage
- External surfaces, priority to pedestrians.

Housing Our Aging Population: Plan for Implementation (HAPPI 2)

Key Areas

Government inquiry into the implementation of the HAPPI Report.

Comments

The inquiry urges the government to boost the adoption of the HAPPI Report through its various departments and agencies:

- Homes and Communities Agency
- Department of Health

- Department of Communities and Local Government
- Local Planning Authorities
- Housing Departments/Adult Care Services.

Lifetime Homes

Key Areas

Lifetime Homes incorporates 16 standards that a new dwelling should achieve to be designated a Lifetime Home:

- Parking (width or widening capability)
- Approach to dwellings from parking
- Approach to all entrances
- Entrances
- Communal stairs and lifts
- Internal doorways and hallways
- Circulation space
- Entrance-level living space
- Potential for entrance-level bed space
- Entrance-level w.c. and shower
- W.c. and bathroom walls prepared for grab rail fixing
- Stairs and potential through floor lift in dwellings
- Potential for fitting hoist
- Bathrooms
- Glazing and window handle height
- Location of service controls.

The London Housing Design Guide

The London Housing Design Guide (LHDG) gives space standards for all new residential development in London. The Lifetime Homes standards are referenced in the LHDG, and it is expected that all units achieve the Lifetime Homes criteria or have full wheelchair provision.

Standards for wheelchair housing are also given in the LHDG, although this is superseded by the recent changes to Part M.

Habinteg Wheelchair Housing Design Guide

The Habinteg guide (www.habinteg.org.uk) gives standards and guidance for the design of housing for use by wheelchair users. The guide gives recommendations as well as requirements. This standard has been absorbed into Part M of the building regulations and is very similar to Part M4(3) Wheelchair User Dwellings.

Building Regulations Part M 2015 Edition Volume 1: Dwellings

This amendment to Part M of the building regulations effectively absorbs the Lifetime Homes standard and the Habinteg guide. From 1 October 2015, local authorities will be obliged to use these three standards, rather than any Disability Discrimination Act guidance that they may have developed.

The three standards are:

- M4(1) Category1: Visitable dwellings
- M4(2) Category2: Accessible and adaptable dwellings
- M4(3) Category3: Wheelchair user dwellings.

These relate to pre-existing guidance as follows:

- M4(1) – Brings in minimum standards for level access, doors and w.c. provision
- M4(2) – Effectively absorbs the Lifetime Homes Standard
- M4(3) – Effectively absorbs the Habinteg Wheelchair Housing Design Guide.

Housing and Communities Agency (Now Homes England): Design and Quality Standards

Key Areas

Precise guidance for the design and quality standards that must be met by affordable housing providers who get funding from the Homes and Community Agency.

Comments

Standards include, amongst others, space standards that must be achieved within set size bands. Reference is made to Lifetime Homes and Building for Life.

Caveats

- This summary provides an overview of standards which may be applicable in the UK.
- It is not exhaustive or exclusive. Designers should refer to the original source documents from the approved agency or to the relevant nationally applicable standards rather than relying on this summary
- Applicable design standards are subject to continuous change and revisions
- Please make sure that up-to-date documents are used
- To achieve access for all, designers should consider the needs and aspirations of all users and work with the statutory and advisory framework outlined
- New design guidance is being produced continuously by a range of agencies
- Appraisal methodologies are all subjective to some extent. There is no substitute for professional expertise and experience.

Summary

Designers and other professionals who are working in the built environment can help people living with dementia to live well. The approach outlined in this publication is holistic, based on an awareness and understanding of the challenges for those living with dementia, and wide reaching, dealing with the whole environment, including neighbourhoods and town centres.

There is also a finely grained consideration of detail involved, including specifications of finishes and furnishings. Small choices can make a big difference.

The intent of Design *for* Dementia is *aspirational*, raising standards in the design of housing and the public realm to respond to the challenge of the increasing numbers of the population who will live with dementia. But there is also something for everyone in this approach. Many of the lessons learnt about the effect of the environment on those with dementia can benefit everyone.

Things like reduced clutter in pavements, wayfinding in the public realm and stimulus to all the senses would benefit us all.

Design *for* Dementia does not deal with the design considerations indicated by dementia in isolation from the needs and aspiration of others. We are designing for all abilities and for all disabilities through the same process. While tick boxes and point-scoring systems are a good way of auditing designs, they do not in themselves produce good design.

The authors would rather encourage designers to be thoughtful and consider the problems of those with dementia and to work in participation with dementia action groups such as SURF and DAA and local communities, using their creative skills to develop richly stimulating designs. Their creative skills are needed to produce safe, secure, convivial, community-empowered neighbourhoods and the responsive living environments that society needs.

The working methods used to research this book are based on participation with those living with dementia, carers, professionals, academics and an inter-disciplinary team of designers. This experience is a resource which is hard to tap into but which, through the participatory approach employed, has been richly rewarding and enjoyable for all involved. The fun factor is always a vital ingredient!

The methods used, including photo cue cards, sandplay and hands-on modelling, are described in Chapter 5, and the detailed evaluation of the living labs and their outputs is fully demonstrated.

A full-size, fully functional demonstration project has been built at the BRE's Innovation Park, Watford, and is described and evaluated in Chapter 6. Meanwhile, all the members of the team have been inspired to create designs which respond to the needs and aspirations of those living with dementia. Whether they are involved in designing buildings, landscapes, interiors or the urban environment, they now use their awareness and design skills to focus on creating dementia-friendly and sustainable neighbourhoods for the future.

References

Bentley, A.M., and McGlynn, S., 1985. *Responsive Environments*. Butterworth Architecture: Oxford.

Hazen, T., and McManus, M., 2012. Activities and outside space. *Designing Outdoor Spaces for People with Dementia*. Hammond Press and the Dementia Services Development Centre: Stirling.

Mitchell, L., and Burton, E., 2012. Dementia-friendly neighbourhoods – a step in the right direction. *Designing Outdoor Spaces for People with Dementia*. Hammond Press and the Dementia Services Development Centre: Stirling.

Pollock, A., and Marshall, M., 2012. *Designing Outdoor Spaces for People with Dementia*. Hammond Press and the Dementia Services Development Centre: Stirling.

11 The Way Forward

Bill Halsall, Eef Hogervorst and Mike Riley

Introduction

There may not be a pharmaceutical treatment for dementia soon, given the last decades of largely unsuccessful treatment trials. Currently prevention is the best and cheapest option. This is prevention at three levels: primary: along the life course, secondary (when people have developed prodromal stages of dementia) and tertiary (once people have dementia). The last two are both about preventing progression to more severe dementia stages. While lifestyle changes ('what is good for the heart is good for the brain') are now better known as important preventative factors, there are other less-known factors. However, lifestyle changes such as exercising, reducing risk for head injury and falls and eating better diets can be supported by the environment to alter this to better cater to optimising lifestyles at home and outside in the garden, as outlined in Chapter 10.

More recently, other preventative aspects are being given more attention, which can also benefit from good design. For instance, sleep deprivation, noise and chemical pollution also need to be considered, as they can play an important role in development of dementia. For instance, design should focus on sleep-promoting and accommodating environments, allowing darkening of rooms, daylight in the morning, good temperature regulation and so on. New soundproofing regulations will further reduce stress and promote sleep. Chemical outdoor and indoor environments are also a focus, but regulations are often not enforced, unfortunately. Ultimately, design needs to be a discussion between architects, builders, policy makers, those who commission projects and those who will live there.

With ageing, variation in performance, ability and needs increase and so having these discussions at an early stage with all stakeholders to adapt and personalise the environment indicate that guidance rather than strict regulation may be the way forward. Where some aspects are generic, many of these are already covered by building regulations Part M (non-slip floor, level access, etc.).

This book has attempted to give dementia-inclusive guidelines through examples. It follows from the University of Stirling's long history of dementia-inclusive design, originally promoted by people like Mary Marshall. Through the design process of the Chris and Sally's House demonstration project, we attempted to use a solid evidence base for the design choices. That evidence base was not always present and for the Chris and Sally House was sometimes hampered by poor availability/supply of materials.

Philosophy and Approach

The fundamental premise of Design *for* Dementia is that through careful design of both the interior domain and the exterior public realm, the quality of life for people living with dementia can be improved and that their capacity can be sustained for longer, enabling them to live more independent lives instead of over-relying on institutional care.

DOI: 10.1201/9781003306054-11

The COVID-19 pandemic of 2020–23 has brought the issue of elderly care into sharp focus, as thousands of vulnerable people living in care homes have suffered severe illness and premature deaths. In an ageing society, how can elderly and vulnerable people be best cared for? There is a strong belief that ageing in place may be better for some elderly people than institutional care, at least for a period of time. This does not mean that we should ignore the need for high-quality extra care and specialist residential care accommodation. In fact, it means the opposite. A spectrum of care is needed to deal with individuals' needs and requirements. But let us not forget about their aspirations! Familiar neighbourhoods, supportive communities and sense of place and belonging are important.

It is a complex picture. Social attitudes may reflect that dementia is a problem being dealt with elsewhere, either by the health service or by social services. People may feel that the epidemic of dementia affects only a small minority of people who are cared for in an institutional setting, rather than at home.

In fact, around 70–80% of people living with dementia live in their own homes; they live in the same neighbourhoods and use the same facilities in the town centre as everyone else. What can be done to help them live safely and securely and comfortably within their own homes, streets and towns?

This book goes some way to answer this question from the perspective of design. The authors have researched different aspects of the subject of living with dementia both from an academic research perspective and from a practical implementation point of view.

Physical projects, such as the demonstration project Chris and Sally's House, built at the BRE's Innovation Park in Watford, have been pivotal to developing understanding from a very practical point of view of how Design *for* Dementia can be achieved, and the academic research which forms the basis of the design work provides a strong body of evidence to support the practical guidance put forward in this book.

The research described in the book, as well as the design guidance put forward, should inform the design of housing, new and refurbished as well as publicly accessible buildings like shops, offices and commercial and entertainment buildings.

The design guidance also includes reference to specialist care facilities and to the public realm we all share.

Projects which should involve these considerations are:

- New build housing
- Remodelling or refurbishing housing
- Neighbourhood revitalisation projects
- Town centre developments
- Public realm improvements and traffic schemes
- New masterplans and urban design projects
- Health buildings, hospitals and health centres
- Residential care projects
- Extra care schemes
- Sheltered housing
- Specialist facilities
- Design of parks and open spaces
- Individual home and garden improvements.

The design of the public realm, parks and streets should also consider the needs of all users of the built environment, including people who may be cognitively impaired as well as those who are physically disabled.

In pursuit of this approach – ageing in place – the necessary support systems and management structures need to work in parallel to the Design *for* Dementia philosophy and approach. The engagement of the care sector is fundamental to the process.

We have not been very successful after many decades of development of trying to develop a drug for medical treatment for dementia. Rather the focus should be on prevention of developing dementia at all stages to help people maintain independence for as long as possible. Personas can indicate overall changes in needs during the dementia journey, but there is a need for a tailored approach rather than 'one size fits all', to be sensitive to individual needs and preferences, taking into account people's history. The Know Me toolkit from Delft University can help with this. From our work with visitors to Chris and Sally's House, it became clear that changes to the home need to be made when people are still able to deal with the stress of renovation. Therefore, major structural alterations should be implemented as early as possible in the last home. Potential alterations include:

- wet rooms
- providing level thresholds
- soundproofing rooms for washing machines
- non-slip floors
- easy-to-use kitchens
- open plan living arrangements
- enlarging windows.

Other aspects that create a calming environment could include soft furnishings, removing all loose rugs and getting rid of sharp corners of furniture. Removing mirrors and painting can be done later. Ultimately, sadly, much is determined by people's ability to afford most of these changes. Unfortunately, the poorest are most likely to develop dementia earlier and suffer for longer, as well as being least able to alter their environments. Therefore, governmental policy should create new guidelines to support all new homes in the UK to be dementia resilient. This will result in a decreased need for costly care homes, and hopefully technology in the future in these homes will also create less need for caregivers. Whether this reduction in contact with real people will result in greater wellbeing remains to be investigated.

Design

Through practice, HLP have realised that as well as a demand for full Design *for* Dementia standards, there is also a place for dementia-compatible design approaches. This entails designing homes for life which may not be fully 'kitted out' for dementia at the construction stage, but which have inbuilt compatibility for future adaption. Most obviously, this includes fixing positions for hoists or grab rails, but also includes space allocation for future lift provision (see Lifetime Homes Standards), wider doorways, demountable doors, knock through panels and so on. Most importantly, in terms of 'long life loose fit' approaches to design, is space itself. The Chris and Sally's House demonstration project illustrated how many design solutions can be achieved even within a relatively small and constrained shell, but in principle, a very small dwelling has less future potential than a larger one.

The key design drivers are an open plan for ease of spatial perception and navigation and visual linkage between spaces, such as the view to the loo. These dementia-compatible features are achievable within the design of a house which is not particularly designated for dementia but represent a forward-looking investment in built form which will be more conducive to housing an ageing society and represent a sound social investment into the future. We cannot continue to waste the earth's resources in building new and then knocking down and replacing when it becomes apparent that not enough forethought has been put into design. Design for longevity is a basic green design principle, minimising carbon emissions and energy waste into the future.

The housing stock of the UK consists of largely older properties, and rates of new build housing construction are very low, constituting the housing problem, so it is fairly obvious that our efforts must also go into imaginative reuse of older building structures. The Chris and Sally's House project demonstrates that, in spite of all the constraints, an older property can be reimagined as a dementia-resilient home which can happily be lived in by anyone, without it being stigmatised as a special needs dwelling or an institutionally designed care home. Simple choices, correctly made, actually cost nothing or very little except knowledge and expertise. For example, the use of colour and tonal values represented by LRVs is just the cost of a coat of paint.

The choice of floor finishes and colours that mitigate the risk of falls costs nothing if there was a need for floor finishes anyway. Avoidance of black mats anywhere could avert risk of falls, hospital admissions and potential loss of mobility leading to further decline in health and capacity. Mats come in many colours and tonal values and can easily be coordinated with floor finishes. Similarly, strategically designed natural light is beneficial for those living with dementia but also good for everybody. A view to green reduces stress for anyone.

The Environment

Environmental factors should be part of every design decision, including zero-carbon agendas and the protection of the natural environment. The approach outlined in this book is compatible with this green agenda. As previously stated, design for longevity of buildings is inherent in the basic philosophy. Giving new life and function to older buildings also fulfils the purpose of minimising unnecessary consumption of materials and wasting the embodied energy of building structures. Reduction of demolition material sent to landfill is also an environmental benefit. Housing for older people requires reliable and consistent heating (and cooling), as well as good ventilation to reduce carbon dioxide build-up in the dwelling. Additional thermal insulation in walls, floors and roofs was included in Chris and Sally's House together with underfloor heating and responsive heating controls to reduce energy wastage.

There is increasing worldwide concern about the decline of the natural environment, habitat destruction, loss of species and climate change. Interaction with nature is an important stimulus for people living with dementia and everyone else. The Design *for* Dementia garden includes key design features to attract wildlife, in particular bird life and pollinators to provide interest and stimulus throughout the year. Designs for new neighbourhoods or revitalisation masterplans should include firm proposals for increasing net biodiversity as part of the planning process. These proposals can include the design and provision of sensory gardens with sensory planting mixes to enhance bio-diversity as well as the sensory experience of gardens and open spaces for local residents.

Designing Facilities for Dementia Care

Designing facilities for dementia care is a complex task that requires a multidisciplinary approach. The field of dementia care is constantly evolving, and new trends are emerging that aim to improve the quality of life for people with dementia and their caregivers. However, it is important to critically evaluate these trends to ensure that they are effective and evidence based.

One trend in designing facilities for dementia care is the use of technology, such as virtual reality and robotics, to support people with dementia in their daily activities. While technology can be a useful tool, it is important to consider the potential limitations and ethical concerns, such as privacy and accessibility. Additionally, it is important to ensure that the technology is easy to use and understand and that it is appropriate for the individual's cognitive abilities.

Another trend in designing facilities for dementia care is the use of the built environment to promote engagement, reminiscence and social interaction. This includes the use of natural light, colour and contrast, as well as the incorporation of sensory elements such as smells, textures and sounds. It is important to note that while these elements can be helpful in creating a stimulating and engaging environment, they should be used in conjunction with other strategies to support the well-being of people with dementia.

A third trend in designing facilities for dementia care is the use of a green care or therapeutic garden approach. This approach aims to provide an outdoor environment that is safe and accessible for people with dementia and that promotes engagement with nature. While this approach has the potential to improve the well-being of people with dementia, it is important to ensure that the gardens are designed and maintained in a way that is safe and accessible for people with dementia.

In conclusion, while new trends in designing facilities for dementia care have the potential to improve the quality of life for people with dementia and their caregivers, it is important to critically evaluate these trends to ensure that they are evidence based, appropriate, and inclusive of different needs and abilities. It is also important to involve professionals in geriatric care, dementia care and architecture in the design process to ensure that the facilities are tailored to the unique needs of people with dementia.

Use of New Technology

Another aspect that is important when designing for the future is the increased reliance on technology. Technology in the home could increase quality of life. Examples are wearable vests for medical screening (blood pressure, etc.), mood-sensing radios and other innovative developments. Already our lives are infused with digital technology, from fridges to Alexa. However, with fewer carers and the increasing digitisation of society, it is important to be mindful of digital poverty and digital exclusion of many. As society changes, hopefully more will be digitally literate, but cost is a factor that is difficult to overcome in an increasingly wealth divided society. Technology should not overtake the importance of human contact, but, as always, personalisation, ability and preference should be key when discussing these potentially exciting and life-altering developments.

One of the main challenges and requirements for assisted living is how to monitor the movement of occupants around a dwelling without invading their privacy. One obvious solution is to install cameras, and with the advances in motion detection, tracking a person around a house would be straightforward, but this is a major intrusion into their privacy and so is not a solution. A solution that is already used is a wearable alarm, usually worn around the occupant's neck, and if they get into difficulty, a button can be pressed and help will be called. This system is simple and works for people who have mobility challenges, but is not useable for people living with neurological challenges such as dementia, as the occupant must place it on for it to be used. This is true of most wearables unless they form part of the person's usual clothing, an approach that is being investigated by Liverpool John Moores University. Within the property, one option would be to place a conductive mesh underneath the floor covering that could be spaced every 1 m as a grid allowing the detection of motion within the room or space, and lack of motion would indicate potential difficulties the occupant could be facing, and alerts could be raised. Taking this notion one step further would be to learn a person's movement within a home and then look for variations that could indicate problems and call for assistance. Again, this is something being explored by LJMU. One other element that has been developed at LJMU is to simply look at the variation of electrical current being used in a house and, using machine learning, identify what circuit or appliance has been activated, and by coupling this to the carpet sensors, it should be possible to have a more complete picture of the occupants' activities. This multisensor approach to create sensor fusion could mean that not only could the movements of the occupant be determined, but activity that could result in harm to the occupant can be predicted and controls put in place either to reduce risk or alert activation and response.

Augmented and Virtual Reality

Augmented reality (AR) and virtual reality (VR) are technologies that have the potential to support building design for people with dementia. These technologies can be used to create immersive and interactive environments that can help to improve the quality of life for people with dementia.

One way that AR and VR can be applied to building design is through the use of virtual walkthroughs. This involves creating a virtual representation of the building, which can be explored using VR technology. This can be especially useful for people with dementia, as it can help them to become familiar with the layout of the building and to understand how to navigate it. Additionally, virtual walkthroughs can be useful for caregivers, as they can use them to familiarise themselves with the building and to identify potential hazards.

Another way that AR and VR can be applied to building design is through the use of virtual reality simulations. This involves creating virtual scenarios that simulate real-life situations, such as going to the doctor or shopping for groceries. These simulations can be used to help people with dementia to practice and improve their skills and to provide them with a sense of independence.

AR and VR can also be used to create virtual environments that are tailored to the individual's needs and preferences. This can include creating virtual environments that are based on the individual's memories, such as a virtual representation of their childhood home, or a virtual environment that simulates a place of interest such as the beach. This can help to reduce feelings of isolation and confusion and can also provide a sense of familiarity and comfort.

It is important to note that the use of AR and VR in building design for dementia sufferers should be done in consultation with professionals in geriatric care, dementia care and architecture. The technology should be tailored to the individual's cognitive abilities and should be easy to use and understand. Additionally, the use of AR and VR should be integrated with other strategies, such as simple and easy-to-navigate floor plans, good lighting and contrasting colours and easy-to-use controls.

AR and VR have been used to engage with communities as part of broader-based multi-media consultation strategies. Feedback from this is good.

If the participants are people living with dementia, special care should be taken as the experience, while stimulating, can cause disorientation and nausea. Disclaimers and permissions are advised if necessary. In the case of people with dementia, medical supervision should be sought. As far as mediums for design participation, the use of cue cards, physical models and sand trays, as described in Chapter 5, may be more effective and safer.

Figure 11.1 illustrates augmented reality being used as part of a consultation event as part of the design process for a community building. The participants use handheld smart phones or iPads to visualise the building as a 3D model on a physical baseboard. They can manipulate their devices to view the proposed building from different directions or angles or, indeed, explore the interior, without any physical model making involved. Advantages of this method are that the digital image is directly linked to the 3D model, and the design can be easily modified in response to feedback. The technology is dependent on wireless connectivity on location.

Figure 11.2 shows virtual reality being used as part of a broadly based multi-stranded and multi-media planning consultation event. The participants are pedalling in the pedalo (a real one)

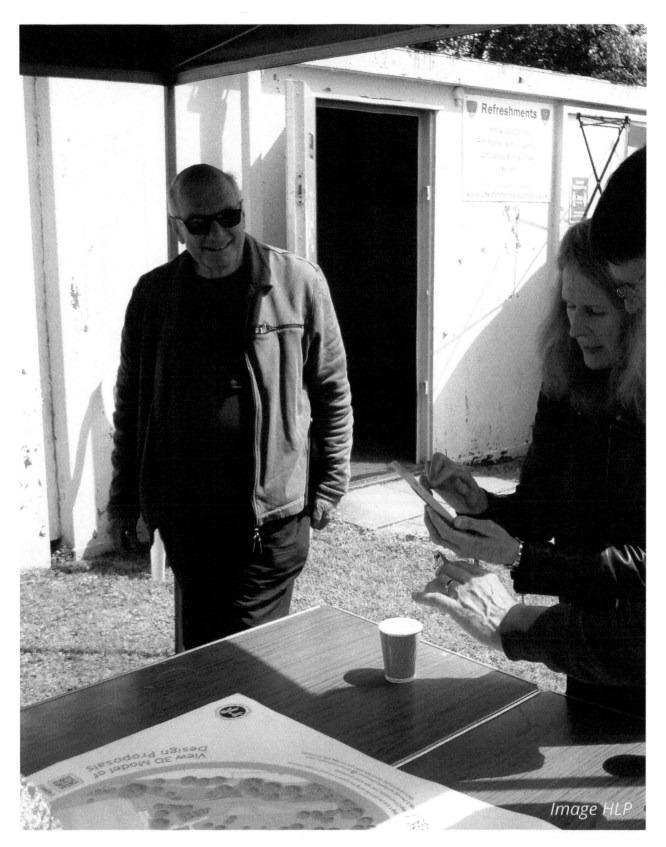

Figure 11.1 Consultation event in Cheltenham

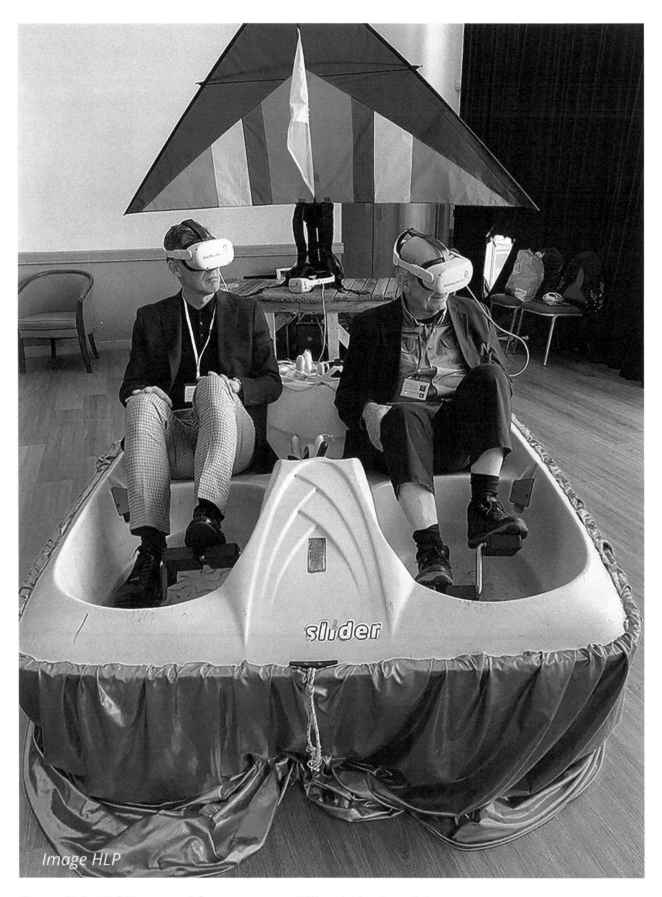

Figure 11.2 AR/VR as a tool for engagement; Bill and Alan in pedalo

but are visually experiencing designs which form a new waterfront development through the VR headsets. The experience is quite realistic and immersive. Participants can feed back comments on their experience verbally or by writing Post-It notes. They may also be able to operate a virtual questionnaire within the three-dimensional environment.

The experience is a bit like a fairground ride and can be very stimulating. The method communicates design intentions well. However, it can also be a disorienting experience and cause nausea. Special care would be needed in its application involving people with dementia, and care should be taken to obtain consent beforehand, if possible, from a medical practitioner.

Artificial Intelligence and Sensor Technologies

The Alzheimer's Society (2019) has carried out work into the use of artificial intelligence as a means of assisting people affected by dementia.

Artificial intelligence takes computer technology forward to a point where it can replicate the functioning of the human brain. Research shows that AI could help people living with dementia in three ways: (i) earlier diagnosis, (ii) understanding how dementia symptoms develop and (iii) helping people to live at home for longer.

Sensors around the house can be used to monitor behaviour and alert carers if something which may present a risk is happening or a deterioration in health is being experienced. Gait may be an indicator of a change in condition and progression of the disease. However, the privacy of the person involved must be respected at all times, and permission to carry out monitoring should be in place. There is no substitute for personal contact and genuine human care.

Sensor technology has been used to assist in producing a controlled environment for someone with dementia, ensuring that carbon dioxide levels, temperature and humidity are adjusted to suit the resident (see Chapter 7).

The use of home technologies such as Alexa has also been put forward as a way of assisting older people and people with dementia to control their home by voice. This technology may suit some people with some conditions. Consideration should be given to the fact that some people with dementia experience hallucinations and may hear voices that are not there. Disembodied voices from devices such as Alexa could create further confusion and disorientation.

Robots

Whilst there is currently no cure for dementia, technology (Smith and Simkhada 2019) and cultural programmes are beneficial non-pharmacological interventions that can improve the lives of people living with dementia. Robots provide a technology that can play a significant role in the provision of social care. Within this context, they have already been used to support care delivered to people living with dementia. Informal trials have shown positive effects such as becoming more talkative (Alzheimer's Society (2019)). However, the therapeutic effect of the robot is not clear. The notion of a robot co-carer system to assist a human carer is attractive, as it allows a social robot to be used for tasks at which it excels. The robot is not intended as a replacement for a human carer but more as an assistant, to help with tasks such as recording, interaction via cognitive stimulation therapy, companionship and monitoring/checking.

The Pepper robot is a popular humanoid social robot which has been used to good effect for interaction with people living with dementia. The robot stands 120 cm tall and provides a child-like, friendly means of social interaction. The robot is equipped with a speech recognition system and an emotion engine, which is used in conjunction with a series of sensors to identify characteristics such as laughter in a voice and facial expressions of joy, disgust, surprise or fear, as well as specific characteristics such as age, gender and ethnicity. In addition to identifying characteristics, the robot can store such characteristics and detect changes over a period of time. People living with dementia will benefit from services that provide information, a sense of connection and a feeling of safety, such as reminding of appointments or medication intake, dietary intake, personal health and home environment status checks.

Cognitive stimulation therapy is an effective therapy for people living with dementia which improves cognition and quality of life. A Pepper robot can be used to deliver a cognitive stimulation therapy programme based on social interaction and cultural activities, such as experiences from the House of Memories application (Neiva Ganga and Wilson 2020). Typical activities within such a programme could include:

- Games and puzzles – Tic-tac-toe, 8-puzzle
- Sounds and music – Background/foreground, context
- My life – Weddings, births/deaths, ancestry
- Food – Recipes, tastes, cooking, internationalisation
- Current affairs – Politics, global/domestic, people
- Faces and places – Family, famous people
- Word associations – Guess the word, rhyming words
- Being creative – Doodling, painting, colouring, patterns
- Categorising objects – According to context and/or history
- Orientation – Maps, travel, shapes
- Using money – Purchases, budgets, change left over

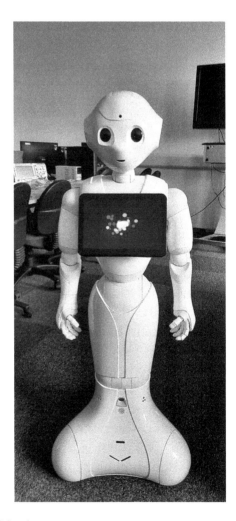

Figure 11.3 Pepper the humanoid robot

- Number games – Odd/even, ordering, next in sequence
- Word games – Simple crosswords, guess the word.

In addition to social interaction and cognitive stimulation therapy, social robots can also be used for dementia assessment in a realistic setting such as a memory clinic, which is a service used to assess the stage of dementia using a series of tests. The robot would not only provide cost savings but would also support standardised, uniform testing required in clinics at a national level.

Integration of Design

Chapter 10 outlines design guidance that can be used to create dementia resilient environments. Other guides such as Stirling University's Dementia Design Audit Tool provide assessment methodology for the design of facilities and environments for people living with dementia.

Chapter 10 also provides an overview of other standards and guidelines that must be negotiated to achieve successful project designs.

It is clear that for designers there is a multiplicity of rules and regulations as well as 'tick boxes' to be negotiated. Much discussion has gone on about the potential of an equivalent to Part M of the Building Regulations aimed at design for dementia. The inherent difficulty with this is that while wheelchair accessibility is easily comprehensible as a principle (if sometimes more difficult to design in practice), there are over a hundred different types of dementia, and each individual may respond differently because of inherent personality and context. It would be very different to regulate on a 'one size fits all' basis. There could well be unintended consequences. Maybe some very simple rules, such as 'no black mats' or consistent directional paving, could be applied, but otherwise it seems difficult to imagine how every individual's needs could be formulated into a regulatory framework. There are also pitfalls in the 'tick box' approach to design. Focusing entirely on dementia design risks a silo approach, potentially over-bureaucratic, narrow and unresponsive to the wide range of design parameters involved in producing good design. Good design should not be defined by a 'tick box' approach. We should be aiming for good design which fulfils all the requirements, not looking for a design that ticks all the boxes and therefore qualifies as good design. The design process is multifaceted and should be based on an integrated holistic approach to provide a quality environment for human life, respecting and rejoicing in the natural environment and stimulating joy for everyone.

Alain De Botton in his book, *The Architecture of Happiness*, references Ludwig Wittgenstein, the great philosopher, who abandoned academia for 3 years in order to construct a house for his sister Gretl in Vienna. He concluded, 'You think philosophy is difficult, but I tell you, it is nothing compared to the difficulty of being a good architect'.

We are all seeking a paradigm, but in reality, we are dealing with a layering of many paradigms. If that weren't difficult enough, the paradigms are shifting all the time, while our buildings are expected to last indefinitely. In designing to address the needs of particular groups in the community, we cannot ignore all the other groups. Engagement from an early stage is vitally important, and understanding people's needs and aspirations is more use than blind obedience to a rule book. Design for dementia is one layer in the analysis and an important part of design methodology, but ultimately design as a response to the human condition is a bigger canvas, and a rigorous design process based on sound evidence-based principles and thorough analysis is the best guarantee of success.

In any case, many of the principles put forward in this book are not just good principles of design for dementia but also provide a sound foundation for design for everyone. The richness of the experience of a sensory garden can provide a stimulus through all the senses for someone living with dementia, but we can all enjoy that sensory stimulus. (Perhaps all gardens should be sensory gardens.)

Organising spaces to be easily navigable is a good general design principle. A view to green reduces stress for everyone, not just for people living with dementia. The more rigorous analytical approach used to design for dementia is a good design discipline, and the experiential philosophy of design, which underlines the thinking in this book, is valid in any design of the built environment.

Implications for NHS and Social Care Systems

A continuing debate about overstretched health and social care services focuses on the large number of older people in 'the system'. There may be a shortage of hospital beds available, and older people with or without dementia may be occupying hospital beds at great expense. Some of these older people may be well enough to leave hospital, but there is no good alternative available for them. As a result, there may be a shortage of hospital beds available for more serious cases. The approach described in this book has the potential to ease the crisis in two ways.

First, by providing better facilities in the community like specialist care facilities, extra care schemes and residential care homes. Older people, whether living with dementia or not, could be cared for in more appropriate accommodation with professional carers and medical staff, less expensively and closer to their support network. If individual homes can be better designed for dementia, then older people occupying hospital beds, with the right support, could move back to their own homes and live well with dementia, ageing in place and retaining their capacity and a degree of autonomy for longer.

Second, more general availability of dementia-resilient dwellings and homes adapted for dementia within neighbourhoods, villages, towns and cities would potentially reduce the need for hospitalisation in the first place by, for example, reducing slips, trips and falls and other accidents at home through well designed, carefully considered and well supported Designed *for* Dementia places to live.

Implications for the Industry

The design and construction of a proportion of new dwellings within new developments which are to Design *for* Dementia standards and the building in of dementia compatibility to general needs housing developments would obviously ease the health and social care crisis for older people as well as those with cognitive impairment in the medium to long term. Existing homes converted or adapted to accommodate the specific needs of individuals would also aid in a more compassionate and respectful approach to tackling cognitive and well as physical impairment within society.

The housing industry and the building industry, as well as the health and care systems, would also have to respond to make this possible. Such schemes built to good standards are already becoming available but sometimes to standards which are below the best standards described in this book. This is because it is perceived as expensive and providing little financial return to the developers. Lack of awareness is also an issue – not just lack of awareness of the problem but lack of awareness that anything can be done through the medium of building processes or procurement. Raising awareness is always an issue and one that this book hopes to address.

As regards costs, clearly there is a cost, just as there was a cost to achieving 'Lifetime Homes' standards or to working to Part M of the building regulations. The building industry has historically not responded well to new imposed standards, citing complications and cost as reasons for not building to increased standards. However, to be fair, affordability of housing is also a factor. Many people are struggling to afford housing of any kind. On the other end of the market, people seem prepared to spend significant sums on new kitchens and bathrooms within their existing homes every 10 years or so. Could these new bathrooms and kitchens be dementia compatible as well as responding to the latest aspirational fashion statement?

Will industry ever respond to the concept and application of Design *for* Dementia standards in the same way as it has been forced to respond to the revised Part M of the building regulations? The new Part M was introduced in 2016 and has had a significant effect on housing design standards. The standards are controlled at the planning applications stage, and the numbers of dwellings to Part M4.1, M4.2 or M4.3 required for a particular development are determined through the planning process.

This has been largely beneficial, but as with any regulatory approach, there can be a 'law of unintended consequences', for example, by producing designs with lifts and corridors or deck access which may bring other management issues, such as maintenance and security. Part M's central focus is accessibility to dwellings for people in wheelchairs, and the physical manoeuvrability issues are related to physical design requirements such as wider doors, turning circles and charging points. The requirements of people living with dementia or with other cognitive issues are more complex, not as easily quantifiable and extremely varied from person to person. An alternative approach may be to try to get Design *for* Dementia into best practice?

Part M fulfils its purpose in focusing designers and planners on physical disability, specifically design for wheelchair accessibility. Other impairments, physical or cognitive, are not on the agenda. Designers and educators should be focusing on the bigger picture, aspiring to achieve a comprehensive philosophy of neurodiversity and an integrated approach to the design of the built environment.

The University of Stirling's Dementia Design Audit tool is an alternative approach. It includes a workbook which assists designers with a checklist approach and is used as an assessment method. The Stirling Dementia Design Audit tool aims to 'design to develop a better quality of life for people living with dementia'. Its application is aimed at extra care schemes, care homes and residential care projects, rather than neighbourhoods, town centres or general housing, and the next step must surely be to tackle the wider environment: the public realm as well as the private domain so that people living with dementia can experience a better quality of life at home. On the other end of the spectrum are tools like Know Me, described in Chapter 4, a tool developed to personalise design as much as possible together with people with dementia. The personas described in Chapter 6 were developed to show designers the variation between people with dementia but also within, with changes in symptoms affecting design needs and focusing on flexibility of design.

Ultimately, design needs to be a discussion between architects, builders, policy makers, those who commission the build and those who need to live there. Costs vs wishes and needs need to be weighed up. With ageing, variation in performance, ability and needs increases, and so having these discussions at an early stage with all stakeholders to adapt and personalise the environment indicate that guidance rather than strict regulation may be the way forward. Where some aspects are generic, many of these are already covered by Part M (non-slip floor, level access, etc.), and it is thus questionable whether we really need a Part M+. This book has attempted to give dementia-resilient guidelines as examples. It follows from Stirling's long history of dementia-friendly design originally promoted by people like Mary Marshall.

With Chris and Sally's House, we attempted to use a solid evidence base for the design choices. That evidence base was not always present and sometimes hampered by availability/supply of materials. This is exaggerated in some – but perhaps not all – people with dementia. Compromises had to be made. If any lessons were learned, these were about continued communication and personalisation, acknowledging the person-centred approach as a focal point for designing for dementia.

The Supply Chain

A key component of Design *for* Dementia revolves around the importance of LRVs in creating appropriate tonal contrasts between adjoining surfaces, helping people living with dementia in their visual orientation and navigation of their surroundings. This design technique also guides the choice of floor finishes to ensure that the tonal values are coordinated to avoid visual confusion and avoidable trips and falls.

Light reflectance values can be measured with a light reflectance meter, and some suppliers will quote LRV references in their product specifications, for example, paint, fabrics and furniture aimed at the care home market.

Some of the products which would be beneficial for people living with dementia, such as cupboards and drawer units with non-reflective glazed fronts, are not generally commercially available at present and would have to be supplied by a specialist.

While suppliers to the care home market have adapted to the LRV methodology, these suppliers of furniture, furnishings and finishes are not generally available on the high street. Many materials, particularly natural materials such as wood, stone or wool, are inherently inconsistent anyway. Paint LRVs may depend on their application or consistency of mixing to achieve the stated LRV.

Improvements in the supply chain will come in response to market demand, so the issue may be how the market can be mobilised or activated to generate the shift required in the supply chain to make suitable products available to people and their families and carers who want to live well with dementia at home.

Delight

In Chapter 5, we referred to Vitruvius's firmness, commodity and delight. Much of this book has been concerned with the medical needs and practicalities in creating living environments, both interior and exterior, which can help people living with dementia to live better, retaining their capacity and independence for longer through good design.

The design guidance outlined largely fits into Vitruvius's 'firmness' – structure of building and spaces, and 'commodity', appropriateness and functionality of the design. But let us not forget beauty, pleasure and delight. Within the design principles described in Chapter 10 (Figure 10.1), we have identified 'comfortable and stimulating' as a key principle.

Providing a stimulus as well as comfort can be achieved through stimulating all the senses: smell, touch, taste, sight and sound. In this way we can gain pleasure from our surroundings and help stimulate responses in the brain. This is a shared experience as part of the common human experience of being alive. People living with dementia and older people in general are not excluded from these stimuli. Although the colours may fade, hearing may begin to fail and our sense of smell may not be as acute, we can still enjoy sensory stimuli as we age.

Use of colour, for example, can be a very good tool in the design toolbox.

As our vision may fade, maybe the colours should be brighter and more vibrant? We shouldn't condemn older people to a life of grey and beige. More imaginative colour schemes can enhance the sensory experience as well as assisting in defining spaces and objects through light reflectance value contrasts.

The sense of smell and taste may not be a normal part of an architect's design palette, but in the context of a garden, community park, kitchen or café can evoke sensation, soothing and relaxing or simple enjoyment, perhaps prompting recall of times, places, people and events from the past. A spa can be introduced into schemes to help with providing calm and relaxation. Loud noise can be particularly difficult for people living with dementia, the sounds amplified by their condition. Cafeteria-style dining experiences can be particularly distressing because of reverberation from hard surfaces, so the acoustic properties of spaces and surface finishes should be carefully considered. Hearing aids may be essential both to enhance the sound environment for older people and also to assist sociability and communication.

Touch is important to older people and part of the human contact that should be a fundamental part of care.

A more imaginative, considered and empathetic approach to design is indicated to enrich the quality of older life and provide people living with dementia with relief, relaxation and enjoyment.

A Regulatory Framework for Design for Dementia

Any attempt to regulate Design for Dementia must consider four things:

1. Dementia manifests in different ways. There are many different types of dementia. Individuals can be affected in different ways and have very different needs. The building regulations (Part M) deal with the design of buildings for physical disability and are generally focused on wheelchair accessibility. The physical requirements for the use of wheelchairs are well known and can be defined by consistent dimensions. Statuary regulation of this kind depends on the ability to define precise metrics. The intent is to avoid any ambiguity or confusion and to minimise scope for interpretation or individual choice or judgement
2. Cognitive impairment is more difficult to define in terms of precise metrics and the need for training for such assessments. Additional requirements would be generic in applicability, leaving little room for personalisation, different cultural and educational backgrounds or for individual involvement and consultation
3. In terms of the working of the design process, building regulation approval takes place quite late in the process; by this time, most design decisions have already been made. Design considerations regarding the needs of people living with cognitive impairment should start at an early stage to fully reflect the potential that design could have in creating dementia inclusiveness in the environment
4. Within the design of the wider environment, the needs and requirements of all groups within the community should be taken into consideration, including, for example, partially sighted, autistic or hearing-impaired people. There is a need to recognise and embrace neurodiversity of all kinds to produce a true neurodiversity-inclusive approach to the design of our shared environments.

The tick-box approach can help designers, but there are many different tick boxes to be negotiated through the design process, some with conflicting criteria. There are other methodologies, such as 'Healthy Cities' modelling tools based on urban determinants of health, used on master planning and urban design projects. Design determinants for dementia, cognitive impairment and neurodiversity could be integrated into this type of planning framework so that they are integrated as a fundamental part of design and planning strategies from the earliest stage.

Conclusion

On balance, it seems that regulation for Design for Dementia, cognitive impairment and neurodiversity fits better into the planning framework and stages for approval through the established process. In the same way that the planning application process requires such documents as design and access statements, drainage strategies, acoustic surveys or ecological reports, then it could also require statements on cognitive impairment, including dementia and neurodiversity in general. This would allow for local context to be considered and design strategies established based on consultation with local groups from an early stage. In this way, inclusive design parameters could be agreed on and then followed through to implementation consistently, holistically and ensuring that better-integrated design solutions can be flexibly and responsively carried through into the more detailed design stages of a project.

Within this work, we have attempted to bring together some key themes that describe and contextualise the nature and impacts of dementia and the challenges and opportunities for designers, carers and people with dementia to create and maintain environments that allow individuals with dementia to live well. This is an ongoing journey.

Maybe this book will help?

References

Alzheimer's Society, 2019. How can a robot, support people affected by dementia? www.alzheimers.org.uk/blog/how-can-robots-support-people-dementia.

Neiva Ganga, R., and Wilson, K.M., 2020. Valuing family carers: The impact of House of Memories as a museum-led dementia awareness programme. *International Journal of Care and Caring*. ISSN 2397–8821.

Smith, G.M., and Simkhada, B., 2019. Co-creating the living well with dementia message. *Issues in Mental Health Nursing*. ISSN 0161–2840.

Index

Note: **Boldface** page references indicate tables. *Italic* references indicate figures.

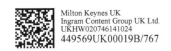